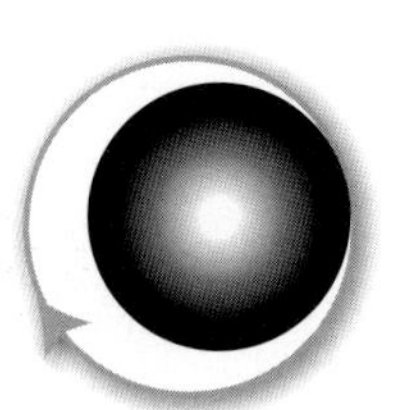

Core Clinical Cases in Medical and Surgical Specialties

Core Clinical Cases
Titles in the series include:

Core Clinical Cases in Basic Biomedical Science
Author: Samy A. Azer

Core Clinical Cases in Medical and Surgical Specialties
Edited by Steve Bain & Janesh K. Gupta

Core Clinical Cases in Medicine and Surgery
Edited by Steve Bain & Janesh K. Gupta

Core Clinical Cases in Obstetrics & Gynaecology 2nd Edition
Authors: Janesh K. Gupta, Gary Mires & Khalid S. Khan

Core Clinical Cases in Paediatrics
Authors: Andrew Ewer, Timothy G. Barrett & Vin Diwakar

Core Clinical Cases in Psychiatry
Authors: Tom Clark, Ed Day & Emma C. Fergusson

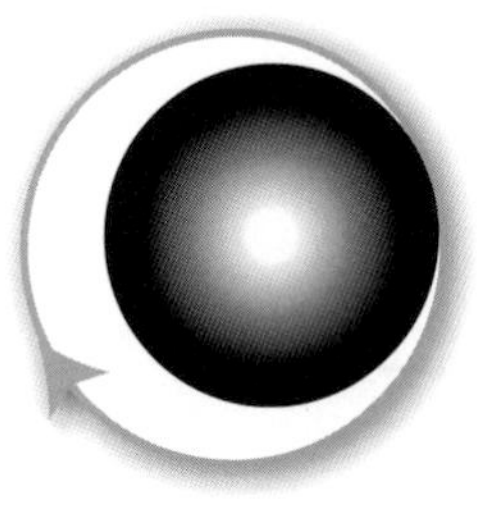

Core Clinical Cases in Medical and Surgical Specialties

a problem-solving approach

Edited by

Steve Bain MA MD FRCP
Professor of Medicine (Diabetes), University of Wales, Swansea, & Honorary Consultant Physician, Swansea NHS Trust, Singleton Hospital, Swansea, UK

Janesh K. Gupta MSc MD FRCOG
Clinical Senior Lecturer/Honorary Consultant in Obstetrics and Gynaecology, University of Birmingham, Birmingham Women's Hospital, Birmingham, UK

Core Clinical Cases series edited by

Janesh K. Gupta MSc MD FRCOG
Clinical Senior Lecturer/Honorary Consultant in Obstetrics and Gynaecology, University of Birmingham, Birmingham Women's Hospital, Birmingham, UK

Hodder Arnold

A MEMBER OF THE HODDER HEADLINE GROUP

First published in Great Britain in 2006 by
Hodder Education, a member of the Hodder Headline Group,
338 Euston Road, London NW1 3BH

http://www.hoddereducation.com

Distributed in the United States of America by
Oxford University Press Inc.,
198 Madison Avenue, New York, NY10016
Oxford is a registered trademark of Oxford University Press

Whilst the advice and information in this book are believed to be true and accurate at the date of going to press, neither the author[s] nor the publisher can accept any legal responsibility or liability for any errors or omissions that may be made. In particular, (but without limiting the generality of the preceding disclaimer) every effort has been made to check drug dosages; however it is still possible that errors have been missed. Furthermore, dosage schedules are constantly being revised and new side effects recognized. For these reasons the reader is strongly urged to consult the drug companies' printed instructions before administering any of the drugs recommended in this book.

British Library Cataloguing in Publication Data
A catalogue record for this book is available from the British Library

Library of Congress Cataloging-in-Publication Data
A catalog record for this book is available from the Library of Congress

ISBN-10: 0 340 81572 8
ISBN-13: 978 0 340 81572 4

1 2 3 4 5 6 7 8 9 10

Commissioning Editor: Georgina Bentliff
Project Editors: Heather Smith and Clare Weber
Production Controller: Jane Lawrence
Cover Design: Georgina Hewitt

Typeset in 9 on 12 pt Frutiger Light Condensed by Phoenix Photosetting, Chatham, Kent.
Printed and bound in Malta.

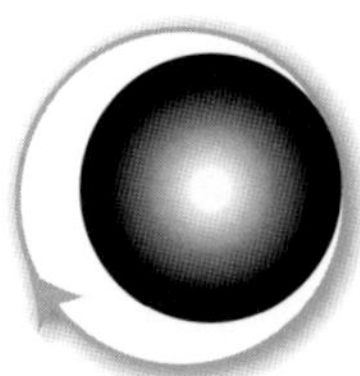

Contents

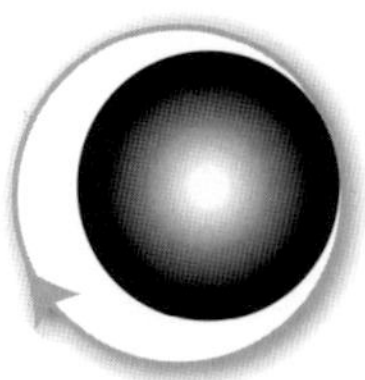

List of contributors

Alan P. Doherty MBBS BSc MD FRCS (Urol) FEBU, Consultant Urological Surgeon, Queen Elizabeth Hospital, Birmingham, UK

Adrian Drake-Lee MMed PhD FRCS, Consultant ENT Surgeon, University NHS Trust, Queen Elizabeth Hospital, Birmingham, UK

Chris Ellis MB FRCP DTM&H, Consultant in Infectious Diseases, Birmingham Heartlands Hospital, Birmingham, UK

Christopher Fegan MBBS MD FRCP FRCPath, Consultant Haematologist, Llandough Hospital, Cardiff, UK

Suresh Ganta FRCS, Specialist Registrar in Urology, Birmingham, UK

Desirée Murray FRCS(Ed) FRCOphth, Lecturer in Ophthalmology, Department of Clinical Surgical Services, University of West Indies, Trinidad, West Indies

Ian Pallister MBBS MMedSci (Trauma) FRCS (Tr&Orth), Morriston Hospital, Swansea, UK

Daniel Rea MBBS BSc PhD FRCP, Senior Lecturer in Medical Oncology, University of Birmingham, Birmingham, UK

Nevianna Tomson MBChB MRCP, Specialist Registrar in Dermatology, Addenbrookes' Hospital, Cambridge, UK

Stuart Weatherby BSc MBChB MRCP MD, Consultant Neurologist, Derriford Hospital, Plymouth, Honorary University Fellow to the Peninsula Medical School, UK

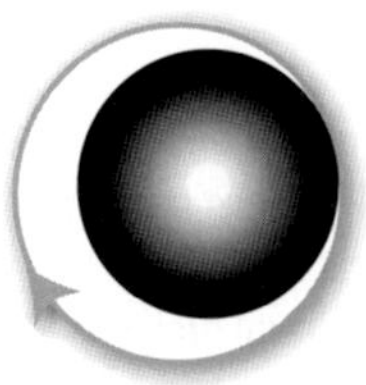

Series preface

'A History Lesson'

Between about 1916 and 1927 a puzzling illness appeared and swept around the world. Dr von Economo first described encephalitis lethargica (EL), which simply meant 'inflammation of the brain that makes you tired'. Younger people, especially women, seemed to be more vulnerable but the disease affected people of all ages. People with EL developed a 'sleep disorder', fever, headache and weakness, which led to a prolonged state of unconsciousness. The EL epidemic occurred during the same time period as the 1918 influenza pandemic, and the two outbreaks have been linked ever since in the medical literature. Some confused it with the epidemic of Spanish flu at that time while others blamed weapons used in World War I.

Encephalitis lethargica (EL) was dramatized by the film *Awakenings* (book written by Oliver Sacks, who is an eminent Neurologist from New York), starring Robin Williams and Robert De Niro. Professor Sacks treated his patients with L-dopa, which temporarily awoke his patients, giving rise to the belief that the condition was related to Parkinson's disease.

Since the 1916–1927 epidemic, only sporadic cases have been described. Pathological studies have revealed an encephalitis of the midbrain and basal ganglia, with lymphocyte (predominantly plasma cell) infiltration. Recent examination of archived EL brain material has failed to demonstrate influenza RNA, adding to the evidence that EL was not an invasive influenza encephalitis. Further investigations found no evidence of viral encephalitis or other recognized causes of rapid-onset parkinsonism. MRI of the brain was normal in 60% but showed inflammatory changes localized to the deep grey matter in 40% of patients.

As late as the end of the 20th century, it seemed that the possible answers lay in the clinical presentation of the patients in the 1916–1927 epidemic. It had been noted by the clinicians at that time that the CNS disorder had presented with pharyngitis. This led to the possibility of a post-infectious autoimmune CNS disorder similar to Sydenham's chorea, in which group A β-hemolytic streptococcal antibodies cross-react with the basal ganglia and result in abnormal behaviour and involuntary movements. Anti-streptolysin-O titres have subsequently been found to be elevated in the majority of these patients. It seemed possible that autoimmune antibodies may cause remitting parkinsonian signs subsequent to streptococcal tonsillitis as part of the spectrum of post-streptococcal CNS disease.

Could it be that the 80-year mystery of EL has been solved relying on the patient's clinical history of presentation, rather than focusing on expensive investigations? More research in this area will give us the definitive answer. This scenario is not dissimilar to the controversy about the idea that streptococcal infections were aetiologically related to rheumatic fever.

With this example of a truly fascinating history lesson, we hope that you will endeavour to use the patient's clinical history as your most powerful diagnostic tool to make the correct diagnosis. If you do you are likely to be right 80–90% of the time. This is the basis of all the Core Clinical Cases series, which will make you systematically explore clinical problems through the clinical history of presentation, followed by examination and then the performance of appropriate investigations. Never break that rule.

Janesh Gupta
2006

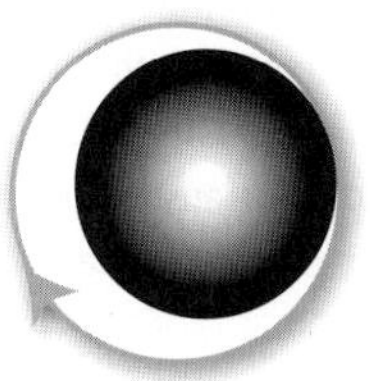

Preface

Why core clinical cases?

In undergraduate medical education there is a trend towards the development of 'core' curricula. The aim is to facilitate the teaching of essential and relevant knowledge, skills and attitudes. This contrasts with traditional medical school courses, where the emphasis was on detailed factual knowledge, often with little obvious clinical relevance. In addition, students' learning is now commonly examined using objective structured clinical examinations (OSCEs), which again assess the practical use of knowledge, rather than the regurgitation of 'small print'.

Core cases in Medical and Surgical Specialties cannot be an exhaustive list of all of the cases which could be regarded as 'core', largely due to the massive scope of these specialties. However, the volumes do present examples which can be used to train the reader in a realistic way of approaching medical and surgical problems. This should help develop a learning strategy for fifth-year medical students to prepare for final examinations, as well as providing useful revision for pre-registration house doctors taking on a new area.

Why a problem-solving approach?

In practice, patients present with clinical problems, which are explored through history, examination and investigation progressively leading from a differential to a definitive diagnosis. Traditionally, textbooks present the subject matter according to a pathophysiological classification which does not help solve real-life clinical scenarios. We have, therefore, based this book on a problem-solving approach. This inculcates the capacity for critical thinking and should help readers to analyse the basis of clinical problems. Of course we accept that the divisions within medicine and surgery are arbitrary, but the areas covered by the specialties are so huge that chapter headings give a steer as to which system will be involved. However, the reader should remember to include other systems in their differential diagnosis, akin to the real life situation where a patient is referred to a neurology clinic with fits but turns out to have a cardiovascular cause for their symptoms.

How will this book inspire problem-solving traits?

The short case scenarios presented in these books are based on common clinical cases which readers are likely to encounter in undergraduate medicine and surgery. These are grouped according to the various subspecialties within medicine and surgery. Groups include varying numbers of cases, each of which begins with a statement of the patient's complaint followed by a short description of the patient's problem. For each case, using a question and short answer format, the reader is taken through a problem-solving exercise. There are two types of problem-solving case in this book: one type deals with the development of a diagnostic and therapeutic strategy, whilst the other deals with the development of a counselling strategy. 'Core' information about the subject matter relevant to the patient's problem is also summarized, as this information is helpful for answering the questions. The format of the book enables the cases to be used for learning as well as for self-assessment.

In the cases that deal with diagnostic and therapeutic strategies, the reader is questioned about the interpretation of the relevant clinical features presented, so as to compile an array of likely differential diagnoses. They may then be asked to identify specific pieces of information in the history and to select an appropriate clinical examination which will narrow down the differential list to the most likely diagnosis. This emphasis is important because, in clinical practice, history and examination result in a correct diagnosis in 80–90% of cases. Following this, readers are asked to suggest investigations which would be required to confirm or refute the diagnosis. Once a diagnosis has been reached, readers develop a treatment plan. In general terms, this should first consider conservative non-invasive options (e.g. the important option of doing nothing), followed by medical and surgical options.

In clinical practice, any therapeutic strategy has to be conveyed to patients in a manner that they can understand. Therefore we have included problems that will challenge the reader to develop a counselling strategy. These counselling cases will help and encourage readers to communicate confidently with patients. This generic learning strategy is followed throughout the book with the aim of reinforcing the skills required to master the problem-solving approach.

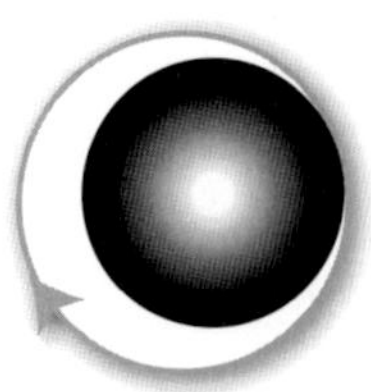

Abbreviations

17-OHP	17-hydroxyprogesterone
5FU	5-fluorouracil
5-HT	serotonin (hydroxytryptamine)
A&E	accident and emergency
ACE	angiotensin-converting enzyme
ACh	acetylcholine
AEDs	anti-epileptic drugs
AFBs	acid-fast bacilli
AFP	α-fetoprotein
AIDP	acute inflammatory demyelinating polyneuropathy
ALT	alanine aminotransferase
ALP	alkaline phosphatase
ANA	antinuclear antibody
AP	anteroposterior
ARDS	adult respiratory distress syndrome
ARMD	age-related macular degeneration
AST	aspartate aminotransferase
ATLS	Advanced Trauma Life Support
BCC	basal cell carcinoma
BCG	Bacillus Calmette–Guérin
BCR	bulbocavernosus reflex
BIPP	bismuth iodoform paraffin paste
BMI	body mass index
BPH	benign prostatic hyperplasia
CEA	carcinoembryonic antigen
CIDP	chronic inflammatory demyelinating polyneuropathy
CMV	cytomegalovirus
CNS	central nervous system
COC	combined oral contraceptive pill
COMT	catechol-*O*-methyltransferase
CRP	C-reactive protein
CSF	cerebrospinal fluid
CT	computed tomography
CVA	cerebrovascular accident
DCR	dacryocystorhinostomy
DIC	disseminated intravascular coagulation
DRE	digital rectal examination
DSD	detrusor–sphincter dyssynergia
DVLA	Driver and Vehicle Licensing Agency
DVT	deep venous (or vein) thrombosis
EBV	Epstein–Barr virus
ECG	electrocardiogram
EEG	electroencephalography
EMG	electromyography
ENT	ear, nose and throat
ESR	erythrocyte sedimentation rate

ESWL	extracorporeal shock wave lithotripsy
ETEC	enterotoxigenic strains of *Escherichia coli*
FBC	full blood count
FDPs	fibrinogen degradation products
FFP	fresh frozen plasma
FNA	fine-needle aspiration
FSH	follicle-stimulating hormone
FVC	forced vital capacity
GCS	Glasgow Coma Score
G-CSFs	granulocyte colony-stimulating factors
GFR	glomerular filtration rate
GI	gastrointestinal
GN	glomerulonephritis
GnRH	gonadotrophin-releasing hormone
Hb	haemoglobin
HbA1c	glycated haemoglobin
β-hCG	β-human chorionic gonadotrophin
HIV	human immunodeficiency virus
HPV	human papilloma virus
HRCT	high-resolution computed tomography
HSV	herpes simplex virus
ICA	internal carotid artery
ICP	intracranial pressure
ICSI	intracytoplasmic sperm injection
Ig	immunoglobulin
INR	international normalized ratio
ISC	intermittent self-catheterization
ITU	intensive therapy unit
IUCD	intrauterine contraceptive device
IVF	in vitro fertilization
IVIG	intravenous immunoglobulin
IVU	intravenous urogram
JVP	jugular venous pressure
LDH	lactate dehydrogenase
LEMS	Lambert–Eaton myasthenic syndrome
LFTs	liver function tests
LH	luteinizing hormone
LHRH	luteinizing hormone-releasing hormone
MAG-3	technetium-99m-labelled mercaptoacetyl triglycine
MCV	mean cell volume
MCH	mean cell Hb
MND	motor neuron disease
MPs	malarial parasites
MRA	magnetic resonance angiography
MRI	magnetic resonance imaging
MRSA	methicillin-resistant *Staphylococcus aureus*
MS	multiple sclerosis
MSU	midstream specimen of urine
Nd:YAG	neodymium:yttrium–aluminium–garnet

NSAIDs	non-steroidal anti-inflammatory drugs
PA	pernicious anaemia
PCA	posterior communicating artery
PCNL	percutaneous nephrolithotomy
PCR	polymerase chain reaction
PCV	packed cell volume
PIN	prostatic intraepithelial neoplasia
PRV	polycythaemia rubra vera
PSA	prostate-specific antigen
PTH	parathyroid hormone
PUJ	pelviureteric junction
PUK	peripheral ulcerative keratitis
PUO	pyrexia of unknown origin
PUVA	psoralen and UVA
PVD	posterior vitreous detachment
RAST	radioallergosorbent test
RBC	red blood cell
RD	retinal detachment
RP	retinitis pigmentosa
RR	respiratory rate
SCC	squamous cell carcinoma
SIADH	syndrome of inappropriate antidiuretic hormone secretion
SIRS	systemic inflammatory response syndrome
SLE	systemic lupus erythematosus
STI	sexually transmitted infection
SUDEP	sudden unexplained death in epilepsy
SVCO	superior vena caval obstruction
TB	tuberculosis
TCC	transitional cell carcinoma
TED	thyroid eye disease
TIA	transient ischaemic attack
TSS	toxic shock syndrome
TURBT	transurethral resection of the bladder tumour
TURP	transurethral resection of the prostate
U&Es	urea and electrolytes
UTI	urinary tract infection
UV	ultraviolet
VZV	varicella-zoster virus
WBC	white blood cell
WCC	white blood cell count
XGPN	xanthogranulomatous pyelonephritis

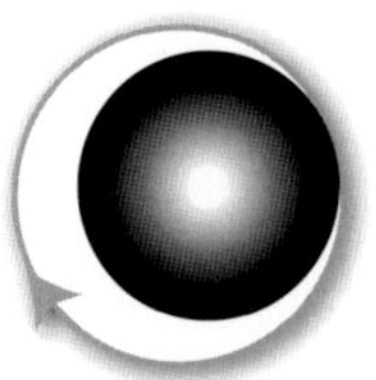

Acknowledgements

Many thanks to Dr David Nicholl, Consultant Neurologist at Queen Elizabeth Hospital Neuroscience Centre, Edgbaston, Birmingham and City Hospital, for helpful comments on the manuscript for Chapter 6.

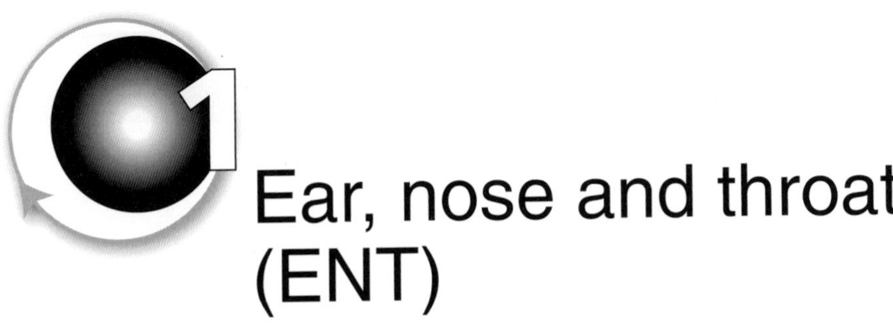

1 Ear, nose and throat (ENT)

Adrian Drake-Lee

NOSE: EPISTAXIS

? Questions for each of the clinical case scenarios given

Q1: What is the likely differential diagnosis?
Q2: What additional features in the history would you like to elicit?
Q3: What investigations would be most helpful and why?
Q4: What are the treatment options?

Clinical cases

CASE 1.1 – Adult with nosebleed.

A 60-year-old retired man, who is on warfarin for a deep vein thrombosis (DVT), presents with a profuse epistaxis to the accident and emergency (A&E) department. There is no other significant history. Examination shows that the patient is actively bleeding from the left side of the nose.

CASE 1.2 – Child with nosebleed.

A 7-year-old girl presents with intermittent bilateral epistaxis to the ENT clinic. Examination of the nose reveals dilated veins anteriorly, but no obvious signs of any other pathology.

OSCE Counselling Cases

OSCE COUNSELLING CASE 1.1 – What advice should you give to an adult male who is coming into hospital and has had his nose packed?

OSCE COUNSELLING CASE 1.2 – A single mother has a child aged 3 years with profuse intermittent nosebleeds, which occur at night.

The mother is concerned that her child might bleed to death. Can you assure her that this will not be the case?

Key concepts

- Epistaxis is commonly the result of a localized nasal condition.
- Epistaxis may be caused by a systemic problem.
- Treat the condition locally and then investigate the patient.

Answers

CASE 1.1 – Adult with nosebleed.

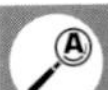

Q1: What is the likely differential diagnosis?

A1

The differential diagnosis in any patient with epistaxis is to determine whether the problem is coming from a local condition or as part of a systemic disease. The vast majority of cases have no underlying pathology locally, except dilated vessels on the anterior septum in younger adults. A nasal tumour may present with unilateral epistaxis, although this is not profuse unless it erodes into an artery. The differential diagnosis of systemic diseases includes any lesion that might interfere with coagulation. Diseases of the bone marrow, liver and drugs may cause problems with clotting.

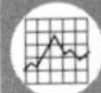

Q2: What additional features in the history would you like to elicit?

A2

The additional feature in the history that would be useful is to take a history of bruising or bleeding elsewhere in the body. A full general medical history should be taken on any adult who presents with epistaxis once the condition has been treated. Therapy may interfere with clotting and the two most common drugs are aspirin and warfarin.

Q3: What investigations would be most helpful and why?

A3

The investigations are undertaken after the patient has been assessed and active bleeding stopped if he or she is admitted to hospital. The pulse and blood pressure should be checked. A full blood count (FBC) should be undertaken at the time of bleeding and 24 h later to assess the degree of blood loss. A clotting screen, particularly prothrombin time and partial thromboplastin time, or an international normalized ratio (INR) should be performed to see whether the patient is over-anticoagulated.

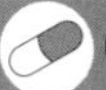

Q4: What are the treatment options?

A4

The priority is to arrest haemorrhage and resuscitate the patient should he be shocked and collapsed. Once the patient has been admitted the local treatment includes packing the nose with a variety of substances, including BIPP (bismuth iodoform paraffin paste) packing under local anaesthesia. If the nose is packed the patient does require admission to hospital. Occasionally, it is possible to treat such patients with cautery to the blood vessel if it can be identified. This may be undertaken using an endoscope to view the blood vessel. If the patient has been over-anticoagulated, correction of this is also required. If the pack remains *in situ* over 48 h antibiotic prophylaxis is required because a secondary sinusitis may develop. All patients with packing should be admitted to the hospital because hypoxia, confusion and inhalation of a pack may occur. Occasionally, operations are required such as correction of septal displacement so that the nose can be packed very tightly under a general anaesthetic. Packing the nose is an uncomfortable procedure and should be undertaken under local anaesthesia.

CASE 1.2 – Child with nose bleed.

Q1: What is the likely differential diagnosis?

A1

The differential diagnosis is the same as for Case 1.1. However, it is exceptionally rare for systemic disease to present with epistaxis in a child, although acute leukaemia may present in this way. The most common cause is dilated vessels in Little's area where the internal and external carotid arteries anastomose.

Q2: What additional features in the history would you like to elicit?

A2

The additional features in the history are those in Case 1.1. Bruising and other bleeding problems should always be asked about in children with epistaxis. A full history of nasal symptoms such as crusting of the anterior nose should also be asked about.

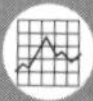

Q3: What investigations would be most helpful and why?

A3

Unless there is systemic disease it is considered that no investigations are required. Occasionally, an FBC is needed if the patient has bled actively and often. Anaemia is very rare from epistaxis in children.

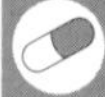

Q4: What are the treatment options?

A4

The treatment in children is slightly different from that in an adult as a child often has vestibulitis. A course of Naseptin cream (chlorhexidine hydrochloride) to the anterior nasal vestibule on both sides may settle any infection and resolve the condition because the child then picks the nose less frequently. Simple cautery with silver nitrate is often effective in over half the cases, and can be undertaken with or without local anaesthesia. If the child is aged under 5 years, it is better to perform cautery under general anaesthesia so that it can be done effectively. Parents should be warned that children with epistaxis tend to get further bleeding in half of all cases.

OSCE Counselling Cases – Answers

OSCE COUNSELLING CASE 1.1 – What advice should you give to an adult male who is coming into hospital and has had his nose packed?

The patient should be advised that he will be in hospital between 2 and 3 days. The packing will be in place for 1–2 days and may be painful when removed. The patient should also be advised that there might be some fresh bleeding and clots when the packs come out. It is important to stress that a few simple investigations will be done to check the clotting status and this may require treatment as well.

OSCE COUNSELLING CASE 1.2 – A single mother has a child aged 3 years with profuse intermittent nosebleeds, which occur at night.

It is important to stress that the bleeding always looks a lot worse than the actual amount lost. A simple analogy – that a cup of coffee or a glass of wine looks more when spilt – will often suffice. It is also worthwhile stressing that children often rub the blood on their face while they are having nosebleeds. Counsel the mother that it is perfectly easy to stop most nosebleeds by sitting the child up, asking him to breathe through the mouth, and squeezing the cartilaginous part of the nasal septum between the thumb and forefingers for between 3 and 5 minutes. Advise that cautery will be undertaken under a general anaesthetic if she wishes for surgical treatment because this is the most effective way to control the symptoms. Stress also that it possible to try to control the nosebleeds by using Naseptin cream to control any vestibulitis.

UNILATERAL NASAL DISCHARGE

? Questions for each of the clinical case scenarios given

Q1: What is the likely differential diagnosis?
Q2: What additional features in the history would you like to elicit?
Q3: What investigations would be most helpful and why?
Q4: What are the treatment options?

Clinical cases

CASE 1.3 – Child with unilateral discharge.

A child aged 2 years presents with a 1-week history of unilateral nasal discharge.

CASE 1.4 – Adult with head injury.

A 24-year-old man who had a head injury a month previously with slight concussion has a loss of sense of smell and a unilateral clear discharge from the left side of the nose. Q4 is not applicable in this case.

OSCE Counselling Cases

OSCE COUNSELLING CASE 1.3 – The child with a unilateral discharge.

The mother is concerned about the risk of a general anaesthetic in a child. How can you reassure her that the child is not in any danger?

OSCE COUNSELLING CASE 1.4 – The adult with a CSF leak.

The patient wonders why he needs an operation because the amount of cerebrospinal fluid (CSF) is only a few drops every few minutes.

Key concepts

- Unilateral mucoid nasal discharge in a child is a foreign body.
- Unilateral nasal discharge should be investigated.
- Unilateral clear nasal discharge is CSF until proved otherwise.

Answers

CASE 1.3 – Child with unilateral discharge.

Q1: What is the likely differential diagnosis?

A1

A foreign body.

Q2: What additional features in the history would you like to elicit?

A2

Ask the parent if the child put anything into his nose. Remember that other children may have put an object into the child's nose. Examination may show the foreign body and it is rare that this can be hooked out in the outpatient department.

Q3: What investigations would be most helpful and why?

A3

No investigations are required for a mucoid or purulent discharge. The child should be examined in the operating theatre.

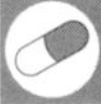

Q4: What are the treatment options?

A4

The treatment is to examine the child in theatre to exclude a foreign body. If none is found the child may have unilateral sinusitis and a washout can be undertaken at the time. The child should be put on the next available operating list and the nose examined under general anaesthesia. The foreign body is usually easily found and removed. The discharge may take a few days to settle, particularly if there is some granulation tissue in the nose. If this is florid it can be removed at the same time.

CASE 1.4 – Adult with head injury.

Q1: What is the likely differential diagnosis?

A1

The chief worry is a CSF leak. This is the diagnosis of exclusion because sinusitis may occur.

 Q2: What additional features in the history would you like to elicit?

A2

Ask if there have been any other episodes of discharge before the head injury. If so this changes the probable diagnosis. Although spontaneous CSF leaks do occur, they are relatively rare. Ask the standard history for the nose episodes of blockage, running, sneezing, etc. Adults rarely put foreign bodies up their nose unless they are mentally disturbed or have a learning disability.

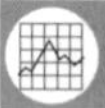 Q3: What investigations would be most helpful and why?

A3

Collect the fluid to measure Tau protein (β-transferrin). Computed tomography (CT) of the paranasal sinuses and magnetic resonance imaging (MRI) of the anterior cranial fossa should be undertaken. The treatment is simple: the CSF leak should be closed surgically. The patient should be given prophylactic antibiotics and operated on as soon as possible. This may be undertaken endoscopically.

OSCE Counselling Cases – Answers

OSCE COUNSELLING CASE 1.3 – The child with unilateral discharge.

Stress that the risk of general anaesthesia is very small. Say also that the child is in excellent hands and they are used to dealing with children and their problems. Some children are frightened about needles and local anaesthetic creams will make the process pain free. If a child prefers, gas may be used instead. About 8 per cent of children have asthma and most volatile agents are bronchodilators.

OSCE COUNSELLING CASE 1.4 – The adult with a CSF leak.

The risk of meningitis is high and serious complications could result, including the death of the patient. It is much better to close the leak when the patient is well and the risk of complications small. The patient has to be counselled that there are very slight risks that when the CSF leak is being repaired he could have a loss of sense of smell if this has not occurred before. If the leak has been present for a month as in this case spontaneous closure is highly unlikely because it normally occurs within 2 weeks of the injury.

NASAL OBSTRUCTION

? Questions for each of the clinical case scenarios given

Q1: What additional features in the history would you like to elicit?
Q2: What should one look for in the examination?
Q3: What investigations would be most helpful and why?
Q4: What are the treatment options?

Clinical cases

CASE 1.5 – Child with nasal obstruction and snoring.

A child aged 7 presents with blocked nose and snoring at night. The mother asks that the adenoids be removed to improve the symptoms.

CASE 1.6 – Adolescent with nasal trauma.

A 17-year-old teenager had trauma to his nose 6 months previously and comes to the clinic with his father. He requests surgery to sort out his nasal obstruction.

OSCE Counselling Cases

OSCE COUNSELLING CASE 1.5 – A mother asks whether a cat should be destroyed if this causes allergic rhinitis.

OSCE COUNSELLING CASE 1.6 – What advice should you give to the boy in Case 1.6 who wants to continue playing football and judo?

Key concepts

- Bilateral nasal discharge is often the result of allergy rather than an adenoid problem.
- Treat allergy medically.
- Treat septal deformity by surgery when contact sport has ceased.

Answers

 CASE 1.5 – **Child with nasal obstruction and snoring.**

 Q1: What additional features in the history would you like to elicit?

A1

Determine whether the nasal obstruction fluctuates from side to side or is continuous. Ask whether obstructive apnoea is present at night. It is much more common in children aged under 4 years. Other nasal symptoms include sneezing attacks, or clear or mucoid running nasal discharge. Older children and adults may complain of postnasal drip, changes in the sense of smell and facial pain. Asthma and rhinitis coexist.

 Q2: What should one look for in the examination?

A2

Watch the child in the clinic. If a child is breathing through his or her nose, the adenoids cannot be hypertrophied. Adenoid hypertrophy causes permanent nasal obstruction and these children sit with their mouths open. It is important to examine the tonsils because large tonsils may cause mouth breathing. The tip of a child's nose turns up easily to help when looking at the mucosa. A purple colour suggests allergy. Place a metal spatula under the nose and observe the misting pattern.

 Q3: What investigations would be most helpful and why?

A3

Undertake allergy testing and a radiograph of the postnasal space.

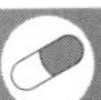 Q4: What are the treatment options?

A4

If the child has an obvious allergic rhinitis the standard treatment is avoidance of the allergen, if at all possible, followed by medical treatment. Surgery has little part to play. The radiograph of the postnasal space will confirm adenoid enlargement. Enlarged adenoids may be removed surgically.

CASE 1.6 – Adolescent with nasal trauma.

Q1: What additional features in the history would you like to elicit?

A1

Take the same history as for Case 1.5, but always ask about contact sport. Never advise nasal surgery except for manipulation of a fracture when the risk of re-injury is high.

Q2: What should one look for in the examination?

A2

Examine the bony pyramid of the nose and make sure that this has not been fractured. Look at the cartilaginous septum to see whether this is displaced at either side. Turn the tip of the nose up to see whether the front part of the septum has been dislocated outwards.

Q3: What investigations would be most helpful and why?

A3

Undertake allergy testing on all patients who have bilateral nasal obstruction because many will have an allergic rhinitis. It is rarely necessary to undertake any other investigations.

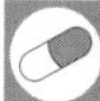

Q4: What are the treatment options?

A4

Surgery should not be undertaken until 18 years of age because the nose is growing. Avoid septal surgery if the child plays a contact sport.

OSCE Counselling Cases – Answers

OSCE COUNSELLING CASE 1.5 – A mother asks whether a cat should be destroyed if this causes allergic rhinitis.

Frequently children are not concerned about their nasal symptoms but the parents are. The cat is more important than the symptoms. The cat should be excluded from the bedroom. If the child is severely disturbed by the symptoms it may be necessary to re-house the pet. The cat must go if it causes severe asthma.

OSCE COUNSELLING CASE 1.6 – What advice should you give to the boy who wants to continue playing football and judo?

Stress that surgery on the septum makes the structure weaker and more prone to further damage. Should another injury occur cosmetic deformity could be extreme and exceptionally difficult to correct. The septum can be corrected at any time, because nasal obstruction is not a life-threatening condition. Boys are often worried about the shape of their nose. Explain that personality is more important than the shape of the nose with prospective partners. Patients and their relatives will usually accept this type of decision.

LANGUAGE DELAY AND DEVELOPMENT

? Questions for each of the clinical case scenarios given

Q1: What additional features in the history would you like to elicit?
Q2: What should one look for in the examination?
Q3: What investigations would be most helpful and why?
Q4: What are the treatment options?

Clinical cases

CASE 1.7 – Parents are worried about a 1 year old who is not speaking.

CASE 1.8 – A mother comes with a child of three and a half who is badly behaved and also not talking well.

OSCE Counselling Cases

OSCE COUNSELLING CASE 1.7 – What would your advice be to a mother who is concerned about the education and development of this child with hearing aids?

OSCE COUNSELLING CASE 1.8 – What advice would you give to a mother who is concerned about swimming and grommets?

Key concepts

Language delay may be the result of sensorineural hearing loss or caused by middle-ear disease.

- Assess development.
- Treat moderate bilateral sensorineural hearing loss with a hearing aid.
- Treat bilateral profound hearing loss by cochlear implantation.
- Children may swim with grommets *in situ*.

Answers

CASE 1.7 – Parents are worried about a 1 year old who is not speaking.

Q1: What additional features in the history would you like to elicit?

A1

Determine whether the child is at risk of developing sensorineural hearing loss. Risks include prematurity, jaundice, hypoxia or a difficult birth, and infections either during pregnancy or post partum, e.g. measles or rubella. Ask whether the child babbled and responded to sound when younger. Also ask about the developmental milestones during the first year, and the age of sitting, crawling and use of a spoon. Sometimes language delay is the result of a general developmental delay, so is it important to exclude this.

Q2: What should one look for in the examination?

A2

Observe the child while he is sitting in the clinic and see whether he responds to sound when people move around behind him. If the child is crying the quality of the cry can also be assessed in the clinic. Examine the ears to make sure that there is no congenital cause for the hearing loss. The position of the ears on the skull may give this away. The external ear canals can be abnormal as well. Make sure that the eardrum and middle ear are normal and that there is no glue ear.

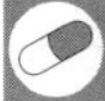

Q3: What investigations would be most helpful and why?

A3

Simple distraction testing can be carried out by trained staff in the audiology department. A tympanogram will demonstrate an effusion. A sensorineural hearing loss can be investigated by cochlear echoes and brain-stem responses. These tests require sedation but can be undertaken after a feed in some younger children.

Q4: What are the treatment options?

A4

The treatment is to identify the cause of the problem. If the child does have bilateral severe sensorineural hearing loss, it is important to provide hearing aids so that language development can occur as quickly as possible. If the child has a profound sensorineural hearing loss a cochlear implant should be considered. The earlier that surgery is undertaken the better. If surgery is undertaken before the age of 2 years, the child stands a very good chance of developing normal language.

CASE 1.8 – A mother comes with a child of three and a half who is badly behaved and also not talking well.

Q1: What additional features in the history would you like to elicit?

A1

Ask whether language development was normal up to 2 years. Also ask whether the child has any older brothers and sisters, because language may be slower in later children. Exclude recurrent acute otitis media and discharging ears in a child of this age. There may occasionally be a sensorineural hearing loss, particularly if the child has had meningitis, so a full past history should be taken.

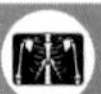

Q2: What should one look for in the examination?

A2

A full ENT examination should be undertaken. However, the most likely cause at this age is glue ear (otitis media with effusion).

Q3: What investigations would be most helpful and why?

A3

Children of this age may be old enough to undertake a pure-tone audiogram but may require conditioned response audiometry. Children are conditioned to remove a toy from a container when they hear a sound. Accurate thresholds can be determined well in this way at different frequencies. However, both ears are assessed together using this technique. Language should develop normally even if one ear is deaf. Impedance audiometry will exclude glue ear.

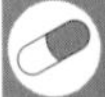

Q4: What are the treatment options?

A4

A child with glue ear and language delay should have ventilation tubes (grommets) inserted. Behavioural problems reinforce this. It is normal practice to observe the condition to see whether it resolves over a 3-month period. As many of these children have been seen at least 2 or 3 months before their ENT clinic visit the effusion is usually previously documented.

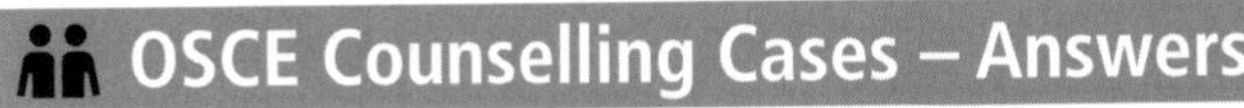

OSCE COUNSELLING CASE 1.7 – What would your advice be to a mother who is concerned about the education and development of this child with hearing aids?

Stress that many children who have hearing aids accept them well. Older children will use them in the classroom setting. Explain that most children with hearing aids will be educated in a normal school with no additional support. Emphasize that special education can be provided if necessary. The hearing aid service in most areas in the UK is reasonably well developed, with teachers of deaf people entering the school to assess children with hearing aids, in order to ensure that educational needs are met. The child should fulfil his or her full potential and even go to university if desired. (The best centres have multidisciplinary teams, which incorporate teachers, social workers, the doctor and audiology support services.)

OSCE COUNSELLING CASE 1.8 – What advice would you give to a mother who is concerned about swimming and grommets?

There is much controversy about swimming and grommets. Work from Australia would suggest that the prevalence of discharge is no greater in children who swim with grommets than in those who do not. A child should not dive or jump into water. Hair washing is more risky because the soap or detergent reduces the surface tension and makes middle-ear contamination and discharge more likely. Advise parents to protect the ears in younger children and ask the child to make sure that water and soap do not run into the ear during a shower or bath.

ADULT EAR DISEASE

? Questions for each of the clinical case scenarios given

Q1: What is the likely differential diagnosis?
Q2: What is the important finding on examination?
Q3: What additional features in the history would you like to elicit?
Q4: What are the treatment options?

Clinical cases

CASE 1.9 – Ear discharge.

A 25-year-old man presents with progressive hearing loss of 3 years and recently an intermittent, but scanty, smelly discharge.

CASE 1.10 – Progressive hearing loss.

A woman aged 53 years presents with a 12-month history of a progressive, left-sided, sensorineural hearing loss with occasional tinnitus.

OSCE Counselling Cases

OSCE COUNSELLING CASE 1.9 – What advice would you give to the patient who is having a mastoid exploration?

OSCE COUNSELLING CASE 1.10 – A patient with a unilateral acoustic neuroma wants to know the risk of developing one on the other side. What is your advice to the patient?

Key concepts

- Unilateral discharge with mucus means that there is a perforation.
- Unilateral discharge which smells foul may hide a cholesteatoma.
- Always examine the eardrum.
- A unilateral sensorineural hearing loss needs MRI to exclude an acoustic neuroma.

Answers

CASE 1.9 – Ear discharge.

Q1: What is the likely differential diagnosis?

A1

The differential diagnosis includes otitis externa, or otitis media with a perforation and this may have cholesteatoma. A carcinoma is very rare and is painful.

Q2: What is the important finding on examination?

A2

The external ear canal and drum should be inspected. Start with the better ear and then proceed to the diseased side. Note whether there is any wax or debris in the external canal. This requires removal because the eardrum must be inspected fully. Do not syringe a discharging ear. The history in this case suggests chronic middle-ear disease with cholesteatoma. Cholesteatoma is the presence of squamous epithelium in the middle-ear cleft, which erodes into the structures and may give rise to intracranial complications; this is why it is important to diagnose the condition. Brown/white smelly discharge is seen in the attic and also sometimes in the posterior part of the eardrum.

Q3: What additional features in the history would you like to elicit?

A3

Ask about any hearing loss, pain, discharge, dizziness and tinnitus for each ear. Ask about the relationships between the symptoms. If a patient has a progressive hearing loss together with an intermittent scanty discharge, but no pain, it suggests a chronic middle-ear problem. If there is pain the patient may have either a middle-ear problem or otitis externa. If the discharge is profuse and mucoid, it comes from the middle ear, so the eardrum must be perforated. Middle-ear disease may produce vertigo but the dizzy patient is considered later and you are referred to Cases 1.13 and 1.14.

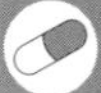

Q4: What are the treatment options?

A4

This patient should have a pure-tone audiogram with air-conduction, bone-conduction and masking thresholds determined.

Imaging: there is a debate about imaging in cholesteatomatous disease. High-resolution computed tomography (HRCT) of the temporal bone may show extension into the semicircular canals towards the brain.

The ear should be examined under the microscope in the outpatient department and the extent of the disease confirmed. If cholesteatoma is present, mastoid surgery is required to eradicate the disease and prevent intracranial complications.

CASE 1.10 – Progressive hearing loss.

Q1: What is the likely differential diagnosis?

A1

Although there is often no cause for a unilateral, progressive, sensorineural hearing loss, an acoustic neuroma must be excluded, i.e. a tumour of the eighth nerve, which either arises in the petrous portion of the eighth nerve or extends into the intracranial cavity by the brain stem. Occasionally, a unilateral sensorineural hearing loss may arise from a viral infection or ischaemia, particularly in older patients.

Q2: What is the important finding on examination?

A2

The external ear canal and drum should be inspected. Start with the better ear and then proceed to the diseased side. Note whether there is any wax or debris in the external canal. This requires removal because the eardrum must be inspected fully. Do not syringe a discharging ear. A patient with a sensorineural hearing loss with no other obvious cause has a normal eardrum.

Q3: What additional features in the history would you like to elicit?

A3

Ask about any hearing loss, pain, discharge, dizziness and tinnitus for each ear. Ask about the relationships between the symptoms. If a patient has a progressive hearing loss together with an intermittent scanty discharge, but no pain, it suggests a chronic middle-ear problem. If there is pain the patient may have either a middle-ear problem or otitis externa. If the discharge is profuse and mucoid, it comes from the middle ear, so the eardrum must be perforated. Middle-ear disease may produce vertigo but the dizzy patient is considered later and you are referred to Cases 1.13 and 1.14.

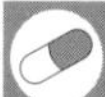

Q4: What are the treatment options?

A4

This patient should have a pure-tone audiogram with air-conduction, bone-conduction and masking thresholds determined.

Imaging: there is a debate about imaging in cholesteatomatous disease. HRCT of the temporal bone may show extension into the semicircular canals towards the brain. The patient with a unilateral sensorineural hearing loss must have MRI undertaken because this defines acoustic neuroma most accurately.

Treatment for an acoustic neuroma is surgical. However, very small lesions can be watched for 6 months or a year to make sure that they are not growing quickly. Surgery often results in complete hearing loss and may also result in a facial palsy. The tumour is usually approached through the inner ear itself because this gives the least morbidity.

OSCE Counselling Cases – Answers

OSCE COUNSELLING CASE 1.9 – What advice would you give to the patient who is having a mastoid exploration?

Stress that the disease may cause a serious problem and even intracranial complications if left untreated. The hearing may be worse after surgery. Explain that there is a very small risk to the facial nerve while undertaking middle-ear surgery. The disease will require some form of follow-up for life if a mastoid cavity is produced during surgery.

OSCE COUNSELLING CASE 1.10 – A patient with a unilateral acoustic neuroma wants to know the risk of developing one on the other side. What is your advice to the patient?

Unless a patient has neurofibromatosis type 2, the risk of developing bilateral acoustic neuroma is incredibly rare. It is possible to hear with one ear perfectly satisfactorily. Problems may occur in localizing sound and discrimination in a crowded environment.

ADULT BILATERAL DEAFNESS

Questions for the clinical case scenario given

Q1: What additional features in the history would you like to elicit?
Q2: What investigations would be most helpful and why?

Clinical case

CASE 1.11 – Adult with bilateral deafness.

A 66-year-old man comes to the department with decreased hearing over the previous 7 years and both ears are the same.

OSCE Counselling Case

OSCE COUNSELLING CASE 1.11 – A patient wants to use a hearing aid but feels that it will exacerbate the condition. What is your advice?

Key concepts

- Presbyacusis may require a hearing aid.
- Hearing aids work if the patient requests them.
- Digital hearing aids may be better than analogue ones.

Answers

CASE 1.11 – Adult with bilateral deafness.

Q1: What additional features in the history would you like to elicit?

A1

Ask about all symptoms as in Case 1.9, to determine whether there are any others. Determine the occupation. Although presbyacusis does occur at this age it may well be exacerbated by a noisy occupation and, although there is much better control of noise levels in factories, many workers do not wear ear defenders. Systemic diseases such as diabetes mellitus and cardiovascular atheroma may exacerbate the ageing changes. Ask whether the patient wants a hearing aid – relatives often want the device rather than the patient. This is a recipe for failure.

Q2: What investigations would be most helpful and why?

A2

Assess the degree of hearing loss in both the low and the high frequencies. The high-frequency component is the element associated with articulation. Patients will often say that they hear what people say but they cannot understand. Most patients who have a moderate hearing loss or greater require a hearing aid but the patient has to accept this before it is worth prescribing one. If a patient is in two minds I suggest that he or she tries one for a period and then returns it if it is unsatisfactory. I also suggest that a further audiometric assessment may be undertaken after a year if a patient is unhappy with a hearing aid. Modern digital hearing aids can be tuned to the hearing loss and so may be more suitable for patients.

OSCE Counselling Case – Answer

OSCE COUNSELLING CASE 1.11 – A patient wants to use a hearing aid but feels that it will exacerbate the condition. What is your advice?

There is no evidence that wearing a hearing aid worsens any sensorineural hearing loss. Stress that the hearing will change over time and become slightly worse irrespective of whether or not a hearing aid is used.

EARACHE

? Questions for each of the clinical case scenarios given

Q1: What is the important finding on examination?
Q2: What should one look for in the examination?
Q3: What investigations would be most helpful and why?
Q4: What are the treatment options?

Clinical cases

CASE 1.12 – **Child with earache.**

A child aged 3 years has an acute earache, which has started that day.

CASE 1.13 – **Adult with earache.**

An adult aged 37 years presents with intermittently painful ears, mostly affecting the right side.

OSCE Counselling Case

OSCE COUNSELLING CASE 1.12 – **A patient wants to swim when you have diagnosed otitis externa. What is your advice?**

Key concepts

- Otitis media may be treated conservatively if mild.
- Do not poke the ears in otitis externa.
- Pain may be referred to the ears from the jaw or the neck.

Answers

CASE 1.12 – Child with earache.

Q1: What is the important finding on examination?

A1

Ask if the child has a respiratory infection. How severe is the pain? This can be gauged by asking whether the child is kept awake at night, holds his ear and wants to go to bed. Ascertain whether the child has any other ear symptoms as in the previous questions. Enquire about constitutional symptoms. The most likely diagnosis is acute otitis media. Other structures may refer to the ear and a teething child may have pain, which can be difficult to distinguish from a middle-ear problem.

Q2: What should one look for in the examination?

A2

Examine both ears and see whether one sticks out more than the other. A child might have a more severe problem such as acute mastoiditis. There is swelling behind the ear and it is pushed forwards and slightly downwards. Examine the better ear first. Children often have a pink eardrum when they have a cold. If both ears look the same, acute otitis media is unlikely. If there is pus behind the drum, it is pushed forwards. This is most obvious in the posterosuperior region and this is the most common site of rupture. If the eardrum has not been examined, the diagnosis of acute otitis media is presumptive.

Q3: What investigations would be most helpful and why?

A3

No investigations are required for simple acute otitis media.

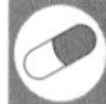

Q4: What are the treatment options?

A4

There is much debate about the need for antibiotic chemotherapy in acute otitis media. There are very obvious flaws in the clinical trials that are evident to those with even a slight knowledge of ENT. Basically, if the child is well and has little in the way of constitutional symptoms, no treatment is required. If the child has mild discomfort, treat with analgesia, because the condition will settle in the vast majority. If the child is unwell and the eardrum bulging dramatically, treat with antibiotics such as amoxicillin at the appropriate dose for the weight and age of the child. If the child is vomiting, the first dose should be given intramuscularly. Erythromycin is a suitable alternative if the child is sensitive to penicillins. Intracranial sepsis follows acute ear infections very occasionally.

CASE 1.13 – Adult with earache.

Q1: What is the important finding on examination?

A1

Ask the patient whether there are any other symptoms in addition to the pain as in the earlier scenarios. Patients frequently miss itching. The most likely cause of earache in the adult is either otitis externa or referred otalgia. Young adults have temporomandibular problems and questions about chewing and pain will help to determine if this is the cause. Elderly people may have problems with the cervical spine, which also causes a referred otalgia. Otitis externa may go from ear to ear and there is a period of irritation followed by self-inflicted trauma and secondary infection. The cycle repeats itself.

Q2: What should one look for in the examination?

A2

Examine the better ear first so that it can be compared with the one causing the problem. If there is debris, this should be removed. The diagnosis of otitis externa cannot be made until the drum has been examined and is shown to be intact. Sometimes there is a secondary otitis externa when there is a perforation, but mucus means that there is middle-ear disease. There are three common types of otitis externa: a furuncle in the hair-bearing area, and diffuse oedematous and diffuse eczematous otitis externa. Examine the temporomandibular joint and neck. Some patients poke their ears if there is pain there and set up secondary otitis externa.

Q3: What investigations would be most helpful and why?

A3

No investigations are mandatory, although an ear swab may help with antibiotic sensitivity. The infecting organism is *Pseudomonas aeruginosa* in most cases.

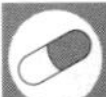

Q4: What are the treatment options?

A4

Treatment is meticulous oral toilet. It is possible to syringe the ear to clean it, but keep this to a minimum. Once the debris is removed treatment with Locorten-Vioform or some other drops is helpful. Tell the patient to keep the ear dry and not to poke it. If the problem does not settle easily referral to the ENT department may be required. Patients with diabetes need careful monitoring because they may develop a severe otitis externa called malignant otitis externa. The condition may erode into the cranial cavity, when it is fatal.

OSCE Counselling Case – Answer

OSCE COUNSELLING CASE 1.12 – A patient wants to swim when you have diagnosed otitis externa. What is your advice?

No. The patient should be symptom free for 3 months before re-commencing swimming.

THE DIZZY PATIENT

? Questions for the clinical case scenario given

Q1: What is the important finding on examination?
Q2: What investigations would be most helpful and why?
Q3: What are the treatment options?

Clinical case

CASE 1.14 – Dizziness.

An adult presents with dizziness when she turns her head and rolls over in bed. She says that it comes from the left side of the head.

OSCE Counselling Case

OSCE COUNSELLING CASE 1.13 – The patient with benign positional vertigo in the first attack is obviously worried that there is something sinister going on. What is your advice?

Key concepts

- Dizziness may be unsteadiness or true vertigo.
- True vertigo coming from the labyrinth never causes unconsciousness.
- Vertigo on head movements for a few seconds is benign positional vertigo.
- Episodic vertigo with hearing loss and tinnitus may be Menière's disease.

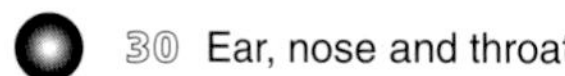

Answers

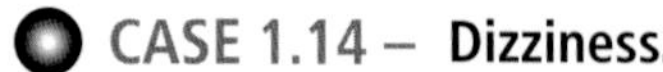

CASE 1.14 – Dizziness.

Q1: What is the important finding on examination?

A1

Determine whether the patient has true vertigo, rather than unsteadiness. Vertigo is the hallucination of movement: either the environment moves or the patient moves. Ask the patient whether she has had similar attacks before and whether the attacks are episodic. Ask how long the attack is. If it is for a few seconds without hearing loss and tinnitus, it is likely to be benign positional vertigo. Menière's disease tends to present with tinnitus and hearing loss, together with the vertigo, over a period of hours. Vestibular neuritis lasts for days and will not be associated with other ear symptoms. Ask about unconsciousness. Patients with peripheral lesions are conscious whereas those with central nervous system problems, which may be vascular in origin, can lose consciousness. Ask whether epileptic attacks occur. A full general history should be taken for all patients with dizziness, including cardiovascular, respiratory, central nervous and gastrointestinal symptoms. Many patients with vascular disease and hypertension feel unsteady when they stand up.

Q2: What investigations would be most helpful and why?

A2

A full but brief neurological examination as well as ENT examination should be undertaken. The pulse and blood pressure should be measured. If a patient has good mobility of the cervical spine, positional tests should be undertaken. The most likely diagnosis here is benign positional vertigo. Details of these may be found in any standard ENT textbook. Investigations include audiometry and occasionally caloric testing. If the diagnosis is benign positional vertigo, no further investigation is required. If there is asymmetrical hearing MRI of the internal auditory meatus should be arranged.

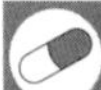

Q3: What are the treatment options?

A3

Treatment for benign positional vertigo is reassurance. The condition is the result of problems in the semicircular canals, and the vast majority of cases resolve spontaneously. Occasionally, physiotherapy and positional exercises may aid the recovery of the condition. As patients find the condition so disabling at times, they are frequently unwilling to undertake these exercises.

OSCE Counselling Case – Answer

OSCE COUNSELLING CASE 1.13 – **The patient with benign positional vertigo in the first attack is obviously worried that there is something sinister going on. What is your advice?**

As it is very easy to make the diagnosis, you can inform the patient that the disease is coming from the inner ear and that he does not have a serious brain condition. Patients are often worried about this and they may not volunteer the information, so mention it. State that the condition is self-limiting but they may have relapses from time to time and take up to 3 months to recover in the first instance. When you undertake a positional test, you can demonstrate that the nystagmus fatigues and that you can localize the side affected. If it is a particular problem, patients should not put that side down in bed; if they do they may well elicit the condition. If they have a lot of problems driving they should not do so until the condition has resolved.

ACUTE FACIAL PALSY

? Questions for the clinical case scenario given

Q1: What is the important finding on examination?
Q2: What additional features in the history would you like to elicit?
Q3: What investigations would be most helpful and why?
Q4: What are the treatment options?

Clinical case

CASE 1.15 – Acute facial palsy.

An adult aged 32 presents with an acute facial palsy on the left side.

OSCE Counselling Case

OSCE COUNSELLING CASE 1.14 – A patient who has an acute Bell's palsy that is partial and occurred 3 days previously is concerned about recovery. What is your advice?

Key concepts

- Assess upper and lower motor neuron function.
- Examine the mouth, external ear and parotid gland.
- Check the eye to make sure that it is protected.
- Try penciclovir 500 mg orally three times daily for 5 days.
- Corticosteroids should be started only in the first 48 h if the Bell's palsy is complete.

Answers

CASE 1.15 – Acute facial palsy.

Q1: What is the important finding on examination?

A1

Check whether it is an upper or a lower motor neuron lesion because upper motor neuron lesions spare the forehead. The vast majority at this age will be lower motor neuron lesions. Try to grade the palsy. If you cannot determine the severity, note whether it is partial or complete. The single most important observation is whether the patient can cover the cornea when she tries to close her eyes. The eye is most at risk from corneal damage with a facial palsy. Lacrimation may well be reduced as well. Examine the ear and the palate because Ramsay Hunt syndrome may present with pain and vesicles on the soft palate, tonsil area, or ear canal and drum. This is the sensory supply of the seventh cranial nerve. The parotid gland should be felt to exclude a lesion in this area. The most likely cause in this age group is Bell's or idiopathic facial palsy.

Q2: What additional features in the history would you like to elicit?

A2

Ask whether the palsy came on suddenly and whether it is painful, particularly pain in the ear. Ask about hearing, taste and lacrimation. A quick neurological assessment and cardiovascular history will exclude these conditions.

Q3: What investigations would be most helpful and why?

A3

A simple case of Bell's palsy requires no investigation except audiometry.

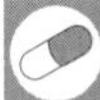

Q4: What are the treatment options?

A4

There is a case for giving a course of penciclovir 500 mg three times a day orally for a week in Bell's palsy. Oral steroids such as prednisolone should be reserved for herpes zoster because there is some evidence that this may help the resolution here, or if the palsy is complete and immediate in Bell's palsy. The most important aspect of treatment is corneal protection. If there is any doubt, the patient should be referred to the eye surgeon. In the meantime artificial tears and tapes should be provided.

OSCE Counselling Case – Answer

OSCE COUNSELLING CASE 1.14 – A patient who has an acute Bell's palsy that is partial and occurred 3 days previously is concerned about recovery. What is your advice?

Stress that virtually every case of Bell's palsy recovers by 6 months. If the palsy is partial and there is good eye closure, the recovery may well be quicker. Some patients are concerned that they have had a stroke and you will be able to reassure them that this is not the case. Others may be concerned that there is something serious going on within the brain, and again you can stress that it is the nerve that supplies face that is affected rather than anything more serious.

THROAT

? Questions for each of the clinical case scenarios given

Q1: What is the important finding on examination?
Q2: What should one look for in the examination?
Q3: What investigations would be most helpful and why?
Q4: What are the treatment options?

Clinical cases

CASE 1.16 – Child with sore throat.

A mother presents with a child who has a recurrent sore throat causing constitutional symptoms.

CASE 1.17 – Adolescent with acute sore throat.

An adolescent aged 17 comes to the surgery with an acute sore throat, feeling unwell.

CASE 1.18 – Smoker with continuous sore throat.

A smoker aged 65 presents with a continuous sore throat, which is progressive, and complains of pain when swallowing.

OSCE Counselling Case

OSCE COUNSELLING CASE 1.15 – A mother wonders when a child may return to school after a tonsillectomy.

Key concepts

- Children have frequent viral respiratory infections.
- Tonsillitis should cause morbidity and school absences for 2 years before a tonsillectomy is performed.
- Adolescents may have infectious mononucleosis.
- Smokers with sore throat and pain on swallowing have a carcinoma.

Answers

CASE 1.16 – Child with sore throat.

 Q1: What is the important finding on examination?

A1

Confirm tonsillitis. Lymphadenopathy may be palpated and is frequent in children, particularly in the jugular digastric region.

 Q2: What should one look for in the examination?

A2

As children have frequent sore throats, determine whether the symptoms are the result of tonsillitis. A normal child will have up to three or four attacks of tonsillitis a year and a further four or five colds in a year. Children should have at least a history of severe tonsillitis for 18 months to 2 years before referral to the ENT surgeon. Ask whether the tonsils swell up and whether they have exudate on them. Determine the length and frequency of the attacks: they should last between 5 and 7 days and cause constitutional symptoms, and there should be six or more attacks a year resulting in school absence. The vast majority of other sore throats are caused by viral infections. The appetite may be affected intermittently and respiratory symptoms may also occur. Occasionally, there is obstructive sleep apnoea in patients with snoring. Sleep apnoea occurs mostly below 4 years of age.

 Q3: What investigations would be most helpful and why?

A3

None is usually required.

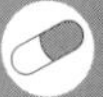 Q4: What are the treatment options?

A4

As the vast majority of infections are viral, no treatment is required. Occasionally, bacterial tonsillitis does occur and if the symptoms are particularly severe and prolonged a 5-day course of antibiotics, such as amoxicillin, may be helpful. Tonsillectomy should not be recommended as the treatment unless the child has at least 10 days of school absence and six or more attacks a year for about 2 years.

 CASE 1.17 – Adolescent with acute sore throat.

 Q1: What is the important finding on examination?

A1

Examine the oral cavity and tonsil region and palpate the neck. Large fleshy tonsils with an exudate encroaching on to the soft palate may indicate infectious mononucleosis. Lymphadenopathy is often particularly severe and may extend from the neck to the rest of the body. Hepatosplenomegaly may occur as well, and pancreatitis and jaundice are rare complications of the condition.

 Q2: What should one look for in the examination?

A2

A similar history should be taken to exclude recurrent tonsillitis. Concentrate on constitutional symptoms and contacts with a similar problem.

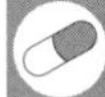 Q3: What investigations would be most helpful and why?

A3

An FBC and serology for glandular fever.

Q4: What are the treatment options?

A4

The vast majority require little more than symptomatic treatment. Occasionally, patients with severe airway problems may require a course of oral steroids to reduce the lymphadenopathy but should be managed in hospital. Very occasionally an urgent tonsillectomy is required for airway management.

 CASE 1.18 – Smoker with continuous sore throat.

 Q1: What is the important finding on examination?

A1

Examine the oral cavity, neck and chest. If you can undertake either a mirror examination or an endoscopic one, it should be performed. The history is highly suggestive of a carcinoma. The tonsil, supraglottic or laryngeal sites are the most likely. Ten per cent of smokers have more than one carcinoma in the aerodigestive tract.

 Q2: What should one look for in the examination?

A2

Particular attention should be paid to the progressive nature of the sore throat, oral intake and respiratory symptoms, including cough, sputum and haemoptysis. The history suggests a supraglottic carcinoma infiltrating the muscle which causes pain on swallowing. This may well not be seen on oral examination.

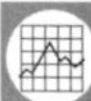 Q3: What investigations would be most helpful and why?

A3

These patients require screening investigations: an FBC, liver function tests, ECG and chest radiograph. Special investigation may include imaging of the neck and chest with CT and MRI. Biopsy the lesion and stage under general anaesthesia.

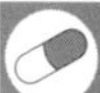 Q4: What are the treatment options?

A4

Staging is the key to treatment. Resection and reconstruction, followed by radiotherapy, offer the best hope. Tumours that extend into the muscle have a poor prognosis. Palliation with radiotherapy and chemotherapy may be all that is possible.

OSCE Counselling Case – Answer

OSCE COUNSELLING CASE 1.15 – A mother wonders when a child may return to school after a tonsillectomy.

Advise that it is usual for a child to stay off school for 2 weeks after surgery. Emphasize that the area has to heal and that there may be a secondary bleed as the slough comes away from the tonsillar fossa. Infection makes this worse, so children should be kept at home during the recovery period. Eating and drinking reduce the risk of infection as well.

DIFFICULTY IN SWALLOWING

? Questions for each of the clinical case scenarios given

Q1: What additional features in the history would you like to elicit?
Q2: What should one look for in the examination?
Q3: What investigations would be most helpful and why?
Q4: What are the treatment options?

Clinical cases

CASE 1.19 – **Lump in throat.**

A woman aged 45 presents with an intermittent feeling of a lump in the throat.

CASE 1.20 – **Problems with swallowing.**

A man aged 68 presents with continuous and progressive problems with swallowing. He is able to swallow liquids but finds solids more difficult.

OSCE Counselling Case

OSCE COUNSELLING CASE 1.16 – **What advice would you give to a patient with globus hystericus who is concerned that he might have a neoplasm?**

Key concepts

- Intermittent dysphagia with a constant weight is benign.
- Continual dysphagia with weight loss is malignant.
- Pain and discomfort are poorly localized in the foregut and may present as a sensation of a neck lump.

Answers

CASE 1.19 – Lump in throat.

CASE 1.20 – Problems with swallowing.

Q1: What additional features in the history would you like to elicit?

A1

Ask the same questions for both cases. Try to unravel whether there is a serious problem for the basis of the complaint. Ask whether there has been any weight change or any symptoms of reflux. The differential diagnosis in these two cases is between globus hystericus and a neoplasm. Neoplasms may arise both outside and within the oesophagus. Compression and direct erosion may come from the thyroid gland and rarely from the thoracic cavity contents and eventual ulceration.

Q2: What should one look for in the examination?

A2

Palpate the neck – there is a physical sign called 'Toynbee's sign'. Move the laryngeal cartilages from side to side over the vertebral column. This produces crepitus in the normal individual and a post-cricoid carcinoma will lift the larynx forwards and crepitus is absent. This also occurs in foreign body or abscesses such as tuberculous cold abscesses. Check for lymphadenopathy. In patients with globus there is no abnormality. In the ENT clinic, nasendoscopy with a flexible endoscope may show pooling of saliva or an abnormality such as a space-occupying lesion.

Q3: What investigations would be most helpful and why?

A3

These include an FBC (sideropenic dysphagia). If a patient is severely dehydrated with neoplasm, urea and electrolytes (U&Es) may be indicated. A barium swallow may show both reflux and neoplasia, but high lesions in the oesophagus do not show up well. Patients with globus should have fibreoptic gastro-oesophagoscopy. Perform a direct endoscopy and biopsy under general anaesthesia if in any doubt. Any tumour should be assessed, biopsied and staged.

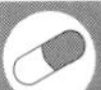

Q4: What are the treatment options?

A4

The management depends on the nature of the underlying lesion and, for globus patients, simple reassurance is often enough. Reflux oesophagitis should be treated appropriately. Reflux is best managed in general practice. Neoplasms require a combination of excision, reconstruction and radiotherapy, or palliation.

OSCE Counselling Case – Answer

OSCE COUNSELLING CASE 1.16 – What advice would you give to a patient with globus hystericus who is concerned that he might have a neoplasm?

Stress that intermittent problems are rarely serious and a stationary weight argues against a serious problem. Say also that the radiological investigation and endoscopy will almost certainly exclude a neoplasm but are not necessary. A hiatus hernia may cause a sensation of a lump in the neck. The primitive foregut extends to the second part of the duodenum and takes its nerve supply with it – it is referred to the neck. Another feature of reflux is spasm of the cricopharyngeus sphincter. An explanation of these anatomical and functional reasons will result in acceptance of the condition and hopefully its cessation.

HOARSE VOICE

? Questions for each of the clinical case scenarios given

Q1: What is the important finding on examination?
Q2: What additional features in the history would you like to elicit?
Q3: What investigations would be most helpful and why?
Q4: What are the treatment options?

Clinical cases

CASE 1.21 – Hoarse voice 1.

A female teacher aged 45 has an intermittent hoarse voice and is concerned that this may affect her job.

CASE 1.22 – Hoarse voice 2.

A 63-year-old heavy smoker presents with a progressive hoarse voice of 6 weeks' duration.

OSCE Counselling Case

OSCE COUNSELLING CASE 1.17 – A woman with an intermittent hoarse voice is worried about her career as a teacher and her voice problem. What advice would you give?

Key concepts

- Intermittent hoarse voice is benign.
- Continual hoarse voice in a smoker is malignant.
- Speech and language therapy should be tried before surgery in benign conditions.
- Smokers may have more than one neoplasm.

Answers

CASE 1.21 – Hoarse voice 1.

Q1: What is the important finding on examination?

A1

Examination is usually uneventful. A flexible nasendoscopy in the clinic may show how the vocal apparatus is working and whether there are any lesions on the vocal cords. Singers' nodules are a sign of vocal misuse and occasionally a unilateral vocal cord polyp may be found. Bilateral diffuse oedema suggests chronic persistent abuse but may be found in conditions such as thyroid disease.

Q2: What additional features in the history would you like to elicit?

A2

Ask about the nature of the job and when the hoarseness comes on. See whether the voice goes back to normal. If it is intermittent and comes on during the day, or during times of persistent voice use, it is benign. Find out about hobbies such as singing. Ask about stress and the voice. Enquire about the symptoms of hiatus hernia and thyroid disease, and also whether the patient smokes or has chest disease such as asthma. Ask about nasal symptoms and snoring because this may dry the throat. Sinusitis is a rare cause of the problem and is often secondary to asthma and coughing.

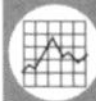

Q3: What investigations would be most helpful and why?

A3

These are rarely needed but do include an FBC and thyroid function tests.

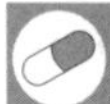

Q4: What are the treatment options?

A4

Vocal hygiene should be practised, such as frequent drinks to keep the larynx moist (not alcohol!). Refrain from smoking if the patient is a smoker. Recent trials have shown that speech and language therapy is effective. Surgery is rarely needed in patients with hoarseness. If the patient has asthma, therapy may improve the voice but sometimes the irritation is the result of the inhalers, or *Candida* species, on the vocal cords.

 CASE 1.22 – Hoarse voice 2.

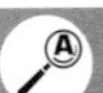 Q1: What is the important finding on examination?

A1

Examination of the larynx will show a laryngeal cancer. This is classified by the TNM (tumours, node, metastases) classification, which helps to determine the treatment.

 Q2: What additional features in the history would you like to elicit?

A2

The history should be taken similar to that in the previous case. The smoking history is most important here. Progressive hoarseness that lasts longer than 6 weeks is most likely to be a neoplasm. Examination of the neck is often uneventful because secondary nodes rarely occur in a simple carcinoma of the larynx as it presents relatively early.

 Q3: What investigations would be most helpful and why?

A3

A chest radiograph should always be taken because secondary neoplasm in the chest occurs in 10 per cent of patients. Similarly, an FBC, U&Es and liver function tests, together with thyroid function tests, may be required before radiotherapy or surgery.

Q4: What are the treatment options?

A4

Treatment depends on the TNM classification. Very small tumours can be lasered off once a biopsy diagnosis has been made. These patients should be followed up closely. The conventional treatment for small tumours is radiotherapy. However, this results in disability to the larynx and pharynx, with dryness and soreness as well as mucositis, and is best given in a fractionated regimen over a 6-week period rather than a shorter one. Larger tumours require surgery and radiotherapy. There is a move at present to more conservative surgery rather than laryngectomy and block dissection.

OSCE Counselling Case – Answer

OSCE COUNSELLING CASE 1.17 – A woman with an intermittent hoarse voice is worried about her career as a teacher and her voice problem. What advice would you give?

Explain that voice care and rest are the most appropriate treatment. Whispering strains the voice more than talking normally. Avoid singing and straining. Stress the value of speech and language therapy, which allows voice training and counselling at the same time. The voice may return to normal.

PAINLESS NECK LUMP

? Questions for each of the clinical case scenarios given

Q1: What additional features in the history would you like to elicit?
Q2: What should one look for in the examination?
Q3: What investigations would be most helpful and why?
Q4: What are the treatment options?

Clinical cases

CASE 1.23 – Painless neck lump 1.

A woman aged 52 has just returned from India and has noticed a painless lump in the midcervical region.

CASE 1.24 – Painless neck lump 2.

A Chinese man aged 33 presents with a painless left jugulodigastric swelling.

OSCE Counselling Case

OSCE COUNSELLING CASE 1.18 – The woman who has had the neck biopsy that shows TB returns to clinic. What advice would you give her?

Key concepts

- Lymph nodes > 2 cm are abnormal.
- Painless neck lumps in Asians are frequently tuberculosis (TB).
- Painless neck lumps in Chinese adults are postnasal space carcinoma metastases.
- Always undertake a fine-needle aspiration sample for cytology before surgery.
- Lymphoma and carcinoma may occur.
- The most common cause is a reactive lymph node swelling.

Answers

CASE 1.23 – Painless neck lump 1.

Q1: What additional features in the history would you like to elicit?

A1

Determine whether there are any night sweats, rigors or any other features of TB such as respiratory symptoms. Ask direct questions about difficulty in swallowing, voice changes or any other constitutional symptoms. Enquire about any family history of TB.

Q2: What should one look for in the examination?

A2

Examination of the neck will often reveal that there is a collection of nodes that are discrete and rubbery, but not attached to the skin or deeper structures. Measure the size because a node > 2 cm diameter is always trouble. A lymphoma may feel the same. A full ENT examination should also be undertaken.

Q3: What investigations would be most helpful and why?

A3

Full blood count, Mantoux and chest radiograph and fine-needle aspiration (FNA) of the neck lump. Undertake excision biopsy with histology and culture after the result of the FNA cytology.

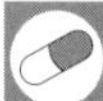

Q4: What are the treatment options?

A4

The treatment depends on the nature of the lesion. The most likely cause of this type of lesion is a tuberculous node. The key point in management is to undertake an FNA before one goes to excision biopsy. Fine needle aspiration can direct the appropriate treatment early on. If TB is suspected an open biopsy with both culture and histology is required. Acid-fast bacilli may be exceptionally difficult to identify on histological specimens and grown only on culture. However, if the diagnosis is suspected, it is important to notify the authorities and to send the patient for appropriate antituberculous chemotherapy.

CASE 1.24 – Painless neck lump 2.

Q1: What additional features in the history would you like to elicit?

A1

Ask which part of China the patient is from because patients from southern China have a high risk of postnasal space carcinoma. Ask about nasal symptoms such as nose bleeding and blockage of the nose. Ask about neurological symptoms such as numbness of the face. Undertake a general history.

Q2: What should one look for in the examination?

A2

Perform a full head and neck examination including full nasendoscopy. It is important to visualize the postnasal space in all patients with upper cervical lesions that might be neoplastic. The cranial nerves should be examined carefully; numbness of the cheek is particularly important, as is any degree of proptosis.

Q3: What investigations would be most helpful and why?

A3

Full blood count, U&Es, liver function tests, radiograph of the postnasal space with CT, FNA cytology of the neck lump and biopsy of the postnasal space.

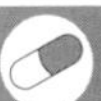

Q4: What are the treatment options?

A4

If the diagnosis is a postnasal space carcinoma, treatment is by radiotherapy plus a neck dissection together with radiotherapy to the neck fields. A third of patients present with nasal symptoms, a third with cervical metastases and a third with intracranial extension. This tumour can be particularly aggressive. It is occurs in a younger age group and is associated with the Epstein–Barr virus (EBV). Levels of the immunoglobulin IgA to EBV may indicate recurrent disease.

OSCE Counselling Case – Answer

OSCE COUNSELLING CASE 1.18 – The woman who has had the neck biopsy that shows TB returns to the clinic. What advice would you give her?

Explain that TB is eminently treatable these days and that the chest physician or infectious diseases doctor will be treating her. Say also that it will be important to screen the family to make sure that no other family members have the disease and that if they do they will have to be treated. This should eradicate the condition and the patient should be well for many years.

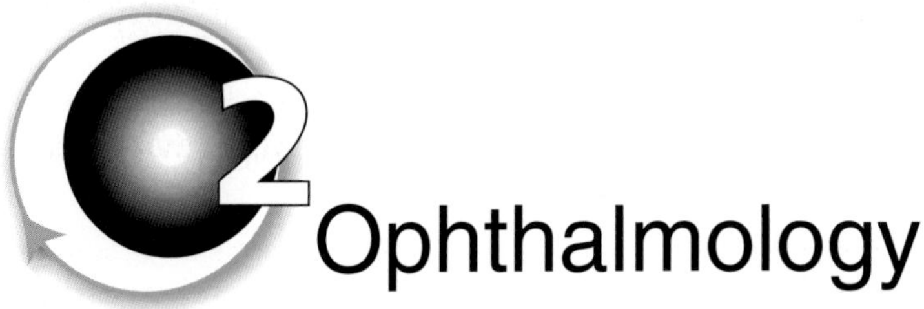

2 Ophthalmology

Desirée Murray

? Questions for each of the clinical case scenarios given

Q1: What is the differential diagnosis?
Q2: What issues in the history support the diagnosis?
Q3: What additional features in the history would you seek to support a particular diagnosis?
Q4: What clinical examination would you perform and why?
Q5: What investigations would be most helpful and why?
Q6: What treatment options are appropriate?

Clinical cases

CASE 2.1 – 'I have pain in my eye and I can't see with it.'

A 65-year-old woman presents with a 1-day history of pain, redness and reduced vision in one eye. She has worn spectacles for reading since the age of 7.

CASE 2.2 – 'I have suddenly lost the vision in one eye, but I have no pain.'

A 50-year-old patient presents with a 1-day history of sudden painless loss of vision. The patient has diabetes and hypertension.

CASE 2.3 – 'I have flashing lights and floaters in one eye.'

A 40-year-old patient gives a 1-week history of sudden-onset flashing lights and floaters in one eye. The patient has worn distance spectacles since the age of 12.

CASE 2.4 – 'My vision has gradually become cloudy and dim, but there is no pain in my eye.'

A 60-year-old patient complains of a gradual deterioration in vision in both eyes over 1 year.

CASE 2.5 – 'I have difficulty seeing at night.'

A 35-year-old patient presents with a 1-year history of difficulty seeing at night. The patient also complains of constriction of the visual field.

CASE 2.6 – 'I have double vision.'

A 60-year-old patient presents with a 1-week history of double vision.

CASE 2.7 – 'I have intermittent loss of vision in one eye for a few seconds and then my vision returns.'

A 50-year-old patient complains of intermittent loss of vision in one eye like a 'cloud' or 'curtain' descending over the vision, which clears after a few seconds.

CASE 2.8 – 'I have intermittent loss of vision in both eyes and then my vision clears.'

A 30-year-old woman complains of episodes of visual loss in both eyes associated with eye movements. She has a 1-month history of intermittent headache.

CASE 2.9 – 'My child's eye has a turn.'

A parent complains that her 2-year-old infant has developed a turn in one eye.

CASE 2.10 – 'My baby has watery eyes.'

A mother complains that her 4-month-old baby has had watery eyes since birth.

OSCE Counselling Cases

OSCE COUNSELLING CASE 2.1 – 'Why am I having difficulty reading since having my cataract surgery?'

A 60-year-old patient recently had uncomplicated cataract extraction with an intraocular lens implant. The patient complains of difficulty reading. The distance vision is good. The patient has not yet obtained new spectacles.

Q1: Can you reassure the patient? Explain why they are experiencing problems with unaided near vision and what can be done to correct the problem.

OSCE COUNSELLING CASE 2.2 – 'Why can't I see as well now as I did after my cataract surgery 18 months ago?'

A 60-year-old patient had successful cataract surgery 18 months ago. The patient complains of gradual reduction in vision in the pseudophakic eye. There is no history of diabetes or hypertension. Ocular examination is normal apart from the presence of posterior capsule opacification.

Q1: What is posterior capsule opacification? Explain this condition to the patient, including its treatment.

OSCE COUNSELLING CASE 2.3 – 'Why am I short of breath since starting treatment for glaucoma?'

This 60-year old-patient has been diagnosed with glaucoma. He was prescribed timolol 0.5 per cent eye drops.

Q1: Is it possible to develop dyspnoea in association with timolol use? Discuss the possible side effects of this eye drop.

OSCE COUNSELLING CASE 2.4 – 'I have recently been diagnosed with glaucoma. Can I still drive?'

Q1: Adequate standards of vision must be met for all drivers. Driving may be continued as long as the patient has been confirmed to meet the visual acuity standard and recommended national guidelines for visual field.

OSCE COUNSELLING CASE 2.5 – 'I have well-controlled diabetes. I have no problems with my vision. I had my eyes checked 1 year ago. When should I next have my eyes examined?'

This 50-year-old patient has had diabetes for 5 years. The patient has normal distance (6/6) and reading (N5) vision with glasses.

Q1: Explain to the patient why he needs a complete eye examination, including dilated funduscopy to screen for diabetic retinopathy, at least once a year, in spite of normal vision. What factors would you consider important when counselling this patient?

OSCE COUNSELLING CASE 2.6 – 'Will laser treatment make my vision worse? My neighbour, who also has diabetes, is now blind following laser treatment.'

This patient has had type 2 diabetes for 10 years. The ophthalmologist has recommended laser treatment for her right eye.

Q1: What factors would you consider important when counselling this patient?

Key concepts

Glossary of terms

Age-related macular degeneration (ARMD)

- Non-exudative ARMD – dry type: age-related macular changes characterized by discrete whitish-yellow spots identified as drusen, pigment changes (hyperpigmentation and hypopigmentation) and atrophy of the retinal pigment epithelium.
- Exudative ARMD – wet type: manifestations of choroidal neovascularization and/or accumulation of fluid or blood beneath the retinal pigment epithelium in a patient with age-related maculopathy.

Amblyopia

Decreased visual acuity without detectable organic disease of the eye.

Anisocoria

Condition in which the pupils of the two eyes are of different sizes.

Astigmatism

This is an optical condition in which the refractive power of the eye varies in different meridians, usually caused by the cornea having a greater curvature in one direction than in another (similar to a rugby ball as opposed to the more even shape of a football). As a result, parallel rays of light do not focus at a point and a distinct retinal image cannot form. It may be associated with long-sightedness, short-sightedness or both.

Cryotherapy

Procedure carried out with a freezing probe.

Cycloplegic refraction

Paralysis of the ciliary muscle by means of drugs, thus allowing measurement of the refractive error uncomplicated by changes in accommodation.

Dacryocystitis

Inflammation of the lacrimal sac.

Dacryocystorhinostomy

Surgical procedure to (re-)establish lacrimal drainage.

Dacryostenosis

Atresia of the nasolacrimal duct.

Degenerative (pathological) myopia

Abnormality in which the axial length of the eye is excessive. The sclera is bared in the region surrounding the optic nerve and the choroid is easily visible.

Electroretinogram

Action potential that follows stimulation of the retina.

Enophthalmos

Recession of the eye within the orbit.

Exophthalmos

Abnormal protrusion of one or both eyes.

Fundus fluorescein angiography

Intravenous sodium fluorescein combined with serial black and white photography to study the retinal circulation.

Hypermetropia/hyperopia/long-sightedness/far-sightedness

This is a condition in which parallel rays of light are brought to a point focus behind the retina, because the eye is too short for its own focusing power.

Hypopyon

Pus in the anterior chamber.

Iridotomy

Opening through all layers of the iris.

Iritis

Inflammation of the iris.

Keratitis

Inflammation of the cornea.

Leukocoria

White pupillary reflex.

Myopia/short-sightedness/near-sightedness

This is a condition in which parallel rays of light are brought to a point focus in front of the retina, because the eye is too long for its own focusing power.

Nasolacrimal duct

Duct that connects the lower end of the lacrimal sac with the inferior meatus of the nose.

Posterior synechiae

Adhesions between the iris and the lens.

Posterior vitreous detachment

Separation of the peripheral vitreous from the retina.

Presbyopia

This is loss of accommodation as a result of loss of elasticity of the lens with increasing age, so that the near point recedes. The inability to focus for near results in most people aged over 40 years needing reading spectacles.

Proptosis

Protrusion of the eyeball.

Relative afferent pupillary defect

This is a transmission defect of the optic nerve demonstrated by the 'swinging flashlight test'. When light is directed into the eye on the normal side both pupils react to light. When light is quickly switched to the abnormal side, the pupil, instead of remaining constricted (from the consensual reaction), dilates despite the light stimulation.

Rods

The light-sensitive elements of the retina that function at low levels of illumination. They are the main photoreceptors of the peripheral retina.

Scintillations

Visual hallucinations with flashing lights occurring in occipital lobe disorders, particularly migraine.

Scleritis

Inflammation of the sclera.

Trabeculectomy

A filtering operation for glaucoma, by creation of a fistula between the anterior chamber of the eye and the subconjunctival space.

Uveitis

Inflammation of the uveal tract.

Answers

CASE 2.1 – 'I have pain in my eye and I can't see with it.'

Q1: What is the differential diagnosis?

A1

- Acute angle-closure glaucoma
- Iritis (anterior uveitis)
- Keratitis – bacterial, viral, autoimmune peripheral ulcerative keratitis (PUK)
- Scleritis/sclerokeratitis.

Q2: What issues in the history support the diagnosis?

A2

The history of having worn reading spectacles since childhood suggests long-sightedness (hyperopia – Fig. 2.1). This increases the risk of developing acute angle-closure glaucoma because patients who are long-sighted have small eyes with crowded anterior segments and narrow drainage angles.

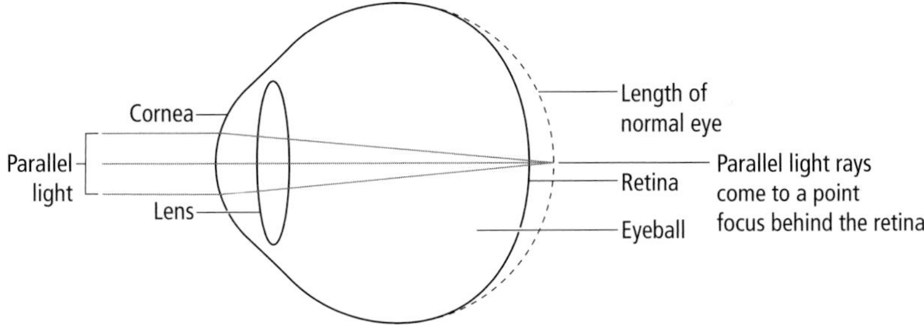

Figure 2.1 Hypermetropia or hyperopia: long-sightedness.

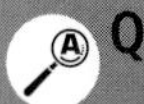

Q3: What additional features in the history would you seek to support a particular diagnosis?

A3

It is important to enquire about symptoms of haloes around lights and intermittent blurring of vision, which suggest previous episodes of increased intraocular pressure with corneal oedema. Previous attacks of angle closure may have resolved spontaneously. Is there any associated nausea and vomiting, as this is often the case in acute glaucoma?

Enquire about photophobia – often quite marked in patients with iritis. Is there a history of rheumatoid arthritis or other autoimmune disorder, which may be associated with PUK or scleritis?

Does the patient wear contact lenses? This may predispose to bacterial keratitis/corneal ulcer. Is there a history of herpetic disease (cold sores or previous herpes simplex keratitis)?

 Q4: What clinical examination would you perform and why?

A4

Visual acuity should be measured. Examine the red reflex. A reduced or absent red reflex is found in corneal oedema. Compare the clarity of the cornea in the affected eye with that in the contralateral eye. Palpate the globe to determine whether the intraocular pressure is elevated, but be gentle because the eye may be quite tender! Examine the cornea with the aid of fluorescein dye and cobalt blue light, looking for staining, which would indicate corneal epithelial erosions, abrasion or ulcer. In patients with herpes simplex keratitis, the corneal ulcer assumes a typical branching pattern known as a dendritic ulcer. Pay attention to the distribution of the redness – circumcorneal injection is typical of iritis (ciliary flush), whereas with scleritis the eye may be diffusely injected or the redness may be localized to one segment of the sclera. Scleral nodules may also be present. Examine the pupil. A constricted pupil may indicate iritis whereas a fixed, mid-dilated, irregular pupil is seen in acute glaucoma. In severe iritis or bacterial keratitis, a hypopyon may be visible in the anterior chamber.

 Q5: What investigations would be most helpful and why?

A5

It is important to examine the contralateral eye to determine whether the drainage angle is narrow. An elevated erythrocyte sedimentation rate (ESR) or packed cell volume (PCV) may indicate an underlying autoimmune or other systemic condition. Do a full blood count (FBC) to check for raised white cell count (WCC; neutrophilia, lymphocytosis or monocytosis). Also do blood glucose to exclude diabetes, because this may sometimes be associated with iritis. A chest radiograph may detect signs of sarcoidosis or tuberculosis (TB).

Q6: What treatment options are appropriate?

A6

If the patient has acute glaucoma, treatment consists of the following:

- Medical treatment: antiglaucoma medications including pilocarpine 4 per cent and intravenous acetazolamide are administered. Pilocarpine eye drops are instilled into the contralateral eye to minimize the risk of that eye developing acute angle-closure glaucoma.
- Laser treatment: Nd:YAG (neodymium:yttrium–aluminium–garnet) laser peripheral iridotomy (Fig. 2.2) is performed when the corneal oedema clears sufficiently. Prophylactic YAG laser peripheral iridotomy is performed in the contralateral eye.
- If there is extensive damage to the anterior chamber drainage angle, ciliary body ablation with the diode laser is sometimes required to achieve a substantial reduction in intraocular pressure.
- Surgical treatment: sometimes glaucoma filtration surgery (trabeculectomy – Fig. 2.3) is necessary to control intraocular pressure.
- Iritis is treated with topical steroid eye drops. Scleritis is treated with oral non-steroidal anti-inflammatory drugs (NSAIDs), topical and/or systemic steroids or steroid-sparing immunosuppressive agents, as indicated. Autoimmune PUK is treated with systemic immunosuppression. Patients with intraocular inflammation should also be treated with cycloplegic eye drops to:

– dilate the pupil to prevent the development of posterior synechiae

– relax the ciliary muscle and reduce ocular discomfort and photophobia.

- Infective keratitis is treated with the appropriate antibacterial or antiviral agent. Bacterial corneal ulcers are treated with intensive topical antibiotics (after corneal scraping for culture and sensitivity). The dendritic ulcer of herpes simplex keratitis is treated with topical antiherpetics such as aciclovir eye ointment.

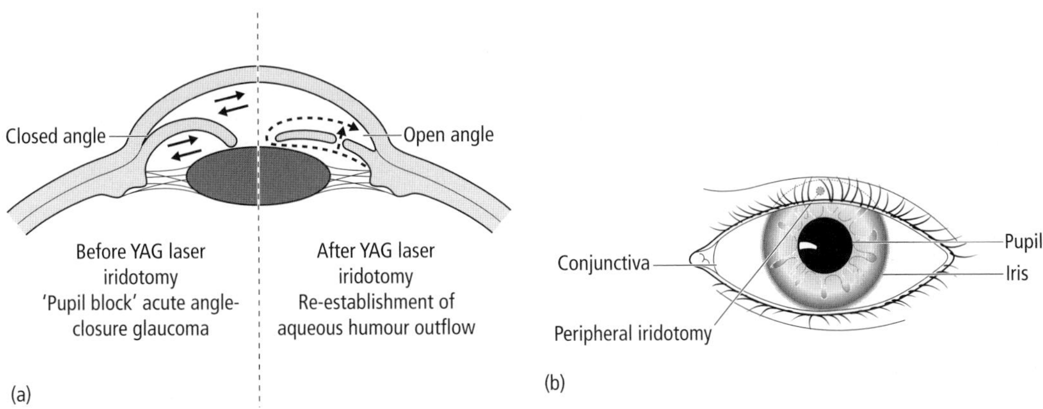

Figure 2.2 (a) Acute angle-closure glaucoma treated by Nd:YAG (neodymium:yttrium–aluminium–garnet) laser iridotomy. (b) Peripheral laser iridotomy.

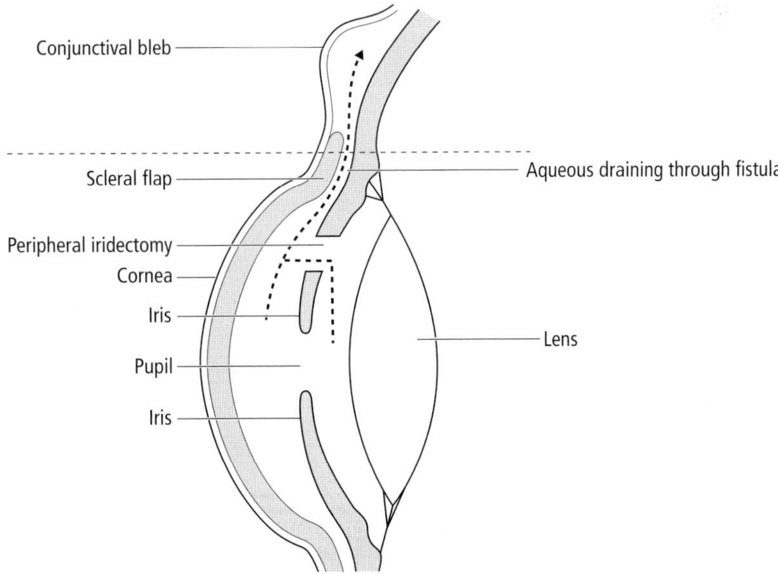

Figure 2.3 Trabeculectomy: glaucoma filtration surgery.

CASE 2.2 – 'I have suddenly lost the vision in one eye, but I have no pain.'

Q1: What is the differential diagnosis?

A1

- Central retinal artery occlusion
- Branch retinal artery occlusion
- Central retinal vein occlusion
- Branch retinal vein occlusion
- Ischaemic optic neuropathy
- Vitreous haemorrhage
- Retinal detachment
- ARMD (wet type).

Q2: What issues in the history support the diagnosis?

A2

The fact that the patient has diabetes and hypertension should alert one to the possibility of diabetic retinopathy, other retinal vascular disease and/or carotid artery disease with embolic sequelae.

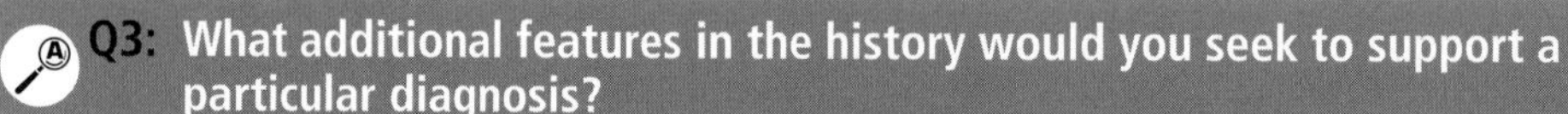

Q3: What additional features in the history would you seek to support a particular diagnosis?

A3

Ask about previous episodes of transient loss of vision, or transient ischaemic attacks (TIAs). Has the patient ever suffered a stroke or heart attack? Has the patient had retinal laser treatment in the past for diabetic retinopathy or macular degeneration? If the patient is short-sighted (myopic – Fig. 2.4) or there is a history of ocular trauma, the risk of retinal

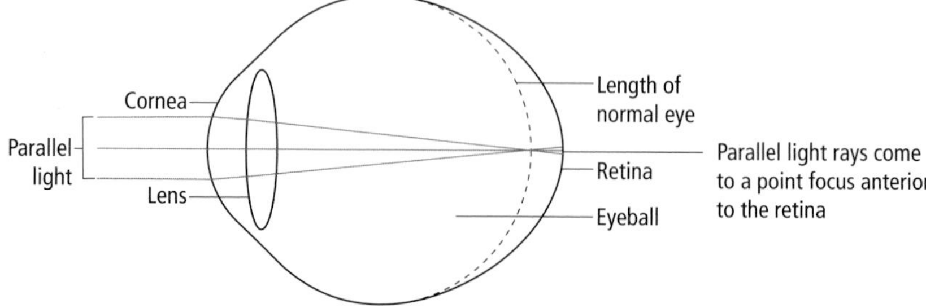

Figure 2.4 Myopia: short-sightedness.

detachment is increased. Enquire about headache, scalp tenderness, proximal myalgia, jaw claudication, anorexia and weight loss – symptoms of giant cell arteritis. The drug history is important. Is the patient on digoxin or warfarin for atrial fibrillation? Does the patient smoke?

Q4: What clinical examination would you perform and why?

A4

Measure the visual acuity. Examine the pupils for a relative afferent pupillary defect (RAPD). Examine the red reflex, which is reduced or absent in vitreous haemorrhage. Perform ophthalmoscopy. Look for evidence of diabetic retinopathy (retinal haemorrhages, hard exudates and cotton-wool spots), retinal vein occlusion (retinal haemorrhages and cotton-wool spots), retinal artery emboli (yellow refractile plaques at the bifurcation of retinal arterioles), 'cherry red spot' at the macula, optic disc swelling and superficial disc haemorrhages or retinal detachment. Macular haemorrhages and hard exudates may also be seen in 'wet' macular degeneration. Examine the cardiovascular system – pulse, blood pressure, cardiac murmur and carotid bruit.

 Q5: What investigations would be most helpful and why?

A5

In the case of ischaemic optic neuropathy or retinal artery occlusion, an ESR, plasma viscosity (PV) and/or C-reactive protein (CPR) should be done to exclude giant cell arteritis. The blood sugar and the lipid profile need to be measured. Do an FBC to check for thrombocytopenia. Carotid Doppler ultrasonography should also be requested to determine the extent of carotid artery stenosis. Electrocardiography and echocardiography may be indicated.

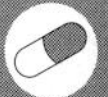 Q6: What treatment options are appropriate?

A6

Treatment is aimed at preventing a similar occurrence in the contralateral eye and reducing the risk of a major cardiovascular event.

- Medical treatment: giant cell arteritis is a medical emergency and the patient must be admitted for treatment with high-dose systemic steroids. Temporal artery biopsy may confirm the diagnosis. Retinal artery occlusions presenting within 4–6 h of the onset of symptoms are ophthalmic emergencies. Urgent referral to the ophthalmology department is needed so that measures can be instituted to attempt to dislodge any retinal artery emboli. Blood pressure, blood sugar and serum lipids need to be controlled if elevated.
- Laser treatment: sometimes laser treatment is indicated for retinal neovascularization secondary to proliferative diabetic retinopathy or ischaemia after retinal vein or artery occlusion. Laser treatment is also indicated for macular oedema after retinal vein occlusion and for some cases of wet ARMD.
- Surgical treatment: temporal artery biopsy may be useful in confirming a diagnosis of giant cell arteritis. The patient should be referred to a vascular surgeon to determine whether carotid endarterectomy is indicated. The patient with a retinal detachment is referred to the ophthalmologist for surgical repair.

CASE 2.3 – 'I have flashing lights and floaters in one eye.'

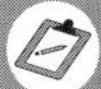

Q1: What is the differential diagnosis?

A1

- Posterior vitreous detachment (PVD)
- Retinal detachment (RD)
- Migraine.

Q2: What issues in the history support the diagnosis?

A2

This history of having worn distance spectacles since childhood is evidence of short-sightedness (myopia – see Fig. 2.4). Myopic patients are prone to PVD at a younger age than patients who are not myopic. They also have an increased risk of developing RD. Fortunately, most patients with a PVD do not develop RD, but the latter can be excluded only by detailed examination of the retina through a dilated pupil. A history of migraine may suggest that diagnosis for the present episode.

Q3: What additional features in the history would you seek to support a particular diagnosis?

A3

Ask about any noticeable visual field defect, often described by the patient as a shadow or dark patch in the peripheral vision. The triad of flashes, floaters and a field defect is very suspicious of RD. A history of ocular trauma increases its risk. Enquire about associated headache, nausea and vomiting suggestive of migraine. Scintillations lasting 15–20 min are virtually diagnostic of migraine.

Q4: What clinical examination would you perform and why?

A4

Visual acuity should be measured, and pupils assessed for RAPD. Dilated funduscopy is performed at the slit-lamp with a contact lens or by using the binocular indirect ophthalmoscope and indentation to visualize the peripheral retina.

Q5: What investigations would be most helpful and why?

A5

Examination of the contralateral eye to exclude asymptomatic retinal breaks or RD is important.

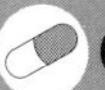 Q6: What treatment options are appropriate?

A6

- Reassurance: PVD in the absence of retinal breaks or RD does not require treatment.
- Medical treatment: migraine usually responds to appropriate analgesics.
- Laser treatment: retinal holes, tears or breaks may be treatable with laser if detected at an early stage.
- Surgical treatment: RD is referred to the ophthalmologist for surgical repair.

CASE 2.4 – 'My vision has gradually become cloudy and dim, but there is no pain in my eye.'

 Q1: What is the differential diagnosis?

A1

- Cataracts
- Age-related macular degeneration (dry type)
- Diabetic retinopathy
- Primary open-angle glaucoma.

 Q2: What issues in the history support the diagnosis?

A2

The gradual and progressive onset of the visual loss is typical of cataract and dry ARMD.

 Q3: What additional features in the history would you seek to support a particular diagnosis?

A3

Is the deterioration in vision for distance, near or both? Cataracts affect both, whereas ARMD and diabetic maculopathy may affect near vision to a greater extent than distance vision. Ask about a history of diabetes and hypertension. Does the patient smoke? Is there a family history of glaucoma?

Q4: What clinical examination would you perform and why?

A4

Measure the visual acuity. Examine the red reflex – this is reduced if there is nuclear sclerotic cataract. Intraocular pressure is measured. Ophthalmoscopy is performed looking for signs of ARMD and diabetic retinopathy, including retinal

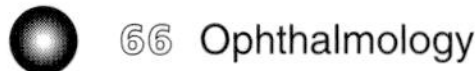

haemorrhages and hard exudates at the macula. Examine the optic disc closely. Note the disc colour, the contour of the disc margins and the cup:disc ratio. The cup:disc ratio is enlarged in primary open-angle glaucoma.

 Q5: What investigations would be most helpful and why?

A5

If diabetic maculopathy is detected, the patient may require fundus fluorescein angiography. Fluorescein angiography may also be helpful in excluding wet ARMD, which may coexist with the dry type. The blood pressure, blood sugar and lipid profile are measured. Visual field analysis is performed if glaucoma is suspected.

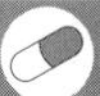 Q6: What treatment options are appropriate?

A6

Unfortunately, there is no effective treatment for dry ARMD. Although prophylactic laser treatment has been tried, there is little evidence that this is of benefit. The Age-Related Eye Disease Study (AREDS) evaluated the effect of high doses of zinc and selected antioxidants (β-carotene and vitamins C and E) and found significant reduction in the risk of progression in patients with advanced ARMD (categories 3 and 4). Specific nutritional supplements are therefore indicated in advanced ARMD. The patient should also be advised to stop smoking. Arrangements for the provision of low visual aids (large-print material, optical aids and non-optical aids) and rehabilitation should be remembered.

- Medical treatment: in most cases, primary open-angle glaucoma is successfully treated with anti-glaucoma eye drops.
- Laser treatment: laser trabeculoplasty is sometimes used in the treatment of glaucoma. Laser treatment is performed for diabetic maculopathy, if there is clinically significant macular oedema.
- Surgical treatment: glaucoma filtration surgery (trabeculectomy – see Fig. 2.3) may become necessary if medical treatment is ineffective or not well tolerated. Visually significant cataract is treated by phacoemulsification and intraocular lens implant.

CASE 2.5 – 'I have difficulty seeing at night.'

Q1: What is the differential diagnosis?

A1

- Retinitis pigmentosa (RP)
- Vitamin A deficiency
- Primary open-angle glaucoma
- Cataracts
- Degenerative myopia.

 Q2: What issues in the history support the diagnosis?

A2

Night blindness (nyctalopia) is a feature of many diseases. Vitamin A is necessary for the conversion of light energy to an electrical signal in the rod outer segments. The rods function at low levels of illumination, so vitamin A deficiency results in night blindness. Difficulty with night vision may indicate an abnormality of rod function and is characteristic of RP. However, any cause of extensive peripheral retinal degeneration, including primary open-angle glaucoma and degenerative myopia, results in peripheral visual field loss and poor night vision. Cataracts cause a general reduction in the amount of light entering the eye and can therefore produce similar symptoms.

 Q3: What additional features in the history would you seek to support a particular diagnosis?

A3

It is important to determine the onset of symptoms. Patients with RP often begin having difficulty with night vision in the teenage years, e.g. they may report having had difficulty finding their way around a cinema or other dark environment. Does the patient have a hearing deficit? Usher's syndrome is a variation of RP that also impairs hearing. Ask about symptoms that may suggest constriction of the peripheral visual field, such as involvement in road traffic accidents. Is the patient myopic (short-sighted – see Fig. 2.4)? Does the patient wear spectacles or contact lenses? The incidence of myopia is increased in RP. Ask about a family history of RP, night blindness, glaucoma and cataracts. Enquire about any history of abdominal surgery involving small bowel resection or liver disease, which may cause malabsorption and hypovitaminosis (vitamin A deficiency).

 Q4: What clinical examination would you perform and why?

A4

Measure visual acuity and assess visual fields to confrontation. Examine the red reflex, which may be reduced in eyes with cataract. Posterior subcapsular cataract often occurs in patients with RP. Check the intraocular pressure. Dilated funduscopy may show the classic appearance of RP with pigment proliferation and accumulation of pigment shaped as bone corpuscles ('bone spicules') in the midperipheral retina. There may be diffuse large areas of chorioretinal atrophy in degenerative myopia. Examine the optic disc carefully for optic atrophy and/or pathological optic disc cupping (enlarged cup:disc ratio). Look for retinal arteriolar attenuation and cystoid macular oedema seen as a dull or absent foveal light reflex, because this may occur in patients with RP.

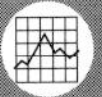 Q5: What investigations would be most helpful and why?

A5

In patients with RP or advanced glaucoma, visual field testing shows marked constriction of the peripheral field (tunnel vision). In RP, the electroretinogram is the most useful electrodiagnostic test. It is reduced in amplitude or non-recordable and helps to confirm the diagnosis. Cataracts are uncommon at such a young age and, if present, fasting blood sugar should be requested to exclude diabetes.

Q6: What treatment options are appropriate?

A6

In patients with RP, the eyes should be examined annually to determine the progression of the disease and to monitor for the development of cataract and glaucoma. Genetic counselling is mandatory. A complete family history and ophthalmological assessment of all family members will help to classify the disease as X-chromosome linked, autosomal dominant or autosomal recessive. Many patients with RP are legally blind in middle age and appropriate counselling must be given in collaboration with a geneticist.

- Counselling: unfortunately there is no treatment for degenerative myopia. Appropriate advice and support need to be organized.
- Medical treatment: there have been many different treatments suggested for RP, ranging from vitamin A in high doses to retinal electrostimulation, but to date none has been effective. Small doses of vitamins A and E may be appropriate but the recommended daily allowance should not be exceeded.
- Primary open-angle glaucoma is treated medically with anti-glaucoma eye drops.
- Laser treatment: argon or selective laser trabeculoplasty is sometimes useful in controlling intraocular pressure in patients with glaucoma.
- Surgical treatment: glaucoma filtration surgery (trabeculectomy – see Fig. 2.3) may be necessary to lower intraocular pressure effectively.
- Visually significant cataract is treated by phacoemulsification cataract extraction and intraocular lens implant.

CASE 2.6 – 'I have double vision.'

Q1: What is the differential diagnosis?

A1

- Isolated oculomotor nerve palsy
- Cerebrovascular accident with cranial nerve palsy
- Increased intracranial pressure (ICP)
- Thyroid eye disease (TED)
- Myasthenia gravis
- Multiple sclerosis
- Orbital tumour
- Orbital inflammatory disease (orbital myositis or pseudotumour)
- Trauma (orbital wall fracture).

 Q2: What issues in the history support the diagnosis?

A2

Diplopia may be caused by a number of possible aetiologies. Monocular diplopia is usually the result of refractive error and/or opacities or irregularities of the optical media, including corneal scarring, cataract, vitreous opacities and macular disturbances. Binocular diplopia may be the presenting symptom of serious underlying neurological, systemic or orbital disease causing misalignment of the visual axes.

Misalignment may be the result of an abnormality of muscle innervation, muscle function or orbital architecture. Ocular motility disorders may result from ischaemic or haemorrhagic brain-stem lesions. There may be involvement of peripheral nerves only, with no central lesion (isolated oculomotor nerve palsy or peripheral mononeuropathy). Aneurysms of the internal carotid artery (ICA) may develop at the junction with the posterior communicating artery (PCA) or within the cavernous sinus. Aneurysms of the ICA–PCA junction account for a significant proportion (over 50 per cent) of all third cranial nerve palsies, as a result of sudden dilatation of the aneurysm or from subarachnoid haemorrhage.

Extraocular muscle involvement is common in patients with dysthyroid eye disease and may be the first sign of the disease. Patients may be hyperthyroid, hypothyroid or euthyroid.

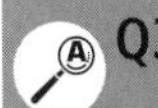 Q3: What additional features in the history would you seek to support a particular diagnosis?

A3

It is important to establish whether the diplopia is monocular or binocular. Monocular diplopia disappears when the affected eye is occluded but is still present when the unaffected eye is covered. Binocular diplopia is no longer present when either eye is covered.

Ask about associated symptoms suggestive of intracranial pathology, malignancy or giant cell arteritis such as headache, jaw claudication, scalp tenderness, neck stiffness, weight loss and/or loss of appetite. A detailed headache history must be elicited to determine whether elevated ICP may be present – exacerbating factors such as whether the headache is worse on waking or on bending, lifting, coughing or straining. Is there a history of trauma? Is the diplopia constant or variable, e.g. is it worse towards the end of the day, suggesting an element of fatiguability?

Determine the meridian of the diplopia – whether the two images are displaced horizontally, vertically or torsionally:

- Horizontal diplopia: the images are 'side by side':

  lateral rectus palsy – cranial nerve VI lesion

  medial rectus palsy – cranial nerve III lesion or internuclear ophthalmoplegia.

- Vertical diplopia: the images are 'one on top of the other':

  superior rectus palsy – cranial nerve III lesion

  inferior rectus palsy – cranial nerve III lesion

  inferior oblique palsy – cranial nerve III lesion

  superior oblique palsy – cranial nerve IV lesion

  TED

  orbital floor fracture.

- Torsional diplopia: the images are 'tilted':

  diplopia is particularly marked in downgaze, e.g. when reading or walking downstairs

  superior oblique palsy – cranial nerve IV lesion.

The past medical history is important: diabetes, hypertension, thyroid dysfunction, multiple sclerosis or myasthenia gravis.

Q4: What clinical examination would you perform and why?

A4

Inspect the patient for a compensatory head posture. Inspect the eyes for an obvious squint, lid retraction, lid lag on downgaze, exophthalmos/proptosis or enophthalmos (orbital floor fracture). Look for ptosis (cranial nerve III palsy). A full anterior segment examination is necessary. Check the pupils for anisocoria (ipsilateral pupil may be dilated in cranial nerve III palsy) or RAPD, which may indicate optic nerve compression from an orbital lesion (markedly enlarged extraocular muscles in dysthyroid eye disease, orbital tumour, orbital pseudotumour). Examine the extraocular movements for limitation of motility. Check smooth pursuit as well as saccades and convergence. In paralytic strabismus, the diplopia is greatest in the direction of action of the palsied muscle, e.g. a patient with right lateral rectus palsy describes two images having horizontal displacement greatest on looking to the right. However, if there is mechanical restriction of eye movement, the reverse may occur and there may be associated pain on attempted eye movement, e.g. a patient with right inferior rectus restriction (TED or orbital floor fracture) describes vertical diplopia that is greatest in upgaze. It may be possible to tire the muscles, a sign suggestive of myasthenia gravis.

Visual fields to confrontation may demonstrate homonymous hemianopia. Funduscopy may reveal papilloedema or optic atrophy.

Neurological examination may reveal associated pyramidal signs or abnormal movements of the limbs:

- Weber's syndrome: cranial nerve III palsy and contralateral hemiplegia
- Benedikt's syndrome: cranial nerve III palsy with contralateral involuntary movements of the limbs and contralateral hemianaesthesia
- Millard–Gubler syndrome: palsy of cranial nerves VI and VII and contralateral hemiplegia.

Q5: What investigations would be most helpful and why?

A5

Arteriosclerosis is a common cause of isolated ocular motor palsy in patients aged 60 or over with systemic hypertension. Check the blood pressure. Blood investigations should include FBC, ESR, fasting blood sugar, fasting lipids, thyroid function tests and acetylcholine receptor antibodies, depending on clinical findings.

Neuroimaging (computed tomography or CT and/or magnetic resonance imaging or MRI) is indicated if intracranial or orbital pathology is suspected.

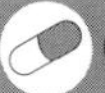 Q6: What treatment options are appropriate?

A6

- Conservative management: relief of diplopia is of major concern to the patient. Temporary prisms incorporated on to the patient's spectacles, or occlusion of one eye, may be necessary until muscle function improves and ocular alignment is re-established. Sometimes permanent prisms are necessary. The patient should be advised to stop driving unless the two images can be aligned.
- Medical treatment: primary treatment of dysthyroid eye disease must include making the patient euthyroid. Corticosteroids and radiotherapy may be necessary if there is keratopathy from corneal exposure or optic nerve compression.
- Many treatment options are available for myasthenia gravis. Initial treatment usually consists of oral pyridostigmine or neostigmine. Systemic prednisolone may be administered together with the anticholinesterase. Azathioprine and plasmapheresis are also effective. Thymectomy in patients with thymoma often results in remission of the disease.
- Surgical treatment: in patients with temporary problems of extraocular muscle innervation or muscle function (e.g. palsy of cranial nerve VI), botulinum toxin may be injected into the overacting antagonist (medial rectus) of the affected muscle (lateral rectus). This induces deliberate temporary paralysis of the medial rectus by chemodenervation until recovery of lateral rectus function occurs.
- Orbital decompression alleviates symptoms and signs of exposure keratopathy or optic nerve compression. Strabismus surgery is sometimes required.

CASE 2.7 – 'I have intermittent loss of vision in one eye for a few seconds and then my vision returns.'

 Q1: What is the differential diagnosis?

A1

Amaurosis fugax (transient visual loss).

 Q2: What issues in the history support the diagnosis?

A2

Amaurosis fugax is reversible visual obscuration lasting less than 24 h. It is a subtype of transient ischaemic attack (TIA). The blindness or partial blindness usually lasts less than 10 min. It may be caused by thromboembolic phenomena, vasospasm, blood hyperviscosity, vasculitis involving blood vessels that supply the visual pathway or intermittent optic nerve compression with gaze-evoked amaurosis. The most common cause of amaurosis fugax is atherosclerosis of the internal carotid or vertebrobasilar system. Amaurosis fugax resulting from involvement of the internal carotid artery system is unilateral.

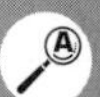

Q3: What additional features in the history would you seek to support a particular diagnosis?

A3

The history is crucial. Visual loss lasting more than 10 min or not returning completely should alert one to the possibility of a retinal vascular occlusion. Ask about symptoms of giant cell arteritis such as headache, scalp tenderness, jaw claudication, anorexia and weight loss.

Q4: What clinical examination would you perform and why?

A4

Patients should have a thorough examination of the cardiovascular system, including blood pressure, pulse, auscultation for a cardiac murmur and echocardiogram. Auscultate for a carotid bruit, which may indicate carotid artery stenosis from atherosclerosis.

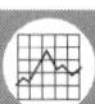

Q5: What investigations would be most helpful and why?

A5

An ESR should be requested to exclude possible vasculitis associated with giant cell arteritis, systemic lupus erythematosus (SLE) or other autoimmune disorder. Carotid Doppler ultrasonography will determine the extent of carotid artery stenosis.

Q6: What treatment options are appropriate?

A6

After a single TIA, a patient has a risk of stroke at 5 per cent per annum and death at 5 per cent per annum.

- Medical treatment: patients with carotid artery stenosis may be treated with anti-platelet drugs such as aspirin or dipyridamole. Anticoagulation with warfarin may be considered if a cardiac source of recurrent emboli is identified or if the symptoms persist despite anti-platelet drugs.
- Surgical treatment: the role of carotid endarterectomy after a TIA has been the subject of much research. Patients should be referred to a vascular surgeon if carotid endarterectomy is indicated.

CASE 2.8 – 'I have intermittent loss of vision in both eyes and then my vision clears.'

Q1: What is the differential diagnosis?

A1

- Migraine
- Increased ICP
- Pseudotumour cerebri (idiopathic intracranial hypertension)
- Amaurosis fugax.

Q2: What issues in the history support the diagnosis?

A2

Migraine is a common cause of visual disturbances in young patients. External compression of blood vessels supplying the visual pathway may also cause transient visual loss. In patients with papilloedema, pressure on blood vessels within the swollen optic nerve head may cause transient loss of vision in one or both eyes. Amaurosis fugax resulting from involvement of the vertebrobasilar system may produce binocular visual obscuration. Episodes usually last less than 1 min.

Q3: What additional features in the history would you seek to support a particular diagnosis?

A3

Establish whether or not the patient has transient visual loss with scintillating scotomata or fortification spectra (coloured zig-zag lines oscillating in brightness) usually lasting 15–20 min but can last as much as 1 h. If so, the diagnosis of migraine is very likely. A personal history or family history of migraine is helpful. Determine the nature of the headache, including exacerbating and relieving factors. Raised ICP often causes headache that is worse on waking and exacerbated by bending, straining and coughing. Is there a history of head trauma? Does the headache follow the visual disturbance?

The drug history is important. Tetracycline, steroid use or withdrawal, nalidixic acid, nitrofurantoin, danazol, ciclosporin and vitamin A in excessive doses are all associated with pseudotumour cerebri. Obesity is also a risk factor.

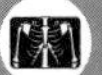

Q4: What clinical examination would you perform and why?

A4

Measure visual acuity. Check for an RAPD. Funduscopy may reveal papilloedema or optic atrophy. In patients with migraine, ophthalmic examination and pupillary reflexes are usually normal. Patients simulating visual deficiency always have a normal examination.

 Q5: What investigations would be most helpful and why?

A5

Request FBC and ESR to exclude anaemia and possible autoimmune disorder or hyperviscosity syndrome. Visual field analysis may detect enlargement of the blind spot. Neuroimaging (CT and/or MRI) may be indicated to exclude a space-occupying lesion, hydrocephalus or dural sinus thrombosis. In patients with pseudotumour cerebri, the cerebrospinal fluid (CSF) opening pressure may be elevated (> 200 mmH_2O) on lumbar puncture and CSF composition is normal. Lumbar puncture should always be performed with extreme caution in patients with papilloedema.

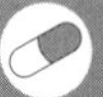 Q6: What treatment options are appropriate?

A6

- Conservative management: pseudotumour cerebri often recovers spontaneously in 3–9 months. In patients with dural sinus thrombosis, the thrombosed intracranial venous sinus usually recanalizes with resolution of the pseudotumour cerebri. Weight loss in obese patients may hasten resolution.
- Medical treatment: in patients with pseudotumour cerebri and persisting headache and/or progressive visual loss, acetazolamide (4 g daily) has been shown to decrease ICP. The administration of oral steroids decreases ICP and promotes the resolution of papilloedema.
- The treatment of migraine involves treatment of the acute attack (analgesics and antiemetics) and prevention of recurrence (β blockers and calcium channel blockers). Prophylactic treatment should be considered in patients with frequent or severe attacks because migraine may rarely be complicated by permanent visual loss or other neurological dysfunction.
- Autoimmune disorders such as SLE need referral to a specialist physician for immunosuppression.
- Surgical treatment: occasionally, lumboperitoneal shunts or optic nerve sheath decompression may become necessary in patients with pseudotumour cerebri.

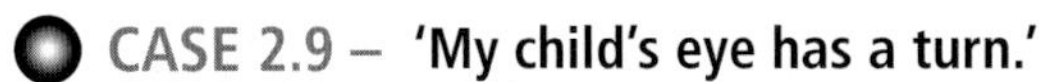

CASE 2.9 – 'My child's eye has a turn.'

 Q1: What is the differential diagnosis?

A1

- Non-paralytic squint
- Paralytic squint
- Retinoblastoma.

 Q2: What issues in the history support the diagnosis?

A2

Squint or strabismus occurs in about 3 per cent of children. Most cases present between the ages of 3 months and 4 years. Most childhood squints are non-paralytic, but paralytic squints may occur. Exclusion of underlying ocular, orbital and/or systemic disease is of the utmost importance.

 Q3: What additional features in the history would you seek to support a particular diagnosis?

A3

The antenatal, perinatal and neonatal history, including history of prematurity, birthweight, birth trauma and developmental milestones, is important. Ask about any family history of refractive errors, amblyopia ('lazy eye'), squint, congenital cataract or retinoblastoma. Is there any previous history of occlusion therapy (patching) of one eye, or squint surgery in the child? Are there any associated neurological symptoms – headache, clumsiness, drowsiness, vomiting?

 Q4: What clinical examination would you perform and why?

A4

Inspect the child for an abnormal head posture, dysmorphic features or hydrocephalus. Examination of the red reflex is extremely important. The red reflex is reduced or absent in cataract or corneal opacification. There may be leukocoria (white pupil) in cataract, retinoblastoma or other posterior segment pathology. Examine extraocular movements for limitation of eye movements indicative of paresis or palsy of a rectus muscle. In children with convergent squints, full abduction of each eye must be demonstrated to ensure that a cranial nerve VI palsy is not present. Dilated funduscopy is essential because conditions such as retinoblastoma may present with strabismus.

 Q5: What investigations would be most helpful and why?

A5

Cycloplegic refraction with cyclopentolate 1 per cent or atropine 1 per cent is mandatory. Ultrasound examination of the posterior segment is performed in cases of media opacity. CT and/or MRI of the brain, eye and orbit may be indicated.

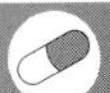 Q6: What treatment options are appropriate?

A6

There is a very close relationship between visual function and ocular alignment in children, and many children with squint develop amblyopia.

- Conservative management: detection and treatment of refractive errors (spectacles) and amblyopia (occlusion therapy of the 'good eye') are important.

- Surgical treatment: ocular realignment by means of strabismus surgery can then be carried out if necessary.
- Retinoblastoma may be treated by chemoreduction and focal therapy (laser photocoagulation and cryotherapy). In some cases, external beam radiotherapy is also needed. Unfortunately, many eyes with advanced disease need to be enucleated.

CASE 2.10 – 'My baby has watery eyes.'

Q1: What is the differential diagnosis?

A1

- Congenital nasolacrimal duct obstruction
- Congenital glaucoma.

Q2: What issues in the history support the diagnosis?

A2

The most common cause of watery eyes in the first year of life is congenital obstruction of the nasolacrimal duct (Fig. 2.5), caused by failure of canalization of its lower end. Abnormalities of facial bone structure may result in dacryostenosis. However, the most significant cause of watery eyes in neonates and infants is congenital glaucoma. In newborns and very young infants and children, large watery eyes associated with photophobia may be signs of congenital glaucoma.

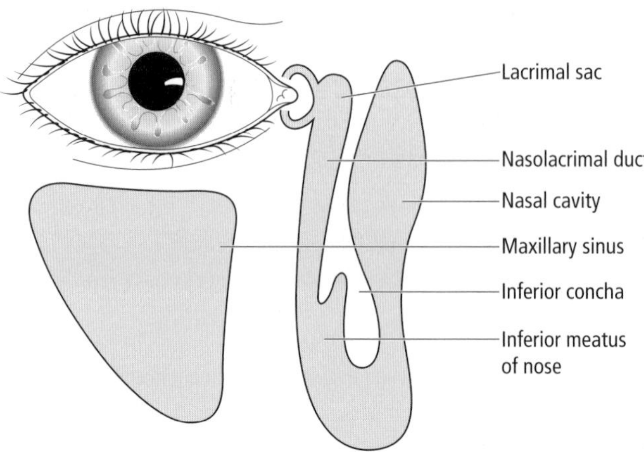

Figure 2.5 Tear passage: nasolacrimal duct.

 Q3: What additional features in the history would you seek to support a particular diagnosis?

A3

The perinatal history is important to exclude a history of birth trauma or forceps delivery. Enquire whether the watering is associated with photophobia and worse in bright lights. Have the parents noticed enlargement of their child's eye(s)? Is there a sticky mucopurulent discharge suggestive of conjunctivitis?

 Q4: What clinical examination would you perform and why?

A4

Press on the area over the lacrimal sac (see Fig. 2.5) and look for regurgitation of mucoid or mucopurulent fluid. This is typical of nasolacrimal duct obstruction. Important signs of congenital glaucoma include enlargement of the eye(s) and corneal opacification. Dilated funduscopy is essential to exclude posterior segment pathology. Cycloplegic refraction should be performed to detect myopia, which may develop as a result of enlargement of the eye(s).

 Q5: What investigations would be most helpful and why?

A5

Examination under general anaesthesia may be necessary to check intraocular pressures, to measure corneal diameters and to perform detailed retinal examination.

 Q6: What treatment options are appropriate?

A6

- Conservative management: delayed canalization occurs in 90 per cent of infants by the first birthday, and any surgical intervention should therefore be postponed until then. Daily massage of the lacrimal sac will prevent accumulation of debris and may reduce the risk of dacryocystitis.
- Surgical treatment: if recanalization does not occur and surgery becomes necessary, a syringe and probe of the nasolacrimal duct are performed under general anaesthetic. Sometimes this needs to be repeated. Rarely, intubation of the duct or dacryocystorhinostomy (DCR) is necessary.
- Congenital glaucoma is very rare and should be managed in specialist centres. Surgical intervention is necessary to achieve successful lowering of the intraocular pressure.

OSCE Counselling Cases – Answers

OSCE COUNSELLING CASE 2.1 – 'Why am I having difficulty reading since having my cataract surgery?'

A1

Cataract surgery leaves the patient presbyopic. There is loss of unaided near vision.

Normally, the lens of the eye changes shape to focus light on to the retina. The ciliary muscle, which is attached to the lens by the zonules, contracts or relaxes to change the shape of the natural crystalline lens, depending on whether the object being viewed is close or far away. The near reflex consists of ciliary muscle contraction (accommodation), convergence and pupillary constriction.

The natural lens becomes cloudy with age and forms a cataract. This natural lens is removed at the time of cataract surgery and replaced with a synthetic lens implant. The lens implant is usually monofocal in design and also cannot change shape in the same way that the natural lens can. As a result, depending on the power of lens implant chosen, light is focused to form a clear image on the retina for either a distant or a near object, but not for both. So, if vision is very clear for distance, it cannot also be clear for close-up. Increasingly, multifocal implants (rather than monofocal ones) are being used to eliminate this problem, but careful patient selection is advised.

The loss of close-up focusing can be corrected by wearing spectacles or a contact lens. Reading spectacles help to focus clearly on objects that are close, such as small print in a book or newspaper. Reading spectacles may be obtained as a separate pair, or incorporated into bifocals, trifocals or varifocals (also known as progressives).

If the cataract in the other eye needs to be operated on, a lens implant can be chosen that allows good near vision with that eye. The dominant eye is then used for far vision and the non-dominant eye for close vision. This is called monovision. However, this difference in focusing power between the two eyes is sometimes not well tolerated.

OSCE COUNSELLING CASE 2.2 – 'Why can't I see as well now as I did after my cataract surgery 18 months ago?'

A1

During a cataract operation, a clear lens implant is placed inside the eye to replace the natural lens that has become cloudy, forming a cataract. The natural lens is encased in a clear capsular bag. The lens implant is placed 'in the bag', which provides support. The implant sits in the same anatomical position as the natural lens that it has replaced.

In some patients, months or years after cataract surgery the capsule thickens up and becomes cloudy. This is not another cataract, although the symptoms may be the same. It is treated quickly and painlessly in the clinic by using a Nd:YAG laser to make a small hole in the capsule.

Only a small hole is needed, so the lens implant still has plenty of support. This small opening allows light to pass into the eye so that the patient sees clearly again.

OSCE COUNSELLING CASE 2.3 – 'Why am I short of breath since starting treatment for glaucoma?'

A1

Timolol is a β-adrenergic blocking agent. It has several potential cardiovascular, respiratory and central nervous system side effects after ocular administration. Patients who are receiving topical ophthalmic timolol should be counselled about and observed for potential side effects.

CARDIOVASCULAR

- Bradycardia
- Arrhythmia
- Heart block
- Palpitation
- Cardiac failure
- Pulmonary oedema
- Cardiac arrest
- Hypotension
- Syncope
- Cerebral ischaemia
- Cerebrovascular accident
- Raynaud's phenomenon.

RESPIRATORY

- Bronchospasm (predominantly in patients with pre-existing asthma or other bronchial disease)
- Respiratory failure
- Dyspnoea
- Cough.

CENTRAL NERVOUS SYSTEM/PSYCHIATRIC

- Depression
- Somnolence
- Insomnia
- Nightmares
- Hallucinations
- Confusion
- Disorientation
- Anxiety
- Nervousness
- Memory loss.

ENDOCRINE

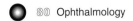

Masked symptoms of hypoglycaemia in patients with diabetes.

OTHER

- Nausea
- Diarrhoea
- Anorexia
- Dry mouth
- Fatigue
- Impotence.

Note that these potential side effects may be amplified by concomitant use of oral β-blocker treatment.

OSCE COUNSELLING CASE 2.4 – 'I have recently been diagnosed with glaucoma. Can I still drive?'

A1

The law states that:

> A licence holder or applicant is suffering a prescribed disability if unable to meet the eyesight requirements, i.e. to read in good light (with the aid of spectacles or contact lenses if worn) a registration mark fixed to a motor vehicle and containing letters and figures 79.4 mm high at a distance of 20.5 m. This corresponds to between 6/9 and 6/12 on the Snellen chart. The minimum field of vision for safe driving is a field of at least 120° on the horizontal measured by the Goldman perimeter using the III4e settings. In addition, there should be no significant defect in the binocular field that encroaches within 20° of fixation above or below the horizontal meridian. Other equivalent perimeters may be used. Poor night vision may also disqualify a patient from driving.

Eyesight complications affecting visual acuity or visual fields are not the only contraindications for driving. Other conditions include, under certain conditions, epileptic seizures, loss of consciousness, TIAs, stroke, angina, myocardial infarction, arrhythmia, syncope, frequent diabetic hypoglycaemic episodes, panretinal laser photocoagulation, drug misuse and dependency, alcohol misuse/dependency and impairment of cognitive function.

It is the responsibility of the driver to ensure that he or she is in control of the vehicle at all times. Advice on fitness to drive can be obtained from the medical advisers at the Driver and Vehicle Licensing Agency (DVLA).

OSCE COUNSELLING CASE 2.5 – 'I have well-controlled diabetes. I have no problems with my vision. I had my eyes checked 1 year ago. When should I next have my eyes examined?'

A1

Diabetic retinopathy is the most common cause of blindness in middle-aged people in the UK. Blindness can often be prevented by early detection and treatment. Diabetic retinopathy may be asymptomatic. This is why at least an annual dilated funduscopy is suggested by the World Health Organization and Diabetes UK. Screening is undertaken to detect disease of any severity and/or to detect disease of sufficient severity to warrant treatment.

All people with diabetes are at risk of retinopathy, even those whose hyperglycaemia is well controlled. However, some factors increase the risk of developing retinopathy, including:

- Duration of diabetes
- Poor glycaemic control
- Hypertension
- Hyperlipidaemia
- Nephropathy (microalbuminuria, proteinuria, renal failure)
- Obesity
- Pregnancy.

OSCE COUNSELLING CASE 2.6 – 'Will laser treatment make my vision worse? My neighbour, who also has diabetes, is now blind following laser treatment.'

A1

Diabetic retinopathy may be non-proliferative or proliferative. Non-proliferative retinopathy may be mild, moderate or severe. Severe non-proliferative diabetic retinopathy is also known as pre-proliferative retinopathy. Proliferative retinopathy can lead to vitreous haemorrhage and traction retinal detachment. Some patients develop diabetic maculopathy, with oedema and hard exudates at the macula, and/or macular ischaemia. Several randomized controlled studies have confirmed the effectiveness of laser treatment for high-risk proliferative retinopathy or clinically significant macular oedema.

Laser is a high-energy beam of light that is focused on the retina, thereby inducing thermal damage – laser photocoagulation. Laser treatment has vastly improved the management of diabetic eye disease. However, there are potential complications following all forms of laser surgery. The treatment is given as an outpatient procedure and is usually painless, although some patients experience significant pain and headache. Macular oedema may occur after panretinal laser, especially if the patient has significant renal impairment. This may cause temporary worsening of vision. There is also a risk of permanent reduction in visual fields and night vision after panretinal photocoagulation. Paracentral scotomata may occur after macular laser treatment.

Sometimes vision continues to deteriorate despite laser surgery. Visual outcome depends on the severity of the retinopathy and the indication for the laser. The patient may have proliferative retinopathy, diabetic macular oedema that is focal or diffuse, ischaemic maculopathy or a combination of these. The aim of laser surgery is mainly to stabilize vision and prevent progressive visual loss. Vision may not necessarily improve. Each patient is different and every eye reacts differently to laser.

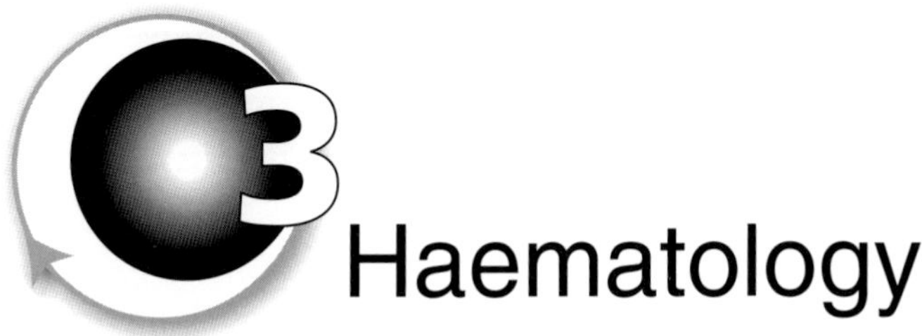

3 Haematology

Christopher Fegan

ANAEMIA

? Questions for each of the clinical case scenarios given

Q1: What is the likely diagnosis and possible differential diagnoses?
Q2: What are the relevant points to elicit from the history?
Q3: What are the possible clinical signs?
Q4: What additional investigations are indicated?
Q5: What is the treatment?
Q6: What is the long-term outcome?

Clinical cases

CASE 3.1 – A 27-year-old woman is referred with palpitations and shortness of breath.

Her haemoglobin (Hb) is 8.2 g/dL (normal 11.5–16 g/dL), white cell count (WCC) 5.2 × 10^9/L (normal 4–11 × 10^9/L) and platelets 513 × 10^9/L (normal 150–400 × 10^9/L). The mean cell volume (MCV) is 69 fL (normal 80–100 fL) and the mean cell Hb (MCH) 23 pg (normal 27–33 pg). She has a life-long history of menorrhagia but has declined therapeutic investigations/intervention. The serum ferritin is 3 ng/mL (normal 6–81 ng/mL).

CASE 3.2 – A 58-year-old woman is referred with a 12-month history of increasing difficulty in walking.

She had been relatively well throughout her life and her only medication was thyroxine 150 μg once daily for hypothyroidism diagnosed many years earlier. Over recent months she has noticed increasing shortness of breath on exertion, although her decreased mobility meant that this was not a particular problem. She worked as a clerical officer, smoked five cigarettes a day but drank no alcohol.

On examination the positive clinical signs elicited were pallor, tachycardia (100/min and regular), decreased sensation in both legs below the knee, absent ankle jerks and upgoing plantars.

Investigations revealed:

- Hb 8.2 g/dL (normal 11.5–16 g/dL)
- MCV 124 fL (normal 80–100 fL)
- WCC 2.4 × 10^9/L (normal 4–11 × 10^9/L)
- Platelets 102 × 10^9/L (normal 150–400 × 10^9/L).
- Urea and electrolytes were normal as were the liver function tests (LFTs) apart from a slightly raised bilirubin of 45 μmol/L (normal < 25 μmol/L) and a lactate dehydrogenase (LDH) level of 2374 U/L (normal 200–500 U/L).

CASE 3.3 – A 78-year-old woman is referred with a 6-month history of general deterioration.

On admission she is confused and her daughter reports that she has been very thirsty for the past 4 weeks. Apart from back pain there had been no other new symptoms. Clinical examination was unremarkable except for signs of dehydration. Her full blood count (FBC) showed:

- Hb 9.5 g/dL (normal 11.5–16 g/dL)
- WCC 4.2 × 10^9/L (normal 4–11 × 10^9/L)
- Platelet count 127 × 10^9/L (normal 150–400 × 10^9/L).

The biochemistry profile revealed:

- Sodium 126 mmol/L (normal 133–147 mmol/L)
- Potassium 4.8 mmol/L (normal 3.5–5.0 mmol/L)
- Urea 17 mmol/L (normal 2.5–7.5 mmol/L)
- Creatinine 201 μmol/L (normal 50–120 μmol/L)
- Total protein 117 g/dL (normal 60–80 g/dL)
- Albumin 28 g/dL (normal 35–48 g/dL)
- Aspartate aminotransferase (AST) 39 U/L (normal < 35 U/L)
- Alkaline phosphatase (ALP) 214 U/L (normal 90–430 U/L)
- Calcium 3.4 mmol/L (normal 2.05–2.6 mmol/L)
- Glucose 4.0 mmol/L.

OSCE Counselling Case

OSCE COUNSELLING CASE 3.1 – A colleague phones asking whether or not to transfuse a 24-year-old Asian woman who is 34 weeks' pregnant with a haemoglobin of 7.8 g/dL secondary to iron deficiency.

Q1: What further information would you require and what are the most salient points you would like to bring to your colleagues attention?

Key concepts

Anaemia is a very common topic because it impinges on all areas of medical care. A basic knowledge of the physiology of red cell production (erythropoiesis) is essential in understanding the causes of anaemia. There are several ways of classifying anaemia, the simplest of which is based on the red cell size: microcytic (MCV < 80 fL), normocytic (MCV 80–100 fL) and macrocytic (MCV > 100 fL), although one can also consider anaemia as either a failure of red cell production or a reduction in red cell survival. The age at which anaemia develops and a good dietary and clinical history, along with the knowledge of how to interpret the data given to you by the FBC, are also essential in narrowing down the differential diagnosis and requesting relevant investigations. The management of anaemia, and in particular the indications for blood transfusion, is a must-know area for any doctor.

Answers

CASE 3.1 – A 27-year-old woman is referred with palpitations and shortness of breath.

Q1: What is the likely diagnosis and possible differential diagnoses?

A1

This woman presents with symptomatic, hypochromic (low MCH)/microcytic (low MCV) anaemia. There are only four conditions giving rise to hypochromic/microcytic anaemia, notably iron deficiency, thalassaemia, anaemia of chronic disease and some rare (usually hereditary) types of sideroblastic anaemia. The low ferritin in this woman indicates that she has iron deficiency anaemia, probably secondary to excess menstrual blood loss.

Q2: What are the relevant points to elicit from the history?

A2

It is likely that the iron deficiency is secondary to the excess menstrual blood loss. However, it is important to ask about diet to ensure that her oral iron intake is adequate and check whether she is taking any non-steroidal anti-inflammatory drugs. Sufficient quantities of dietary iron are found only in meat (red meat rather than pork or chicken) and, therefore, iron deficiency is common in vegetarians. She should also be asked about other routes of bleeding (especially gastrointestinal [GI] or urinary tract symptoms). The platelet count rises in any form of iron deficiency and is not necessarily a sign of blood loss. Oesophageal webs causing dysphagia are a rare associated feature.

Q3: What are the possible clinical signs?

A3

Clinical signs include pallor (difficult sign seen as pale conjunctivae), tachycardia, brittle hair/nails, koilonychia (spoon-shaped nails), smooth atrophic tongue and angular stomatitis.

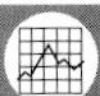

Q4: What additional investigations are indicated?

A4

Depending upon any symptoms elicited from the history one might consider performing a rectal examination, upper and lower GI endoscopy and faecal occult blood estimation. Coeliac disease is also possible, so anti-tissue transglutaminase and/or endomysial antibodies should be requested. Given the long history of menorrhagia, thyroid function tests should also be performed together with consideration of referral to a gynaecologist for more specific tests/investigations.

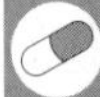 Q5: What is the treatment?

A5

Treatment is with iron. Ideally patients should receive 6 months of ferrous sulphate 200 mg three times daily. Side effects, usually constipation or more rarely diarrhoea, can occur, in which case intramuscular iron can be used; this is, however, very painful! Intravenous iron can be given but may lead to severe anaphylactic reactions. In this patient one could also consider using oral tranexamic acid or the combined oral contraceptive pill to reduce menstrual blood loss.

 Q6: What is the long-term outcome?

A6

On the assumption that menstrual loss is the underlying cause of this anaemia, the outcome should be excellent.

 CASE 3.2 – A 58-year-old woman is referred with a 12-month history of increasing difficulty in walking.

 Q1: What is the likely diagnosis and possible differential diagnoses?

A1

The patient's neurological examination reveals a combination of peripheral neuropathy and an upper motor neuron lesion in the lower limbs. In addition, there are symptoms and signs of anaemia, pancytopenia (i.e. all three cell lineages are reduced) and macrocytosis. All these point to vitamin B_{12} deficiency and a diagnosis of pernicious anaemia (PA) with subacute combined degeneration of the spinal cord and peripheral neuropathy. All dividing cells require vitamin B_{12} and the bone marrow, as one of the tissues with the fastest turnover, is often affected first. The raised bilirubin and LDH are a result of ineffective erythropoiesis within the bone marrow (so-called intramedullary haemolysis). Folate deficiency can give rise to a similar blood picture but neurological deficit does not occur.

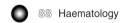

 Q2: What are the relevant points to elicit from the history?

A2

Pernicious anaemia is an autoimmune disease and so a personal and/or family history of other autoimmune diseases should be sought (e.g. type 1 diabetes, thyroid disease, Addison's disease and vitiligo). Has the patient ever undergone any gastric surgery? Rarely there is associated subfertility (but this would not apply in this age group) and visual loss. Vitamin B_{12} is present in foods of animal origin. Daily requirements of vitamin B_{12} are very low so it is very unusual for vegans to develop clinical vitamin B_{12} deficiency but a dietary history should always be taken.

 Q3: What are the possible clinical signs?

A3

The tongue is said to be 'big and beefy' in contrast to the atrophic tongue seen in iron deficiency. The skin has a lemon tinge (caused by the mildly elevated bilirubin). Optic atrophy can also occur and anecdotally patients are often said to be white haired.

 Q4: What additional investigations are indicated?

A4

Measuring the serum vitamin B_{12} levels easily makes the diagnosis. Other useful tests are anti-parietal and intrinsic factor antibodies, which are present in 90 per cent and 60 per cent respectively. It may also be prudent to look for evidence of the other autoimmune disorders that are associated with PA. Historically, a Schilling test was performed to confirm vitamin B_{12} malabsorption but this is rarely performed today because it exposes patients to irradiation and does not usually alter clinical management.

A bone marrow examination would confirm a megaloblastic anaemia but does not distinguish between vitamin B_{12} and folate deficiency, and hence is not routinely performed.

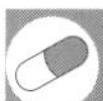 Q5: What is the treatment?

A5

Management is vitamin B_{12} usually given as 1 mg intramuscular injections for six doses over 2 weeks and then every 3 months for life. If required, the response to therapy can be assessed by the rise in reticulocytes and Hb and the fall in LDH.

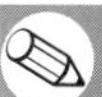 Q6: What is the long-term outcome?

A6

The blood/marrow changes will improve over the following few weeks, but the neurological deficit may take many, many months and if severe at diagnosis may not resolve completely.

 CASE 3.3 – A 78-year-old woman is referred with a 6-month history of general deterioration.

 Q1: What is the likely diagnosis and possible differential diagnoses?

A1

The blood count shows mild pancytopenia and this, taken together with bony pain and hypercalcaemia, could indicate secondary cancer in the bone or possibly a primary haematological cancer of the bone marrow. The total protein is very high and the albumin low, meaning that the globulin level (total protein minus albumin) is very high. Supported by the presence of renal impairment, the diagnosis is likely to be multiple myeloma. When a very high globulin level occurs, a low sodium level is often seen (so-called pseudo-hyponatraemia).

 Q2: What are the relevant points to elicit from the history?

A2

Multiple myeloma is a disease of elderly people and symptoms are often non-specific and attributed to old age. Symptoms caused by anaemia and bony pain (especially back) are typical and myeloma should always be considered with this combination. There are relatively few causes of thirst but the most common are diabetes (mellitus and insipidus), dehydration and hypercalcaemia. Hypercalcaemia also causes the confusion and polyuria that lead to dehydration (this will contribute to the raised creatinine in this patient). Renal impairment in myeloma is caused by dehydration, hypercalcaemia and paraprotein deposition in the kidney.

 Q3: What are the possible clinical signs?

A3

Back pain is common as a result of pressure on spinal nerve roots or pathological fractures. Vertebral collapse can lead to paraplegia. Note that there is usually no enlargement of the liver, spleen or lymph nodes unless secondary amyloidosis has occurred.

 Q4: What additional investigations are indicated?

A4

Multiple myeloma is a cancer of plasma cells. Immunoglobulins are normally produced by plasma cells and therefore a malignant proliferation of plasma cells leads to uncontrolled production of a single type of immunoglobulin (Ig) – so-called paraprotein. The plasma cells proliferate within the bone marrow, damaging normal bone marrow cells and bone and leading to anaemia and other blood cell cytopenias, hypercalcaemia and lytic lesions on radiographs.

The diagnosis of multiple myeloma depends on four tests:

1. Serum Ig estimation and protein electrophoresis.
2. Urinary sample for Bence Jones protein (light chain) analysis.
3. A skeletal survey looking for lytic lesions.
4. Bone marrow examination to assess malignant plasma cell infiltration.

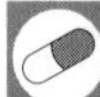 Q5: What is the treatment?

A5

In this case, treatment of the hypercalcaemia would be of most immediate priority because this may reduce the confusion and alleviate symptoms of dehydration. Local irradiation may be indicated for bony pain. The anaemia can be treated with blood transfusion in the short term, possibly with erythropoietin therapy thereafter. Treatment for myeloma consists of chemotherapy with autologous stem cell transplantation for younger patients. Steroids and anti-angiogenic agents also have a role as either upfront or palliative therapy. Regular bisphosphonate therapy reduces the risk of bony fracture and hypercalcaemia.

 Q6: What is the long-term outcome?

A6

The prognosis is poor, with death usually within 2–3 years of diagnosis for patients not fit enough for autologous stem cell transplantation and around 5 years for those who are.

OSCE Counselling Case – Answers

OSCE COUNSELLING CASE 3.1 – A colleague phones asking whether or not to transfuse a 24-year-old Asian woman who is 34 weeks' pregnant with a haemoglobin of 7.8 g/dL secondary to iron deficiency.

This is a common clinical scenario. It is imperative that you treat the patient and not the Hb level, so first you need to know whether the patient is clinically compromised by her anaemia. You also need to know whether or not the patient has been taking iron supplements and if so what dose and for how long. It would also be helpful to know whether this is the first child, or if there have been previous pregnancies, and the plans for delivery of this baby. In addition, it would be reassuring to be informed that this woman and her partner have been screened for thalassaemia and that she has no red cell antibodies that are likely to lead to haemolytic disease of the newborn.

In general terms patients with iron-deficiency anaemia should be treated with iron therapy and not blood transfusion. If the patient cannot tolerate oral iron, consideration should be given to parenteral iron. Adequate iron therapy raises the Hb by about 1 g/dL per week of therapy – within 3 weeks therefore the Hb should be > 10 g/dL in this case. Apart from the usual risks of blood transfusion (reactions, infections, fluid overload), this patient is of Asian origin and therefore blood transfusion has a much higher risk of leading to the development of alloantibodies, which not only may lead to future problems when cross-matching blood but also can predispose to haemolytic disease of the newborn (possibly in this pregnancy, but certainly in future pregnancies). Blood transfusion should be given only if this patient is clinically compromised by her anaemia and there is a need for 'urgent' delivery of the baby or if she is allergic to iron therapy, i.e. previous anaphylaxis with parenteral iron. It would be prudent to genotype the blood for cross-match in order to minimize the risk of alloantibody production; also the patient should be counselled about the risks of blood transfusion, and that, although all reasonable steps have been taken to avoid alloantibodies, nothing can be guaranteed.

ABNORMAL FBC

? Questions for each of the clinical case scenarios given

Q1: What is the likely diagnosis and possible differential diagnoses?
Q2: What are the relevant points to elicit from the history?
Q3: What are the possible clinical signs?
Q4: What additional investigations are indicated?
Q5: What is the treatment?
Q6: What is the long-term outcome?

Clinical cases

CASE 3.4 – A 78-year-old retired mechanic is admitted with increasing left hypochondrial pain of a stabbing character over the previous 12 h.

He had not felt well for 3 months, losing 5 kg in weight and recently noticing night sweats. Clinical examination revealed hepatomegaly of 5 cm and splenomegaly of 15 cm. There was no lymphadenopathy.

The FBC revealed:

- Hb 10.1 g/dL (normal 13.5–18 g/dL)
- WCC 227 × 10^9/L (normal 4–11 × 10^9/L) with prominent eosinophilia and basophilia
- Platelets 741 × 10^9/L (normal 150–400 × 10^9/L).

Urea and electrolytes and LFTs were normal except for a uric acid level of 490 μmol/L (normal 110–420 μmol/L).

CASE 3.5 – A 63 year-old-man presents with a left-sided transient ischaemic attack (TIA).

This follows on from a similar episode 1 week earlier that had been labelled a TIA. After the first TIA the GP performed some blood tests, the results of which are as follows:

- Hb 21.2 g/dL (13.0–16.5 g/dL)
- Red cell count 6.7 × 10^{12}/L (3.8–5.6 × 10^{12}/L)
- Haematocrit 0.61
- WCC 15.3 × 10^9/L (4–10.5 × 10^9/L)
- Increased neutrophils and eosinophils
- Platelets 897 × 10^9/L (150–400 × 10^9/L)
- Sodium 142 mmol/L (135–145 mmol/L)
- Potassium 4.8 mmol/L (3.4–5.0 mmol/L)
- Urea 5.0 mmol/L (2.5–7.0 mmol/L)

- Creatinine 79 μmol/L (50–100 μmol/L)
- Total protein 71 g/dL (60–80 g/dL)
- Albumin 43 g/dL (35–50 g/dL)
- Bilirubin 8 μmol/L (1–22 μmol/L)
- AST 30 IU/L (19–48 IU/L)
- ALP 71 IU/L (30–115 IU/L)
- Cholesterol 3.6 mmol/L (2.5–6.2 mmol/L)
- Triglyceride 1.9 mmol/L (0.1–1.6 mmol/L).

CASE 3.6 – A 23-year-old man is brought into the accident and emergency department (A&E) having become acutely unwell while shopping.

On admission he is barely rousable and unable to provide a history. On admission his Glasgow Coma Score (GCS) is 12 with no obviously localizing signs. His temperature is 39.5°C, his pulse regular with a rate of 130/min and blood pressure 60/35 mmHg. The respiratory rate is 25/min but on auscultation there are no added sounds. Abdominal examination is unremarkable with no obvious tenderness, rigidity or guarding, and bowel sounds are present. An FBC had been performed by his GP 2 days before this episode and showed the following:

- Hb 5.2 g/dL (13.0–16.5 g/dL)
- Red cell count 1.9×10^{12}/L ($3.8–5.6 \times 10^{12}$/L)
- WCC 93.3×10^{9}/L ($4–10.5 \times 10^{9}$/L)
- Neutrophils 0.1×10^{9}/L ($2.0–8.0 \times 10^{9}$/L)
- Platelets 7×10^{9}/L ($150–400 \times 10^{9}$/L).

OSCE Counselling Case

OSCE COUNSELLING CASE 3.2 – What advice would you give a GP who writes to you about a 37-year-old African–Caribbean woman who has had mild fluctuating neutropenia (0.8–1.5 × 109/L; normal 2.0–8.0 × 109/L) over the last 4 years?

Key concepts

The FBC is basically a measure of the quantity and size of the blood cells circulating at that time. If a particular blood cell count is raised, the question is whether this is the result of something inherently wrong with the bone marrow or whether the bone marrow is simply reacting to something else going on within the body, i.e. inflammation, infection or malignancy. The answer may be obvious from the FBC but if not clear a raised C-reactive protein (CRP) typically indicates a reactive process. An invaluable aid to diagnosis is a previous FBC because it may tell you whether the changes are recent or old, e.g. a common scenario is a patient whose Hb rises over a few days during admission. Assuming that the patient has not received an RBC transfusion a reduction in plasma volume, i.e. dehydration, is the usual cause. Likewise, a rapidly falling Hb does not necessarily indicate bleeding. One would expect the Hb to fall in a patient admitted with dehydration once rehydration is complete!

A blood film should be examined to ascertain the exact nature of any cells raised in the peripheral blood, e.g. leukaemia cells.

Low blood counts indicate either a failure of production by the bone marrow or reduced survival of that particular cell. In bone marrow failure one would expect to see all normal blood cells eventually affected, i.e. falling white cells, red cells and platelets. Typically, the neutrophil count falls first because this has the shortest survival in the circulation – 24 hours.

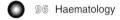

Answers

CASE 3.4 – A 78-year-old retired mechanic is admitted with increasing left hypochondrial pain of a stabbing character over the previous 12 h.

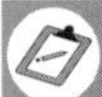

Q1: What is the likely diagnosis and possible differential diagnoses?

A1

This patient presents with hepatosplenomegaly, leukocytosis (with eosinophilia and basophilia) and thrombocytosis. This, taken together with the constitutional symptoms, indicates chronic myeloid leukaemia.

Q2: What are the relevant points to elicit from the history?

A2

During the history, direct evidence of hyperleukostasis should be sought, notably dizziness, headaches and visual loss.

Q3: What are the possible clinical signs?

A3

Splenic infarction leads to acute stabbing pain and this may be elicited on examination. Infarction can occur during splenic enlargement, probably as a result of the very high WCC and hyperleukostasis. In the acute event one may hear a splenic rub. Note that the gradual enlargement of the spleen is not, in itself, usually painful. Other signs of hyperleukostasis are retinal haemorrhages and retinal vein thrombosis.

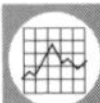

Q4: What additional investigations are indicated?

A4

The diagnosis is easily confirmed by cytogenetic analysis of peripheral blood cells where a translocation between chromosome 9 and 22 is found – the so-called Philadelphia chromosome.

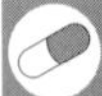

Q5: What is the treatment?

A5

If there are symptoms/signs of hyperleukostasis, leukopheresis should be undertaken to lower the WCC. Immediate care should include analgesia, allopurinol (to prevent acute gout), hydration and chemotherapy. The WCC can be rapidly reduced using hydroxycarbamide (usually) or cytosine arabinoside (rarely required). Having reduced the WCC sufficiently, further therapy should be with imatinib. Interferon-γ or cytosine arabinoside can be added later if there is a poor response to imatinib monotherapy. Patients who present with accelerated phase or blast crisis should be treated with combination therapy, including imatinib, interferon-γ and/or chemotherapy.

The age of this patient makes allogeneic stem cell transplantation from a donor too risky a procedure to be considered.

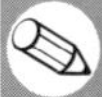

Q6: What is the long-term outcome?

A6

Chronic myeloid leukaemia consists of three distinct phases:

1. Chronic phase: relatively easy to control blood counts with imatinib monotherapy. Patient remains relatively well with few symptoms.
2. Accelerated phase: the blood counts become more difficult to control, often swinging from too low to too high.
3. Blast crisis: the clinical picture becomes more akin to acute leukaemia with increasing constitutional symptoms and marrow failure, i.e. low platelets, anaemia and high WCCs. Further chromosomal abnormalities, in addition to the Philadelphia chromosome, often occur at this stage. Patients at this stage become resistant to conventional therapies and the prognosis is very poor.

With the exception of allogeneic stem cell transplantation, none of the therapies is thought to be curative. Overall survival without transplantation has historically been around 5–6 years but early results with the recently introduced drug imatinib look promising.

CASE 3.5 – A 63-year-old-man presents with a left-sided TIA.

Q1: What is the likely diagnosis and possible differential diagnoses?

A1

This patient is suffering from recurrent TIAs and has a high Hb, red cell count (erythrocytosis), WCC (leukocytosis) and platelet count (thrombocythaemia). This combination is highly suggestive of polycythaemia rubra vera (PRV); in this condition TIAs occur because of high whole blood viscosity caused by increased red cells and also increased platelet 'stickiness'. However, one still needs to consider the common causes of TIAs (systemic emboli resulting from atrial fibrillation, mural thrombus after a myocardial infarction, carotid artery disease).

Q2: What are the relevant points to elicit from the history?

A2

One would be keen to know if the patient had any symptoms suggestive of an alternative underlying condition, e.g. palpitations (atrial fibrillation) or previous chest pain (mural thrombus). Headaches and pruritus are typical of PRV.

 Q3: What are the possible clinical signs?

A3

The patient has an irregular tachycardia (atrial fibrillation), carotid bruits or cardiac murmurs. The spleen is typically enlarged in PRV and there may be plethoric facies and excoriations caused by itching and scratching.

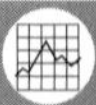 Q4: What additional investigations are indicated?

A4

The patient requires an ECG, carotid Doppler ultrasonography, an echocardiogram and/or computed tomography (CT) of the head depending on symptoms and clinical signs. The combination of a high Hb and splenomegaly is virtually diagnostic of PRV. In the absence of splenomegaly, a high uric acid and/or high vitamin B_{12} level, or a low erythropoietin level, is very suggestive.

The combination of a high Hb and splenomegaly is diagnostic of PRV in the absence of any other cause of polycythaemia, e.g. chronic obstructive pulmonary disease. In the absence of splenomegaly, a clonal bone marrow cytogenetic abnormality or spontaneous peripheral blood or bone marrow erythroid colony growth confirms the diagnosis. High uric acid, white count, platelet count and vitamin B_{12} level, or a low erythropoietin level, is very suggestive of PRV. If the haematocrit is < 0.60 in males or < 0.56 in females the diagnosis of true polycythaemia will need to be confirmed by blood volume studies (directly measuring red cell mass and plasma volume). In equivocal cases oxygen saturation, a chest radiograph and abdominal ultrasonography should also be performed to rule out pulmonary/cardiac/renal causes of polycythaemia.

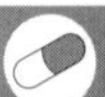 Q5: What is the treatment?

A5

The patient requires urgent hospital intervention to begin red cell venesection. While this is being organized, an anti-platelet agent (aspirin or clopidogrel) should be given.

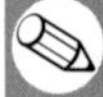 Q6: What is the long-term outcome?

A6

Long-term management includes regular venesection to keep the haematocrit to < 0.45, anti-platelet therapy (aspirin or clopidogrel) and 'mild' chemotherapy, e.g. hydroxycarbamide, to reduce the platelet count to normal levels.

CASE 3.6 – A 23-year-old man is brought into A&E having become acutely unwell while shopping.

 Q1: What is the likely diagnosis and possible differential diagnoses?

A1

The clinical history is one of sudden collapse and shock following what appears to be a relatively short period of ill-health. The differential diagnosis includes acute blood loss, sepsis (including meningitis), pancreatitis, hypoglycaemia, cerebral pathology (fits, thrombosis or haemorrhage) or cardiac problems (infarction, arrhythmia). The patient's blood count shows that there is marrow failure with inability to produce red cells, neutrophils and platelets. This can occur with many conditions but the high WCC (presumably blasts) indicates that the patient has acute leukaemia. This is completely in keeping with the fairly rapid onset of his symptoms.

 Q2: What are the relevant points to elicit from the history?

A2

This would need to be from a third party and would focus on features of anaemia (e.g. lethargy, palpitations, dyspnoea), low neutrophil count (infections) and low platelet count (nose bleeds and bruising). It would also be necessary to exclude other possibilities for his collapse (type 1 diabetes, heavy drinking, epilepsy etc.).

 Q3: What are the possible clinical signs?

A3

Clinically the patient is shocked – low blood pressure, tachycardia, tachypnoea. The high temperature is very suggestive of septic shock precipitated by neutropenia. The most common organisms are Gram-negative bacteria but Gram-positive sepsis is also possible. There may be ecchymoses related to the low platelet count.

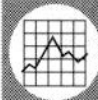 Q4: What additional investigations are indicated?

A4

The patient needs assessment of renal and liver function, calcium, urate, glucose and amylase, arterial blood gases, blood and urine culture, ECG and chest radiograph. Coagulation studies to investigate the possibility of disseminated intravascular coagulopathy (DIC), possibly precipitated by a Gram-negative septicaemia. This diagnosis can be confirmed by measuring fibrinogen degradation products (FDPs). Cerebral imaging should be urgently considered to rule out/confirm intracerebral bleeding.

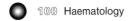

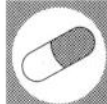 Q5: What is the treatment?

A5

The patient is shocked and therefore raising the blood pressure to allow adequate organ perfusion is essential. Crystalloids are required but correction of the abnormal coagulation with fresh frozen plasma (FFP) and/or cryoprecipitate (which is a better source of fibrinogen than FFP) will also help. Placement of a central venous line to measure central venous pressure and aid fluid replacement and a urinary catheter to assess urine output should be considered. If fluids alone do not adequately raise the blood pressure, inotropes should be instituted. If respiratory failure ensues assisted ventilation will be required.

Platelet transfusions will raise the platelet count and reduce the risk of fatal haemorrhage. The immediate commencement of broad-spectrum antibiotics with activity against both Gram-negative and Gram-positive bacteria is critical if the patient is to survive.

Although the patient is very anaemic this is not the source of shock. Red blood cell transfusions will raise the Hb and potentially aid oxygen delivery to tissues, but this is potentially dangerous because the patient has a very, very high WCC and a sudden increase in intravascular cells via transfusion has a very high risk of precipitating hyperleukostasis, which can be catastrophic. Correction of the anaemia can usually wait until the WCC has been reduced with chemotherapy. If a red cell transfusion is thought to be potentially of benefit this should be given very slowly.

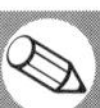 Q6: What is the long-term outcome?

A6

Septic shock associated with neutropenia has a very high mortality rate but, assuming that the patient survives this immediate life-threatening complication, the cure rate for acute leukaemia ranges from 20 to 80 per cent depending on the particular prognostic type.

OSCE Counselling Case – Answer

OSCE COUNSELLING CASE 3.2 – What advice would you give a GP who writes to you about a 37-year-old African–Caribbean woman who has had mild fluctuating neutropenia (0.8–1.5 × 109/L; normal 2.0–8.0 × 109/L) over the last 4 years?

This woman has longstanding isolated but fluctuating neutropenia. The 'normal range' quoted for most haemocytometers is usually based on an Anglo-Saxon white population and therefore may not be appropriate for all ethnic groups. African–Caribbean individuals are well described as having lower neutrophil counts (as low as 0.5×10^9/L) but have no increased infective risk. For this individual the neutrophil count may well be 'normal'. Other causes of isolated neutropenia should be considered, including autoimmune disorders (systemic lupus erythematosus, rheumatoid arthritis, etc.), drugs (angiotensin-converting enzyme [ACE] inhibitors), and familial and chronic benign neutropenia. Systemic problems of the bone marrow are highly unlikely (e.g. cancer – haematopoietic and non-haematopoietic, vitamin B_{12} and folate deficiency) because this condition has not deteriorated over 4 years. A rare cause of neutropenia – cyclical neutropenia – is a possible differential diagnosis but, as the patient has no predisposition to infections, no further investigations are required.

Overall, the GP should be reassured but regular monitoring every 12 months or would be advisable until the diagnosis is clear.

HAEMOGLOBINOPATHIES

? Questions for each of the clinical case scenarios given

Q1: What is the likely diagnosis and possible differential diagnoses?
Q2: What are the relevant points to elicit from the history?
Q3: What are the possible clinical signs?
Q4: What additional investigations are indicated?
Q5: What is the treatment?
Q6: What is the long-term outcome?

Clinical cases

CASE 3.7 – A 3-year-old girl is referred with failure to thrive.

She was the first child born to Asian parents who had recently moved to the UK. There was no family history of note. On examination the girl was pale, slightly icteric, with frontal skull bossing. Pulse was 110/min regular with no obvious added heart sounds. On auscultation the chest was clear. Abdominal examination revealed distension with hepatomegaly 3 cm and splenomegaly 5 cm below the costal margins.

Investigations revealed:

- Hb 5.1 g/dL (13.0–16.5 g/dL)
- MCV 58 fL (normal 80–100 fL)
- MCH 19 pg (normal 27–33 pg)
- WCC 9.1 × 10^9/L (normal 4–11.0 × 10^9/L)
- Platelets 317 × 10^9/L (normal 150–400 × 10^9/L)
- Ferritin 12 ng/mL (normal 6–81 ng/mL)
- Folate 4.1 μg/L (normal 2.1–20 μg/L)
- Vitamin B_{12} 273 ng/L (normal 130–900 ng/L)
- Iron 18 μmol/L (normal 10–30 μmol/L)
- Iron-binding capacity 60 μmol/L (normal 40–75 μmol/L)
- Sodium 142 mmol/L (135–145 mmol/L)
- Potassium 4.8 mmol/L (3.4–5.0 mmol/L)
- Urea 5.0 mmol/L (2.5–7.0 mmol/L)
- Creatinine 79 μmol/L (50–100 μmol/L)
- Total protein 71 g/dL (60–80 g/dL)
- Albumin 33 g/dL (35–50 g/dL)

- Bilirubin 38 μmol/L (1–22 μmol/L)
- AST 65 IU/L (19–48 IU/L)
- ALP 71 IU/L (30–115 IU/L)
- LDH 1584 U/L (normal 200–500 U/L)

CASE 3.8 – An 18-year-old African woman awoke with shortness of breath and bilateral chest pain.

The woman is admitted through A&E. She had been well apart from a cough the previous day, but awoke that morning with shortness of breath and bilateral chest pain. She said she had a similar episode 3 years earlier shortly after arriving in the UK from Nigeria. On examination she was very distressed and tachypnoeic. Her temperature was 39.7°C. General examination was unremarkable apart from the respiratory system and a chronic skin ulcer above the right medial malleolus. The respiratory rate was 36/min with reduced air entry and percussion note at the right midzone. There were widespread bilateral coarse crepitations.

Investigations revealed:

- Hb 6.8 g/dL (13.0–16.5 g/dL)
- MCV 84 fL (normal 80–100 fL)
- MCH 29 pg (normal 27–33 pg)
- WCC 17.1×10^9/L (normal 4 –11.0×10^9/L)
- Platelets 619×10^9/L (normal 150–400×10^9/L)
- Ferritin 45 ng/mL (normal 6–81 ng/mL)
- Folate 6.2 μg/L (normal 2.1–20 μg/L)
- Vitamin B_{12} 416 ng/L (normal 130–900 ng/L)
- Sodium 139 mmol/L (135–145 mmol/L)
- Potassium 4.8 mmol/L (3.4–5.0 mmol/L)
- Urea 11.2 mmol/L (2.5–7.0 mmol/L)
- Creatinine 169 μmol/L (50–100 μmol/L)
- Total protein 64 g/dL (60–80 g/dL)
- Albumin 34 g/dL (35–50 g/dL)
- Bilirubin 42 μmol/L (1–22 μmol/L)
- AST 58 IU/L (19–48 IU/L)
- ALP 71 IU/L (30–115 IU/L)
- LDH 1381 U/L (normal 200–500 U/L)

- Arterial blood gases:
  - pH 7.36 (normal 7.35–7.45)
  - P_{O_2} 6.9 kPa (normal 11.3–14.0 kPa)
  - P_{CO_2} 5.1 kPa (normal 4.7–6.0 kPa)
- Chest radiograph: widespread shadowing, especially at the right midzone.

OSCE Counselling Case

OSCE COUNSELLING CASE 3.3 – If two parents who are carriers of sickle-cell disease have three children, what is the chance of no child being either a carrier or suffering from full-blown sickle-cell disease?

Key concepts

The area of haemoglobinopathies is a test of your knowledge of ethnicity, hereditary diseases, erythropoiesis, paediatrics and hazards/benefits of blood transfusions. In keeping with most fatal hereditary conditions, they are mostly autosomal recessive inheritance but with variable penetrance. Different types of haemoglobinopathies occur in different areas of the world but with globalization they are becoming a more common clinical problem in the UK. Management can be split into preventive, prophylactic and therapeutic.

Answers

 CASE 3.7 – **A 3-year-old girl is referred with failure to thrive.**

 Q1: What is the likely diagnosis and possible differential diagnoses?

A1

There are only four conditions that give rise to hypochromic (low MCH)/microcytic (low MCV) anaemia: iron deficiency, thalassaemia major, anaemia of chronic disease and hereditary sideroblastic anaemia (usually X-linked recessive inheritance, i.e. affects boys). The normal ferritin, iron and iron-binding capacity rule out iron deficiency and anaemia of chronic disease. The raised bilirubin, AST and LDH indicate ineffective erythropoiesis and/or haemolysis, which is characteristic of thalassaemia major. Thalassaemic conditions are found in many different ethnic groups, including Mediterranean, Middle Eastern and Asian.

 Q2: What are the relevant points to elicit from the history?

A2

Thalassaemia major is the result of the inability to produce either α- or β-globin chains as a result of hereditary genetic defects in the respective genes. Thalassaemia major results from the affected individual inheriting two genetic defects – one from each parent, i.e. autosomal recessive inheritance. Over 100 different genetic defects have been described. Very severely affected fetuses may not be viable and result in stillbirths. One therefore needs to ask whether there is any family history of stillbirth or anaemia and if by chance the two parents are related, i.e. consanguineous.

 Q3: What are the possible clinical signs?

A3

Children present with failure to thrive, pallor and shortness of breath (caused by anaemia), mild jaundice (resulting from ineffective erythropoiesis and haemolysis), abdominal distension (hepatomegaly and splenomegaly caused by extramedullary haematopoiesis, haemolysis and later iron overload) and bony enlargement (resulting from marrow hyperplasia – frontal bossing, maxillary and parietal bone enlargement).

 Q4: What additional investigations are indicated?

A4

A blood film will reveal a severe hypochromic/microcytic anaemia with erythroblasts present in the peripheral blood, and with target cells and basophilic stippling. If there is inability to produce either α- or β-globin chains the developing erythroid cell will try to produce other types of Hb to compensate.

Haemoglobin electrophoresis will detect absent or reduced HbA and the presence of abnormal haemoglobins, e.g. HbF, HbH (β4), HbBarts (γ4) and HbA_2. In some patients who are carriers of α-thalassaemia the Hb electrophoresis may be normal and more sophisticated tests such as globin chain synthesis may be required. As the underlying molecular changes are characterized, molecular genetic studies are being increasingly used for diagnostic purposes.

Having identified that a patient has thalassaemia or is a carrier, it will be necessary to screen family members to see whether any are affected. Any identified carriers will require genetic counselling to make them aware of the risk that any as yet unborn child may have of being affected. Advice re antenatal screening or possible termination of future pregnancies needs to be given by counsellors experienced in this field.

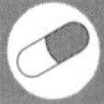

Q5: What is the treatment?

A5

The mainstay of treatment for affected individuals is a red cell transfusion programme. This not only relieves symptoms but also prevents the bony overgrowths that occur.

If children are treated early splenomegaly may not occur. If there is a delay in diagnosis or starting a transfusion programme, splenomegaly and hypersplenism can occur which increases transfusion requirements. In this situation splenectomy can be performed but as a result of infective problems this is usually deferred until after the age of 5 years. Immunization, i.e. with pneumococcal and *Haemophilus influenzae* vaccines, and long-term prophylactic antibiotics will be required in all splenectomized patients.

Among the many risks of blood transfusion is iron overload, which occurs as a result of regular blood transfusions. Each unit of blood contains 250 mg iron and regular monitoring of ferritin to detect early iron overload is required.

This iron accumulation damages normal tissues, e.g. liver, pituitary, heart, gonads, pancreas etc., and desferrioxamine with or without deferiprone is required. Iron excretion by desferrioxamine is increased by vitamin C supplementation. Regular eye and hearing assessments will be required for all patients on long-term desferrioxamine. If organ damage has occurred hormone replacements, e.g. insulin, may be required.

As regular blood transfusions are the mainstay of therapy, immunization against hepatitis B is recommended.

The underlying problem is one of failure of the developing red cells to produce adequate Hb. Haematopoietic stem cell transplantation from a suitable allogeneic donor is hazardous, with many possible pitfalls (including death), but is potentially curative.

Q6: What is the long-term outcome?

A6

Patients who are carriers of thalassaemia have a normal life expectancy. Sufferers of thalassaemia used to die by the age of 20–30 years before iron chelation therapy became widespread. In theory well-chelated patients should have a normal life expectancy, but in reality they often die prematurely. Stem cell transplantation is potentially curative, provided that patients do not succumb to transplantation complications.

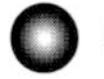

CASE 3.8 – An 18-year-old African woman awoke with shortness of breath and bilateral chest pain.

Q1: What is the likely diagnosis and possible differential diagnoses?

A1

This young African woman presents with respiratory failure and chest pain. The differential diagnosis includes pulmonary embolism, chest infection, asthma and sickle-cell crisis (chest syndrome). The clinical picture is not typical of asthma and the anaemia and biochemical pictures of haemolysis are not explained by pulmonary embolism alone. The clinical examination and chest radiograph are highly suggestive of a chest infection but, again, this alone does not completely explain the clinical picture and blood results. Intractable skin ulceration over the malleoli is a common feature of sickle-cell disease. This patient's clinical presentation and investigations are highly suggestive of a sickle-cell crisis probably precipitated by a chest infection.

Haemoglobin S (HbS) is insoluble and forms crystals when deoxygenated. This distorts the red blood cells, giving them their characteristic shape and blockage of the microcirculation, leading to ischaemia and infarction.

Q2: What are the relevant points to elicit from the history?

A2

Sickle-cell disease has a highly variable clinical course with some patients having a virtually normal life and others succumbing in infancy to crises or infection. It is important to ascertain whether the patient is known to have sickle-cell disease, has had previous crises or if there is a parent or sibling known to have sickle-cell disease or to be a sickle carrier. Precipitating factors known to lead to sickle crises, i.e. hypoxia (altitude), surgery, trauma, cold, infections and dehydration, should be sought.

Q3: What are the possible clinical signs?

A3

Anaemia (pallor, tachycardia, tachypnoea) is universal as a result of chronic intravascular haemolysis.

Acute sickle-cell crisis is caused by acute occlusion of the microcirculation, leading to tissue hypoxia and organ infarction on a background of intravascular red cell haemolysis. Clinical signs are highly variable depending on the predominantly affected organ. Acute pain – bony (long bones, vertebrae, ribs etc.) or abdominal (spleen, liver, gut infarction) – is very common. Splenomegaly is common in young children but ultimately splenic infarction leading to hyposplenism supervenes. Cerebral vessel occlusion can manifest as hemiparesis, paraparesis, fits, loss/reduced consciousness and/or blindness. The combination seen in this patient of fever, leukocytosis, dyspnoea, chest pain and pulmonary infiltrate is often referred to as acute chest syndrome. The clinical and chest radiograph findings are non-specific and hence do not distinguish sickling within the chest from a chest infection.

Chronic sickle-cell disease leads to ischaemic necrosis of joints and secondary arthritic changes. High-output cardiac failure as a result of a combination of chronic anaemia, myocardial and pulmonary microinfarction often leads to premature death. Renal impairment caused by papillary necrosis and proliferative retinopathy is a late manifestation. Hepatomegaly is usually modest, but pigmented gallstones and biliary disease are common. Leg ulcers are a common typical feature.

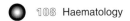

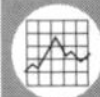 Q4: What additional investigations are indicated?

A4

First one has to confirm the diagnosis of sickle-cell disease – this is most easily done by looking at the blood film. Blood film changes of hyposplenism, i.e. target cells, Howell–Jolly bodies and thrombocytosis will also be seen. The presence of HbS can be confirmed with a Sickledex test and Hb electrophoresis.

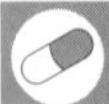 Q5: What is the treatment?

A5

Acute crisis management

General measures to treat any underlying precipitating factor, i.e. analgesia, antibiotics, rehydration and oxygen therapy, are essential. Patients should also be anticoagulated with heparin (unless contraindicated) because they have a very high risk of thrombosis.

Blood transfusion of red cells dilutes HbS, improving microvascular circulation and oxygen delivery; it also temporarily suppresses HbS production. Partial exchange transfusion is usual.

Prophylactic therapy

All patients should be taking oral folic acid.

Regular blood transfusions of red cells to keep the percentage of HbS below 30 per cent will effectively prevent crises occurring. As long-term blood transfusions are potentially very hazardous, this approach should probably be reserved for high-risk periods, e.g. before surgery, or during pregnancy.

The drug hydroxyurea (hydroxycarbamide) increases production of HbF, which has a protective effect on sickling cells and reduces crises.

Antibiotic prophylaxis/immunizations: sickle patients are hyposplenic and should therefore receive pneumococcal and *Haemophilus influenzae* immunization along with life-long penicillin.

Allogeneic haematopoietic stem cell transplantation is potentially curative but high risk. It may have a role in selected patients, e.g. children with strokes.

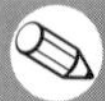 Q6: What is the long-term outcome?

A6

In the developing world many sickle-cell patients die in childhood from crises or infection. With good medical care many patients will survive into middle age.

OSCE Counselling Case – Answer

OSCE COUNSELLING CASE 3.3 – If two parents who are carriers of sickle-cell disease have three children, what is the chance of no child being either a carrier or suffering from full-blown sickle-cell disease?

As sickle-cell disease is an autosomal recessive condition, each parent must have one normal gene and one sickle gene. Thus, each individual child has a one in four chance of not being a carrier and not having sickle-cell disease. Thus, the chance of all three children not being carriers or having full-blown sickle-cell disease is $1/4 \times 1/4 \times 1/4 = 1$ in 64.

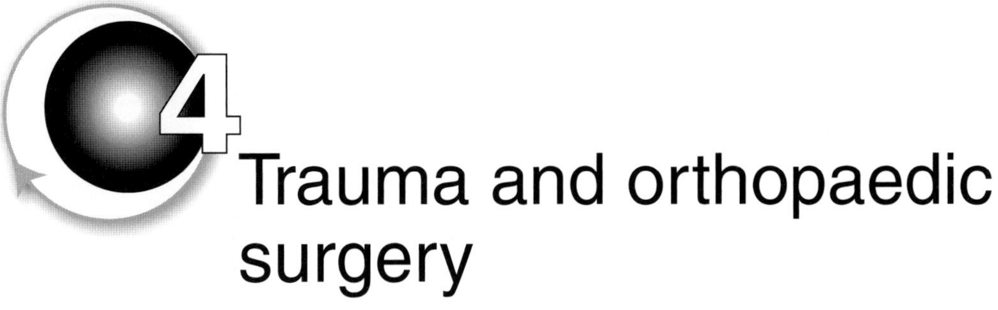

4 Trauma and orthopaedic surgery

Ian Pallister

THE PAINFUL HIP

? Questions for each of the clinical case scenarios given

Q1: What is the likely differential diagnosis?
Q2: What issues in the given history support the diagnosis?
Q3: What additional features in the history would you seek to support a particular diagnosis?
Q4: What clinical examination would you perform and why?
Q5: What investigations would be most helpful and why?
Q6: What treatment options are appropriate?

Clinical cases

CASE 4.1 – The toddler who will not weight bear.

A 15-month-old toddler is referred via the GP because he is refusing to put his right foot down to the ground and walk. Attempts to encourage him to weight bear clearly distress him but, when left to his own devices, although he is slightly off his food and rather unwell, in general terms he will sit and play quietly.

CASE 4.2 – The boy whose knee hurts and who limps after playing football.

A 9-year-old boy is referred with a 3-month history of knee pain, which seems to be related to him playing football or riding his bike. He can usually do the activity for a little while, but then usually comes into the house in some distress complaining of a sore knee and limping quite badly. This has lasted for a couple of days before usually clearing up. The next time he feels inclined to play football or ride his bike the same thing happens.

CASE 4.3 – The teenager with a groin strain.

A 14-year-old girl who is a little overweight presents with what appears to be a groin strain. She is not a keen athlete but was taking part in games doing the triple jump. She experienced pain in the groin 6 weeks ago and this has not got any better. She has been able to weight bear, but reluctantly, and certainly cannot run.

CASE 4.4 – A stiff painful hip in a retired man.

A retired man is referred with a 5-year history of increasing pain and stiffness in his right hip. This has gradually worsened and is no longer responding to simple analgesics.

OSCE Counselling Cases

OSCE COUNSELLING CASE 4.1 – 'Doctor I had my hip replaced 2 months ago; it doesn't hurt but I'm still limping.'

OSCE COUNSELLING CASE 4.2 – 'My knee has been hurting for 2 years. I have had two steroid injections in the last year. Does it mean I need to have my knee replaced?'

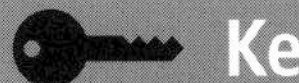

Key concepts

The surgical sieve

Orthopaedics lends itself very well to considering disease types in terms of a surgical sieve. Conditions may be genetic/congenital in origin, developmental, traumatic, inflammatory, infective, neoplastic or degenerative.

Patients in infancy or early childhood are, naturally, more likely to present with problems related to congenital/genetic or developmental abnormalities. As a result of their immature immune status, they are also more likely to have infective problems. Similarly, they are also relatively more likely to have neoplastic problems.

Trauma in terms of straightforward isolated limb injuries increases as children become more active and independent. Injuries peak in the form of severe life-threatening multiple trauma in early adult life. Trauma then becomes less common until the effects of osteoporosis and general infirmity supervene, with patients having falls in what would otherwise be fairly safe surroundings, sustaining fractures of pathologically weakened bones.

Answers

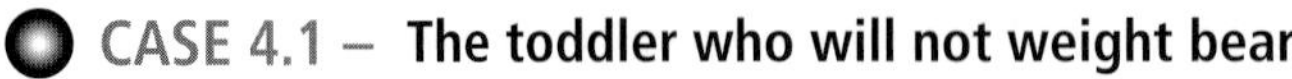

CASE 4.1 – The toddler who will not weight bear.

Q1: What is the likely differential diagnosis?

A1

- Transient sympathetic synovitis of the hip joint (the archetypal cause of irritable hip)
- Septic arthritis of the hip (an acute surgical emergency)
- Osteomyelitis of the proximal femur or pelvis
- Greenstick fracture elsewhere in the right lower limb
- Metastatic neoplasm (exceedingly rare).

Q2: What issues in the given history support the diagnosis?

A2

Irritable hip is the name given to this type of presentation, but it is not a diagnosis. Think of it as a general term for presentation, such as acute abdomen. Sympathetic synovitis is the most common diagnosis, and is usually seen in children of this age a week or so after an upper respiratory tract infection. It appears to represent a form of cross-reaction between viral antigens and the synovium. It is a self-limiting condition with no adverse sequelae. The child has usually recovered from the upper respiratory tract infection, but occasionally the two things happen concurrently. The child will usually sit comfortably and will be interested in playing, eating etc., but will resist attempts to get him to walk.

Q3: What additional features in the history would you seek to support a particular diagnosis?

A3

In septic arthritis the child is usually unwell, off food and wants to lie still. In a classic presentation of a fulminant septic arthritis, the slightest jolt will result in extreme pain. In very young children, however, this can be hard to establish, especially if the child is already distressed.

Osteomyelitis usually has a more indolent and less florid presentation, but is invariably seen in a child whose sleep has been disturbed by the pain and is unwell in other respects.

Greenstick fractures are fairly common in toddlers of this age. A history of the child crying, limping or refusing to weight bear after attempting to kick a football is quite common. The child often twists on the leg supporting the weight, resulting in an undisplaced spiral fracture of the tibia with an intact fibula.

 Q4: What clinical examination would you perform and why?

A4

The child as a whole should be examined, checking the temperature, ears, nose and throat in particular. It is often easier to examine the child while he is being cuddled by a parent. Examine the normal limb first and tickle the child's toes to see how free the movements are. Then, gently examine the problem limb, starting with a tickle and gentle passive movements, before systematic palpation.

In the child who wishes to lie still, it is worth noting the resting position of the affected limb. To relax the capsule in the presence of an effusion, the hip is instinctively held in a slightly flexed and externally rotated position. In septic arthritis or osteomyelitis, the child is often obviously very unwell and pyrexial. A key feature of septic arthritis is that movement of the limb concerned will be excruciatingly painful. In all other circumstances movement may be possible and limited only at the extremes.

Careful clinical examination of the lower limb may reveal localized tenderness in the presence of a greenstick fracture.

 Q5: What investigations would be most helpful and why?

A5

The most important diagnosis to exclude is that of septic arthritis. A blood sample should be taken for full blood count (FBC), erythrocyte sedimentation rate (ESR) and C-reactive protein (CRP). These are usually normal in transient sympathetic synovitis. If the child is pyrexial or otherwise unwell, blood cultures should also be taken at this point in time.

A plain radiograph of the pelvis should be taken, which is usually normal. Subtle changes in the soft tissues around the hip may suggest the presence of an effusion in the hip.

The investigation of choice is that of ultrasonography, which, in skilled hands, readily demonstrates the presence of an effusion; in a cooperative child this can be aspirated.

After careful palpation, radiographs of the area of tenderness will show the presence or absence of a fracture.

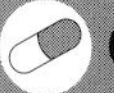 Q6: What treatment options are appropriate?

A6

Transient sympathetic synovitis requires no specific treatment. It usually resolves in 48–72 h and has no long-term sequelae. Simple analgesia and reassurance are all that are required.

Septic arthritis is an acute surgical emergency. Blood cultures should be obtained before emergency surgery to incise and drain the hip joint. Whether this is approached from the front or back is a matter of surgical preference. In a well-established septic arthritis, sometimes a repeated incision and drainage can be required in order to bring an acute suppurative infection under control.

Systemic antibiotics should ideally be commenced once either an aspiration has been performed or surgical specimens are obtained in the operating theatre. Naturally, if a child is endotoxaemic they have to be begun before either of these is performed.

Greenstick fractures in the lower limb are relatively common in toddlers. Plaster of Paris or lightweight polymer cast splintage of the limb is all that is required, and children invariably try to walk on them as soon as the acute pain has gone. This usually happens within a few days of injury. Plaster immobilization is normally needed for only about 3 weeks.

For osteomyelitis, initial radiographs may be entirely unremarkable and magnetic resonance imaging (MRI) or a bone scan may be required to confirm the diagnosis. If diagnosed early enough, antibiotics may be sufficient to obtain resolution. However, once a sequestrum has formed surgical drainage of this is mandatory.

In the rare instance of metastatic neoplasm presenting as an irritable hip, the treatment is naturally directed towards identifying and treating the primary cause.

CASE 4.2 – The boy whose knee hurts and who limps after playing football.

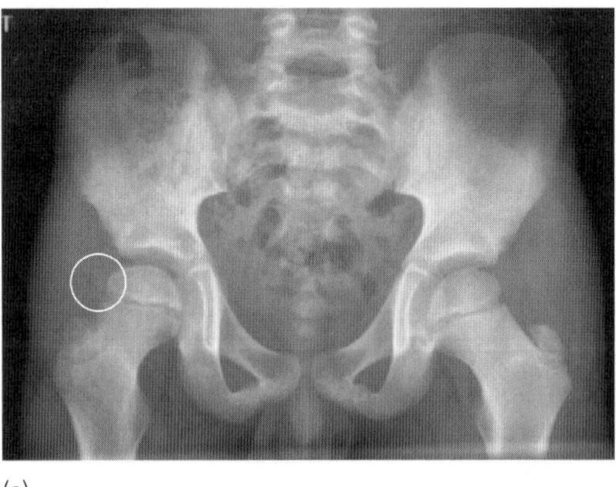

(a)

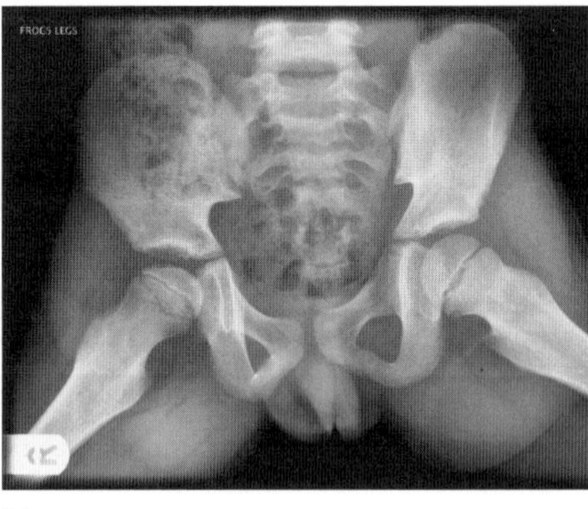

(b)

Figure 4.1 Perthes' disease. (a) Anteroposterior (AP) and (b) frog lateral views of the pelvis are shown. Apart from a small island of calcification lateral to the femoral head (encircled in (a)), the AP view is relatively normal. The frog lateral view shows collapse of the anterior part of the femoral head.

Q1: What is the likely differential diagnosis?

A1

- Perthes' disease
- Transient sympathetic synovitis of the hip joint (the archetypal cause of irritable hip)
- Septic arthritis of the hip (an acute surgical emergency)
- Osteomyelitis of the proximal femur or pelvis
- Greenstick fracture elsewhere in the right lower limb
- Metastatic neoplasm (exceedingly rare).

 Q2: What issues in the given history support the diagnosis?

A2

Perthes' disease is more common in boys and presents usually at school age; although the disease manifests in the hip it commonly presents with referred pain in the thigh or knee. The child is invariably well and otherwise active and has pain provoked by normal childhood activities.

 Q3: What additional features in the history would you seek to support a particular diagnosis?

A3

A family history of Perthes' disease strongly supports the diagnosis.

 Q4: What clinical examination would you perform and why?

A4

The child should be carefully examined from the lumbar spine to the toes. If able to weight bear, the child will invariably walk with an externally rotated leg on the affected side and, when lying supine and actively flexing, the hip will almost certainly rotate externally as it is brought up in flexion (obligatory external rotation).

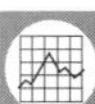 Q5: What investigations would be most helpful and why?

A5

Plain radiographs, anteroposterior (AP) pelvis including frog lateral should be performed. Depending on the stage or grade (severity) of the disease, the femoral epiphysis may show cystic or sclerotic changes. There may be a subchondral fracture, giving a 'head-within-a-head' appearance. The femoral head may show 'at-risk' signs, indicating deformation, with flattening of the head. The hip is therefore at risk of changing from a ball-and-socket joint into a hinge one. In cases of doubt these can be supplemented with either a bone scan or preferably MRI.

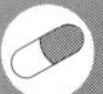 Q6: What treatment options are appropriate?

A6

The goal of treatment in Perthes' disease is to ensure that the child achieves skeletal maturity with a round femoral head in a round hip socket.

The disease has been characterized as an osteochondritis. It is a rather enigmatic condition and, for reasons that are poorly understood, part of the femoral epiphysis or growth centre undergoes avascular necrosis. This naturally leads to softening and potential deformation of the femoral head. The younger the child at presentation and being of male sex are associated with a better prognosis.

Current treatment ranges from osteotomy of the proximal femur or the acetabulum to confining the child to a broomstick cast until the phases of softening, deformation, healing and consolidation of the femoral head have run their course.

CASE 4.3 – The teenager with a groin strain.

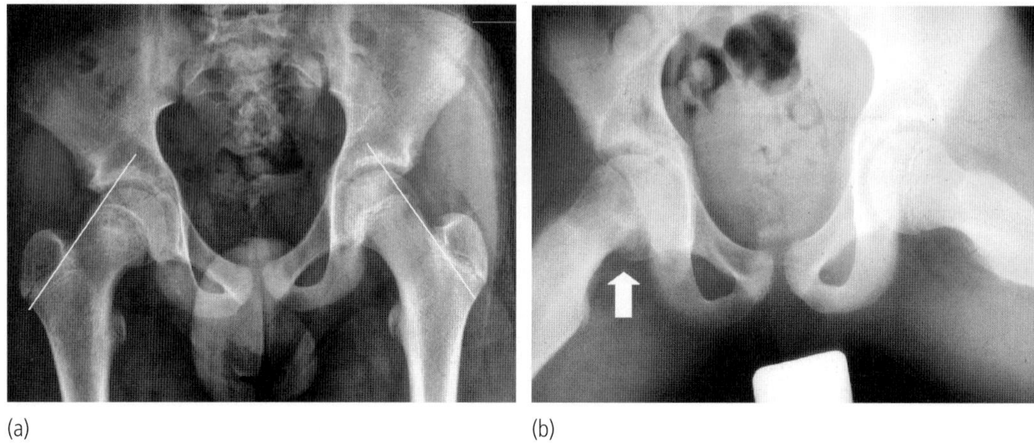

(a) (b)

Figure 4.2 Slipped upper femoral epiphysis: (a) the anteroposterior pelvis radiograph shows little apart from the subtle sign that a line drawn on the lateral aspect of the asymptomatic femoral neck just passes through the edge of the femoral head. When drawn on the symptomatic side, the line misses the femoral head altogether. (b) As the femoral head slips posteriorly, the displacement is best seen on the frog lateral view. As this is a chronic slip, new bone has formed at the posterior margin of the femoral neck in an effort to shore up the femoral head (arrow)

Q1: What is the likely differential diagnosis?

A1

The probable diagnosis is a slipped upper femoral epiphysis.

Q2: What issues in the given history support the diagnosis?

A2

The history given is a typical presentation. Pitfalls in the typical presentation are that there can be no associated apparent traumatic event and, as in Perthes' disease, the pain can be manifest in the thigh or knee.

Q3: What additional features in the history would you seek to support a particular diagnosis?

A3

The incidence of bilateral slip is about 20 per cent and occasionally there is also a family history.

Q4: What clinical examination would you perform and why?

A4

If the patient can walk, careful evaluation of the gait pattern should be performed, paying attention to external rotation, range of active and passive motion while lying supine. Again obligatory external rotation is common even in early slips.

Q5: What investigations would be most helpful and why?

A5

A plain AP radiograph of the pelvis is essential, and thus must be accompanied by a frog lateral. As the femoral head epiphysis slips posteriorly as well as inferiorly, it is thrown into clear profile only on the radiograph when the frog lateral view is obtained. The plain AP radiograph can look deceptively normal even in the presence of a very significant slip, which is very obvious on a frog lateral view.

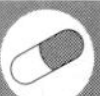

Q6: What treatment options are appropriate?

A6

The child should be admitted and put to bed. The operation of choice is that of fixing the slipped capital femoral epiphysis *in situ* using a cannulated screw. This prevents further slippage and encourages the physis actually to ossify and close. The screw should be left in place until skeletal maturity.

Slips can be classified into acute or chronic, stable or unstable. Although this case did have an apparent acute precipitating cause because of the interval between this occurring and the presentation, it would be classified as chronic. As the child can weight bear it is classified as being stable; if the child cannot weight bear, the slip is unstable. In very acute slips, which have occurred, for example, in a fall from a bicycle in an otherwise normal hip, efforts to reduce the femoral epiphysis and then fix it are advisable. In chronic slips, because of the very rapid nature of remodelling, attempts to effect a reduction are fraught with danger and can lead to avascular necrosis of the femoral head.

CASE 4.4 – A stiff painful hip in the retired man.

Q1: What is the likely differential diagnosis?

A1

- Osteoarthritis of the hip
- Delayed degenerative presentation of:
  - developmental hip dysplasia
  - Perthes' disease
  - slipped capital femoral epiphysis
- Paget's disease
- Metastatic bone disease.

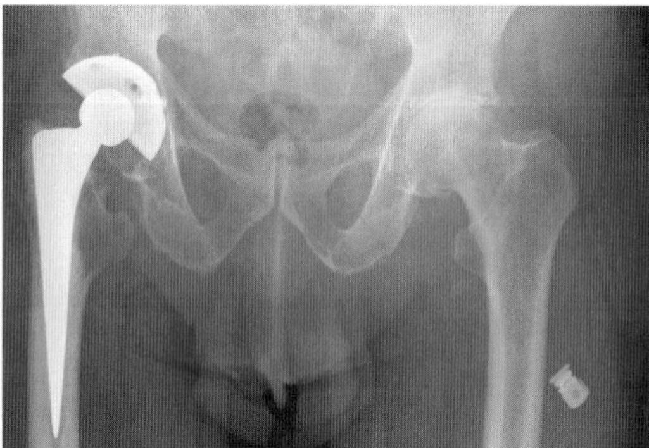

Figure 4.3 Osteoarthritis. Patient shows hip replacement.

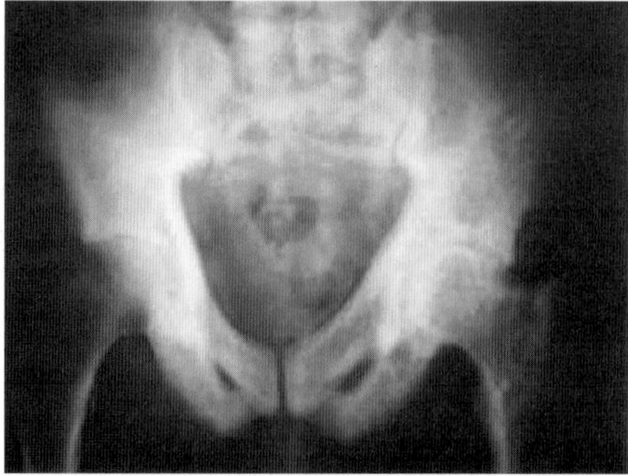

Figure 4.4 Paget's disease.

 Q2: What issues in the given history support the diagnosis?

A2

Typically the start of pain is associated with activity. Stiffness is often worse in the morning and then limbers up with gentle activity. As the day wears on, the pain and stiffness recur.

Simple analgesia and anti-inflammatory drugs are usually of benefit, but as the joint degeneration worsens they invariably become ineffective. It is usually about this point in time that patients start to tolerate the use of a walking aid such as a stick or crutches.

End-stage disease is indicated by pain at night preventing the patient sleeping.

 Q3: What additional features in the history would you seek to support a particular diagnosis?

A3

The absence of a history of problems in childhood goes strongly against a delayed presentation of a childhood problem. Post-traumatic osteoarthritis does occur as a consequence of acetabular or proximal femoral fractures, but these are rare in the general population. The traumatic episode is usually clearly remembered!

Paget's disease often has a similar presentation to that of osteoarthritis, and can also coexist with it. Along with metastatic bone disease, night pain, unrelated to daytime activity, is more common. The disease is a benign tumour of osteoclasts which results in a dramatic increase in bone turnover. As the new bone is woven, it is softer than its healthy lamellar counterpart. Consequently, it may bend or even fracture under normal loads.

Metastatic disease may present in patients who have a known primary (usually prostate, breast, thyroid, kidney, myeloma or lung). Alternatively, the primary may be occult.

 Q4: What clinical examination would you perform and why?

A4

Careful clinical examination, including evaluation of the limb length, gait pattern, and passive and active movements, is required.

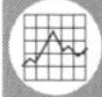 Q5: What investigations would be most helpful and why?

A5

Plain radiographs of the pelvis and lateral view of the affected hip will give the diagnosis. The typical radiological features of osteoarthritis are those of loss of joint space, subchondral sclerosis, and cyst and osteophyte formation, with the possibility of a loss of alignment at the joint. As the hip is a ball-and-socket joint this is usually difficult to appreciate.

Paget's disease can affect one bone or many. It may be limited to the proximal femur, ischium, pubis, ilium or the whole innominate bone. The bone is diffusely sclerotic and thickened, and may have areas that look washed out.

The lesion in metastatic disease is usually lytic and, if destruction continues, a pathological fracture can occur. Occasionally sclerotic metastases are seen.

Q6: What treatment options are appropriate?

A6

The current best available treatment option is that of a total hip replacement or arthroplasty. This is a major operation and consists of replacement of both acetabular and femoral sides of the hip joint. A variety of implants and techniques is available. The technicalities, the choice of which is beyond the scope of this publication, and the long-term results of these are indeed very similar. Total hip replacement affords a good range of painless motion and most patients are capable of abandoning walking aids 6–12 weeks after surgery. Most arthroplasties last 15–20 years before needing revision. Early revision can be needed because of recurrent dislocation or septic loosening.

Skin organisms such as *Staphyloccus epidermidis* are inevitably introduced into the operative field at the time of surgery. These usually cause no problems; however, in a small percentage of patients a slow loosening process occurs with osteolysis around the implants. Revision surgery in this case is normally completed as a staged procedure, which appears to carry the least risk of recurrence of infection.

Aseptic loosening occurs much later and seems to be as a result of the body's own response to wear-and-tear debris from the plastic (polyethylene) acetabular components slowly being abraded by the metal weight-bearing head.

Macrophages attempt to ingest the polyethylene wear particles and this leads to the release of powerful destructive enzymes. Again osteolysis occurs. In such circumstances single-stage revision is usually possible.

In years gone by hip fusion was the mainstay of treatment for patients who would otherwise lead an active life. Patients whose mobility was much more restricted were often treated with excision arthroplasty known as a girdlestone procedure. The femoral head and neck were removed leaving the intertrochanteric area of the femur to articulate with the lateral cortex of the pelvis. This would appear to be a mutilating procedure but it was effective in relieving severe end-stage arthritic pain. Patients were usually able to mobilize with the use of walking aids for distances sufficient for them to be mobile around their own home.

Paget's disease can usually be managed well with non-operative measures as for osteoarthritis. Bisphosphonates are very effective in managing pain that does not otherwise respond.

In occult malignancy the primary should be sought and treated, and local radiotherapy treatment given, if appropriate. Prophylactic stabilization of the bone should be carried out if a fracture is impending.

OSCE Counselling Cases –Answers

OSCE COUNSELLING CASE 4.1 – 'Doctor I had my hip replaced 2 months ago; it doesn't hurt but I'm still limping.'

Various approaches to the hip for hip replacement surgery have been described. One common approach detaches some of the principal abductors of the hip; although these are repaired at the time of surgery, sometimes the repair fails and the abductors avulse from the greater trochanter. When this occurs the patient normally notices a tearing sensation and there is a sudden dramatic deterioration in physical performance; not only that, but the hip often becomes unstable and can dislocate. Fortunately this particular complication is rare.

It is a little more common for the superior gluteal nerve to be stretched during elevation of the abductor muscles. If this occurs and the nerve does not recover, a permanent abductor lurch or Trendelenburg gait can result. However, far more common is simply some postoperative wasting of the same abductor muscles, which recovers with time. Specific physiotherapy can sometimes be needed, particularly in patients who are a little more wary of aggressively mobilizing themselves and getting out and about. Simple reassurance and targeted physiotherapy are usually all that is needed.

OSCE COUNSELLING CASE 4.2 – 'My knee has been hurting for 2 years. I have had two steroid injections in the last year. Does it mean I need to have my knee replaced?'

Knee replacement surgery is a very good option to relieve intractable pain from degenerative joint disease. It is a relatively safe and highly successful procedure, which is carried out thousands of times every year in the UK.

The risks of having serious complications are low but there are no trivial complications from joint replacement surgery. Any problems, such as wound infection, venous thrombosis or wear of the artificial joint, can lead to potentially disastrous consequences. Having said that, 90 per cent of patients have joint replacements that last between 15 and 20 years, and revision surgery is possible for those cases where infection occurs or the artificial joint wears out.

The indications for joint replacement surgery relate to quality of life. It is a question of balancing the small risks of major complications against the benefits of the elimination of pain and restoration of mobility. Patients should be encouraged wherever possible to use simple analgesics or anti-inflammatories if they can tolerate them, to lose weight, to use physiotherapy and exercise, and simple walking aids, such as a walking stick, for long distances. It is certainly a much wiser idea for someone to overcome his pride and use a walking stick than to risk serious complications from joint replacement surgery. Having said that, many people reach an end stage where, if they have been active during the day, the pain is so bad at night that they cannot sleep. When this is happening regularly, joint revision surgery is a reasonable option.

These similar paradigms hold true for hip replacements.

FRACTURES

? Questions for each of the clinical case scenarios given

Q1: What is the likely differential diagnosis?
Q2: What issues in the given history support the diagnosis?
Q3: What additional features in the history would you seek to support a particular diagnosis?
Q4: What clinical examination would you perform and why?
Q5: What investigations would be most helpful and why?
Q6: What treatment options are appropriate?

Clinical cases

CASE 4.5 – The schoolboy with a femoral shaft fracture.

An 8-year-old boy was riding his bike and attempted to do a jump; he fell off the bike landing on an extended right leg, which twisted and gave way beneath him, and he has been brought to hospital by ambulance. He is in a great deal of pain and when he cries out you notice that the right femur bends in the middle. The leg is obviously shortened and externally rotated.

CASE 4.6 – The skateboarding teenager with a broken wrist.

A 14-year-old girl was skateboarding, fell on to an outstretched left hand and has presented with an obviously deformed left wrist with blunting of sensation in the thumb, index and middle fingers.

CASE 4.7 – The young adult with multiple injuries.

A motorcyclist was in collision with a parked van when he attempted to weave in and out of traffic. He has been conscious since the time the ambulance service arrived. He is able to speak and is complaining of pain in the lower abdomen, hips and right lower leg. He has a respiratory rate of 25/min, a heart rate of 120 beats/min and a blood pressure of 90/70 mmHg. There is obvious tenderness in the suprapubic area and there is a wound over the subcutaneous border of the distal right tibia with bone visible. Q2 is not applicable in this case.

CASE 4.8 – The elderly woman with hip fracture.

A 78-year-old woman was being escorted to the bathroom in her residential home when she tripped and fell, injuring her right hip. Her right leg is shortened and externally rotated. She appears fairly comfortable at rest but any attempts at movement or change of position on the bed result in a great deal of pain.

OSCE Counselling Cases

OSCE COUNSELLING CASE 4.3 – 'Doctor I have a pin and plate in my leg. Does it need to be removed?'

OSCE COUNSELLING CASE 4.4 – 'Doctor, with this open fracture of my tibia, am I going to lose my leg?'

Key concepts

Restoration of function is the goal of treatment. Great strides have been made in recent years in refining the management of fractures. The goal is always to restore the patient to normal or as close to normal function as circumstances will allow.

The management of the fracture begins with the evaluation of the patient as a whole. The needs of an 8-year-old child are completely different from those of an 80-year-old adult. Similarly, the range of complications to which each could be subjected is again radically different. Broadly speaking, after a thorough clinical examination of the whole patient, followed by that of the affected limb, an obviously dislocated joint or malaligned fracture in which the skin is threatened from pressure within can be realigned, splinted with a plaster of Paris backslab and then a radiograph taken. In cases of uncertainty the radiograph can sometimes be deferred until after the plaster has been applied. It should always be borne in mind that adequate immobilization is the best form of pain relief for a fractured limb.

Children with fractures tolerate bed rest and immobilization in casts much, much better than adults do. Thus methods can be employed in the management of children's' fractures that have been surpassed by more active intervention in adult injuries.

After evaluation of the soft tissue envelope and establishing the presence or absence of wounds, and the presence of pulses, sensation and movement in the limb distal to the relevant injury, the radiographs can be evaluated usefully. In the fractured bone, the location (diaphysis or metaphysis) can be identified along with the pattern of the fracture – transverse, oblique or spiral. If there are more than two fracture fragments the fracture is comminuted; if there is a soft tissue wound (an open fracture) or nerve or blood vessel injuries, the fracture is described as being complicated. It is especially important, if the fracture is in the metaphysis, to decide specifically whether or not it involves the adjacent joint. Similarly, to evaluate an injured limb it should be possible to see the joint both above and below the fracture to exclude other concomitant injuries or fracture extension lines.

If a fracture involves the joint and is displaced the treatment hinges upon reducing the joint to an anatomical position and holding it rigidly in that position until fracture healing occurs. Other fractures of long bones can be treated well by any method that realigns the limb in terms of length, rotation and angulation, and simply holds it in that position. Fracture union occurs more rapidly in low-energy injuries, which are usually buckle or greenstick fractures in children or spiral fractures in the long bones. Transverse and oblique fractures, those with comminution and also those with overlying soft tissue wounds are high-energy injuries and will require prolonged support to maintain the reduction before union occurs.

Special mention needs to be made of the increasing problems seen in the elderly population suffering the effects of osteoporosis. Fractures of the spine, wrist and proximal femur carry a huge morbidity for the patients who have these injuries. Osteoporotic spinal fractures have no specific management other than prevention. Wrist and hip fractures are very common. Hip fractures are usually seen in the more frail elderly population, and the goal of treatment is to restore the patient to mobility as soon as possible after the injuries. If the patient is immobile surgery is still often the only humane solution because this affords the best and most rapid form of pain relief.

Answers

CASE 4.5 – The schoolboy with a femoral shaft fracture.

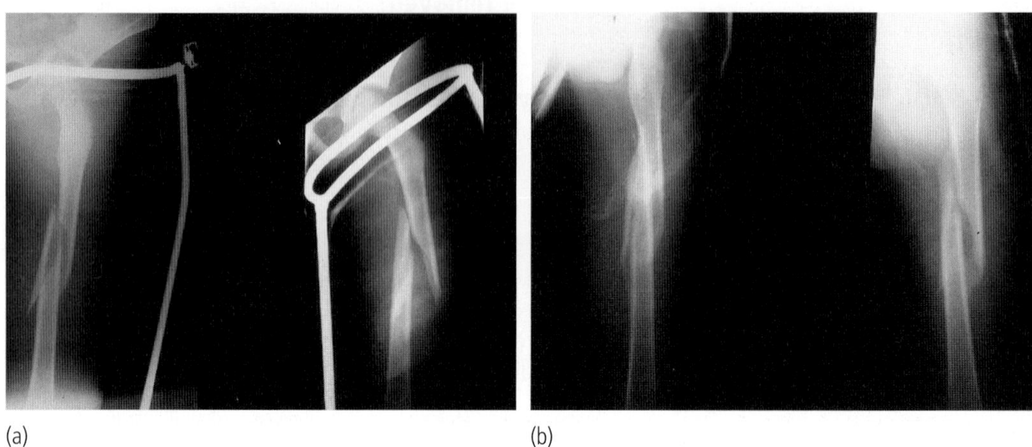

(a) (b)

Figure 4.5 Closed femoral shaft fracture: (a) anteroposterior (AP) and (b) attempted lateral views of the femur showing a multi-fragmentary (or comminuted) spiral fracture of the femoral shaft at the junction of the upper and middle thirds of the shaft.

Q1: What is the likely differential diagnosis?

A1

The appearances described are those typical for a femoral shaft fracture in a child. As the soft tissues are pliable, alarming deformation can appear in the thigh when the distressed child attempts to move. This not surprisingly increases the pain and worsens the situation.

Q2: What issues in the given history support the diagnosis?

A2

The scenario and physical signs described are entirely consistent with sustaining a low-energy fracture such as a spiral fracture of the shaft of the femur. This can be confirmed with plain radiographs after adequate splinting (see below).

Q3: What additional features in the history would you seek to support a particular diagnosis?

A3

Little more can be obtained from the history.

 Q4: What clinical examination would you perform and why?

A4

The rest of the child should be examined rapidly to exclude any further injuries from which the child is being distracted. Once this has been done a Thomas splint should be applied to the leg, having given the child some 'gas and air' to breathe via a facemask and allowing him to be comforted wherever possible by his mother or father. The Thomas splint is applied using skin traction tapes to each side of the leg and the hoop of the splint is slid up the leg, which rests on felt that is attached to the long side bars of the splint to make a kind of cradle. The traction cord is then tied to the end of the splint, and the leg is padded and bandaged to give it further support. This rapidly relieves pain and the limb can be examined for sensation and pulses.

 Q5: What investigations would be most helpful and why?

A5

Plain AP and lateral radiographs of the femur are required. The hip and knee should be visible on the radiographs and this will allow the fracture's location, pattern etc. to be characterized.

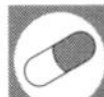 Q6: What treatment options are appropriate?

A6

For children of this age, provided that the application of skin traction can restore the alignment of the limb and rotation can be controlled by careful readjustment of the traction apparatus, such injuries can be managed very well by closed non-operative means. If non-operative management is planned, balanced traction should be applied with the Thomas splint suspended from Balkan beams attached to the patient's bed. Weekly radiographs are required along with meticulous pressure area care. It is a good idea for the radiographs to be requested at the beginning of the week so any adjustments can be made during the subsequent 5 working days. It is important for the child and the parents to understand that frequent readjustments of one part of the traction or another are necessary until callus forms. Spiral fractures are particularly suitable to be treated in this way because they heal quite rapidly. Alarming fracture gaps between the bone ends in femoral fractures in children are of no real consequence provided that the fracture is not distracted (i.e. pulled apart). Rapid healing will occur and most children can be mobilized after spending 6–8 weeks in the Thomas splint. In transverse fractures in which the bone ends are overlapping badly or in cases where the child has other injuries and is otherwise unsuitable for non-operative management, plating has been carried out successfully in children, which carries a relatively low complication risk. Femoral plating does, however, require the plate to be removed at a later date.

Another alternative is to stabilize the fracture using elastic nails. These are slender metal rods that can be inserted from just proximal to the distal femoral epiphysis. One is inserted on each side and these will act as a fairly elastic splint. For fractures of a highly unstable pattern they are not really suitable.

CASE 4.6 – The skateboarding teenager with a broken wrist.

Q1: What is the likely differential diagnosis?

A1

The differential diagnosis rests between a Salter–Harris type II fracture of the distal radius, the most common injury, to a metaphyseal fracture of the distal radius and more rarely a dislocation of the carpus. The presence of blunting of sensation in the median nerve distribution of the hand suggests an associated neuropraxia of the median nerve.

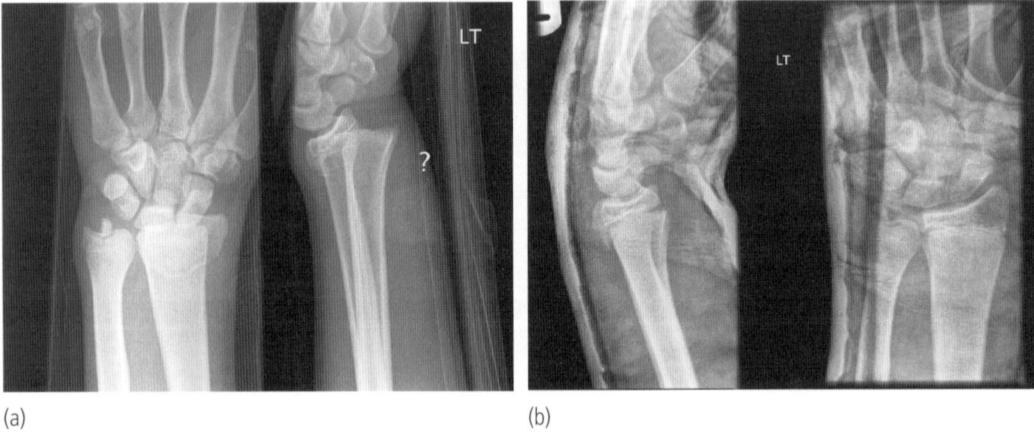

(a) (b)

Figure 4.6 Salter–Harris type II fracture of the distal radius.

Q2: What issues in the given history support the diagnosis?

A2

Radiological evaluation will determine which fracture is present.

Q3: What additional features in the history would you seek to support a particular diagnosis?

A3

Little more can be obtained from the history.

Q4: What clinical examination would you perform and why?

A4

The youngster should be examined to make sure that there are no other undisclosed injuries. If the arm is very obviously fractured a backslab should be applied and radiographs obtained. Detailed physical examination is required to carefully document the nerve vessel and soft tissue injuries associated with fractures, as has been done. In the presence of median nerve symptoms rapid reduction of the fracture is required, and this may also warrant stabilization to allow the carpal tunnel to be decompressed acutely.

 Q5: What investigations would be most helpful and why?

A5

Plain radiographs will give the diagnosis along with the pattern of displacement and allow the patient's fracture management to be planned.

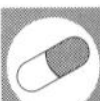 Q6: What treatment options are appropriate?

A6

Whatever the fracture pattern, in the presence of median nerve symptoms reduction should be obtained swiftly. In a compliant patient reduction can be attempted with the use of Entonox for pain relief, once the pattern of the fracture has been defined in these circumstances. However, if access to the operating theatre can be assured within an hour or so it would probably be better to take the patient to theatre.

Fractures of the epiphysis or growth area of bone are described using the Salter–Harris classification.

- Type I is a shear fracture in which the whole of the epiphysis is sheared off. This is very similar to an acute slip of the capital femoral epiphysis.
- Salter–Harris type II fractures are the most common type. Here the whole of the epiphysis is sheared and the triangle of metaphysis remains attached, which is what is seen at the wrist.
- Type III and type IV fractures both involve a split of the epiphysis. In type III it is the detached split fragment of the epiphysis that displaces with no metaphyseal attachment. In type IV there is a split of the epiphysis with a triangle of metaphysis attached.
- A fifth type has since been described and this is a crush injury to the epiphyseal plate. It is usually a retrospective diagnosis because there is very little to see on the initial radiographs. This is rare.

Accurate reduction of Salter–Harris injuries is required along with adequate stabilization. If there is loss of position beyond 7 days from the original manipulation, further manipulations are believed to carry a risk of partial or complete growth arrest and are probably inadvisable.

Early reduction is required and this can, as a result of the irregular surface of the epiphysis, require a great deal more effort than may first be appreciated – hence the wisdom of taking the child to the operating theatre rather than attempting reduction in A&E.

Re-examination of the child's hand after immobilization is essential. The simple intervention of applying a backslab and elevating the limb may relieve some of the median nerve symptoms. In a situation in which the median nerve symptoms are improving, acute carpal tunnel decompression is probably not indicated. If the symptoms are worsening the fracture needs to be reduced and held in such a way that the carpal tunnel can be decompressed.

In most circumstances closed reduction and application of a moulded cast are sufficient to retain the reduced position.

Should any further operative intervention be required, insertion of a smooth K-wire (1 or 2) to transfix the metaphyseal fragment to the intact metaphysis is all that is required to stabilize this type of injury; carpal tunnel decompression can then be carried out without difficulty.

It should be borne in mind that, if the symptoms are severe, complete resolution of median nerve problems is not seen despite a rapid decompression. This can take several weeks to resolve.

CASE 4.7 – The young adult with multiple injuries.

Q1: What is the likely differential diagnosis?

A1

The patient is in hypovolaemic shock. The possible reason is a so-called 'open book injury' to the pelvis caused by the motorcycle's fuel tank jamming up between the patient's legs. He also clearly has an open fracture of the distal right tibia – a serious injury and one that requires prompt treatment.

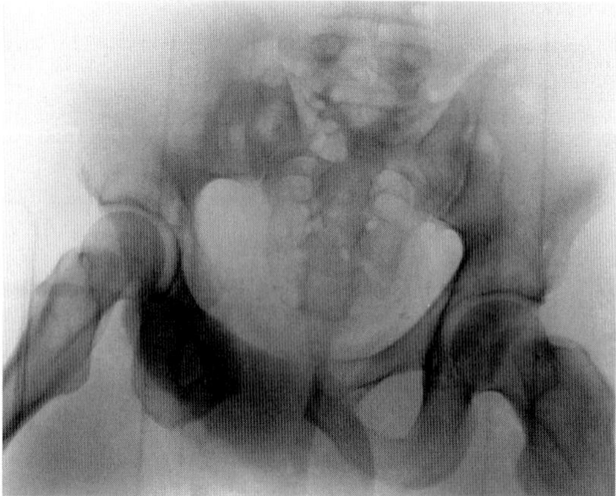

Figure 4.7 'Open book injury' to the pelvis: an external rotation injury (open book injury to the right hemipelvis).

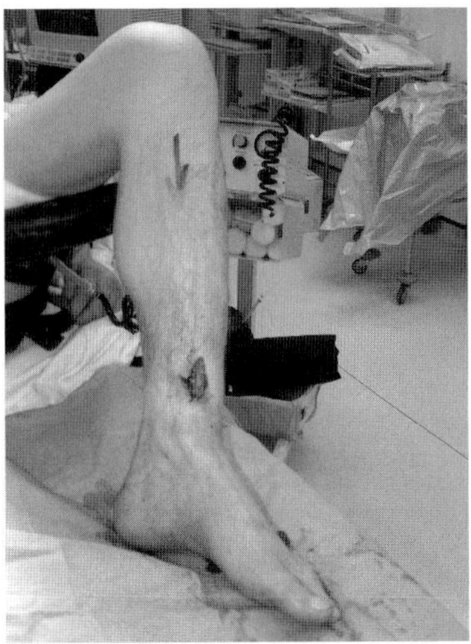

Figure 4.8 Open fracture of the distal right tibia.

 Q2: What issues in the given history support the diagnosis?

A2

Not applicable.

 Q3: What additional features in the history would you seek to support a particular diagnosis?

A3

It would be useful to know whether the patient had lost consciousness, if any witnesses are available to question. It is helpful to know whether the patient is covered for tetanus immunization, whether he has any allergies and, as the patient will require emergency surgery, any significant past medical history and when he had his last meal.

The patient has already been evaluated in terms of the primary survey in accordance with Advanced Trauma Life Support (ATLS) protocols. The purpose of the primary survey is to identify and treat immediately life-threatening problems. The airway is evaluated first; the patient who can talk is preserving his own airway, and the one unable to talk must have his airway preserved for him.

Breathing is evaluated next and a chest radiograph performed at this point in time. Auscultation and percussion are carried out at the apex and in the base. Bear in mind that the patient is supine and not erect as in a classic physician's chest examination. Therefore air will be present on the anterior chest at the apex and fluid (blood) will be present in the posterior chest, which is the base.

The position of the trachea is checked. All patients should have high-flow oxygen supplied and the cervical spine immobilized in a hard collar. Measurement of heart rate and blood pressure is part of the circulation assessment. Tachycardia (a heart rate ≥ 100 beats/min in an adult) is the earliest sign of hypovolaemic shock. Once it is identified a rapid bolus of fluids should be given and the source of haemorrhage sought. Specimens should be sent to the laboratory for cross-matching of 6 units, and full blood count (FBC), urea and electrolytes (U&Es), and a clotting screen done.

A radiograph of the chest will show any subtle signs of a haemothorax developing, and one of the pelvis is mandatory at this point in time whether or not the patient has pain.

 Q4: What clinical examination would you perform and why?

A4

Careful re-evaluation of the patient's response to the fluid bolus is essential. The patient will return to haemodynamic normality and stay there, the tachycardia will return to normal, the pulse pressure will widen or the systolic blood pressure will rise. If the patient remains haemodynamically normal and well perfused with a good urine output, he or she is described as a good responder. Initially, the fluid bolus may produce the benefits, but then when the fluid infusion rate is reduced the patient's observations again decline. This patient would be a transient responder, indicating that the bolus given has not replaced the fluid losses because bleeding is continuing, albeit relatively slowly. In these circumstances it is easy to appreciate the importance of identifying the source of potential haemorrhage so this can be dealt with rapidly. The patient whose observations remain unchanged is a non-responder and imminent exsanguination is likely. Emergency surgery is indicated. While waiting for this to become clear, it is possible to extend the patient's examination and ensure that no injuries from which the patient has been distracted are overlooked. The pelvic injury (an open book) with separation of the symphysis at the front and gaping of the sacroiliac joint at the back should be stabilized by binding the pelvis tightly using a drawer sheet. The hips and knees should be flexed slightly over a rolled-up blanket, with binding around the distal femurs. The open fracture of the tibia should be photographed if a Polaroid camera is available, and the distal circulation and sensation assessed rapidly along with toe movement. The wound should be covered in an antiseptic-soaked swab and the limb immobilized in a plaster of Paris backslab before any radiographs are taken. This limb should remain entirely covered until the patient is in the operating theatre.

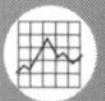 Q5: What investigations would be most helpful and why?

A5

If the patient's condition allows, computed tomography (CT) of the thorax and abdomen may be useful in such circumstances to exclude any serious concomitant injury. However, if the patient is a transient or non-responder emergency surgery is required. Anteroposterior and lateral radiographs of the fractured lower limb will also enable staff to be warned in the operating theatre of the proposed surgery.

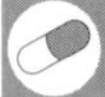 Q6: What treatment options are appropriate?

A6

Once the pelvis has been bound some improvement in the patient's haemodynamic status should be seen. Thorough examinations should be performed of the patient's urogenital triangle, and any signs of urethral injury, such as blood at the meatus, heavy scrotal bruising or a prostate difficult to feel on rectal examination, should be noted. If present one gentle attempt at periurethral catheterization may be made; otherwise this should not be carried out.

The patient should be taken to the operating theatre and the pelvis stabilized using an external fixator. If the patient's haemodynamic status does not improve a laparotomy may be required. This may be directed by the findings on CT in a patient who was in a more stable condition.

As far as the open fracture to the tibia is concerned treatment hinges on the wound being debrided of all dead, devascularized and foreign tissue. The traumatic wound should be extended, all questionable tissue removed and the bones stabilized using either an external fixator or an intramedullary nail.

Experience shows that soft tissue coverage should be achieved within 5 days of such an injury and, once it is clear that the margins of the soft tissue envelope are viable, the bone stabilization should be done as soon as possible.

Experience shows that it is rarely possible to close such wounds primarily and the assistance of a plastic surgeon is required. Local fasciocutaneous rotation flaps, or even free tissue transfers of the latissimus dorsi or rectus abdominis muscles, are often required in these circumstances.

CASE 4.8 – The elderly woman with hip fracture.

Q1: What is the likely differential diagnosis?

A1

The differential diagnosis of fracture of the proximal femur may be:

- intracapsular
- intertrochanteric
- subtrochanteric.

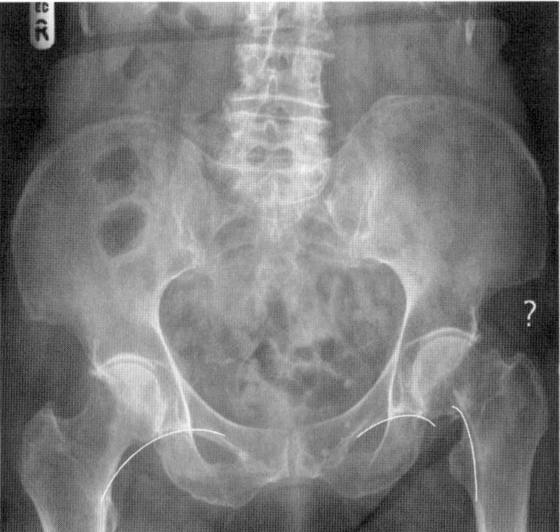

Figure 4.9 The elderly woman with hip fracture: left intracapsular hip fracture.

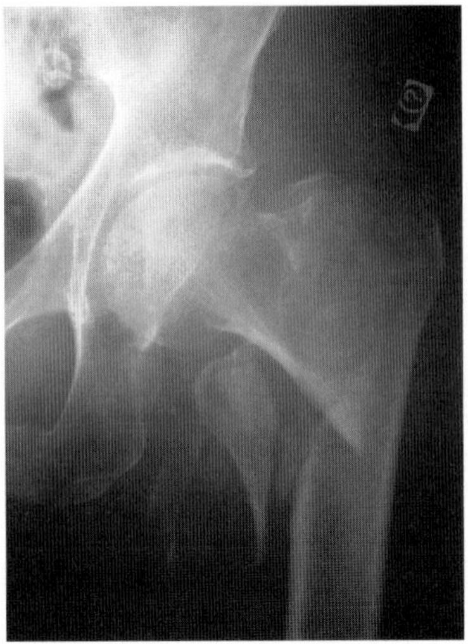

Figure 4.10 The elderly woman with hip fracture: intertrochanteric.

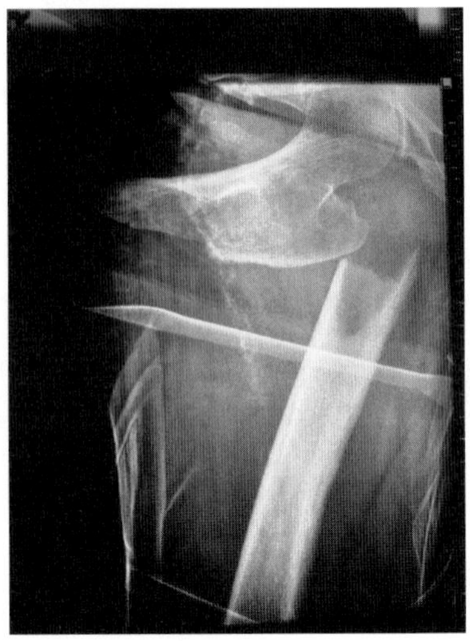

Figure 4.11 The elderly woman with hip fracture: subtrochanteric.

 Q2: What issues in the given history support the diagnosis?

A2

No specific features in the history enable one to differentiate these injuries from each other.

 Q3: What additional features in the history would you seek to support a particular diagnosis?

A3

We have an increasing elderly population, most of whom are female and at high risk of osteoporosis. Similarly the residents of nursing and residential homes represent a high-risk group within this population.

 Q4: What clinical examination would you perform and why?

A4

General clinical examination.

 Q5: What investigations would be most helpful and why?

A5

Preoperative work-up of these patients is essentially to answer the question 'Is this patient as well as possible?' and, if unwell, 'can they actually be made any better?'. Routine bloods are required. If the patient has a pacemaker it needs to be checked preoperatively. Electrocardiogram (ECG), chest radiograph and a cross-match of two units of blood are needed.

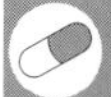 Q6: What treatment options are appropriate?

A6

Treatment options are again tailored to the needs of the individual and the pattern of the fracture. Intracapsular hip fractures are especially problematic when managed by internal fixation. The femoral head has a retrograde blood supply in which the vast majority of blood vessels supplying it are bound to the femoral neck. If the neck is fractured and displaced these vessels are interrupted. In common with other bones with a retrograde blood supply (such as the scaphoid), intracapsular fractures of the femur are fraught with problems of avascular necrosis of the femoral head and also non-union.

In young patients, such as motorcyclists, who sustain a high-energy injury resulting in such a fracture, open reduction and internal fixation are mandatory and should be done as early as the patient's general condition permits.

In an elderly patient, who would not be able to mobilize and is non-weight bearing, a better option is to operate, discard the fractured femoral head and neck segment, and replace this with a hemiarthroplasty. A variety of implants are available that may be secured in the femoral shaft using cemented or uncemented methods. Such implants enable the patients to mobilize as soon as pain permits and functional outcome in the population with restricted activity is usually entirely satisfactory.

Intertrochanteric fractures are extracapsular fractures in the plane between the greater and lesser trochanters. These are entirely suitable for treatment with internal fixation and closed reduction is usually possible using a special operative traction table. Union is usually rapid and pain relief after surgery excellent.

Subtrochanteric fractures are fractures that occur through or distal to the lesser trochanter in essentially a transverse pattern. These fractures are unsuitable for management with plate fixation but lend themselves well to an intramedullary nail. Again rehabilitation tends to follow the same pattern as for intertrochanteric fractures.

Elderly patients cannot tolerate long periods of recumbency. Every effort should be made at the time of their admission to ensure that they are made as well as possible for their surgery. Delays arising from investigations not being carried out when the patient is admitted tend to have a domino effect and a delay of even 24 h in the patient receiving surgery can be problematic.

OSCE Counselling Cases – Answers

OSCE COUNSELLING CASE 4.3 – 'Doctor I have a pin and plate in my leg. Does it need to be removed?'

Removal of metalwork was carried out routinely when operative surgical management of fractures first became an established part of treatment. However, it rapidly became apparent that this creates more problems than it solves.

Most orthopaedic trauma surgeons recommend the removal of metalwork in growing children. This prevents the metalwork becoming embedded in the growing bone, altering its mechanical properties and resulting in stress fractures, which present a very difficult surgical problem because of the presence of the embedded metalwork.

Removal surgery, however, is prone to have problems with wound healing as a result of infection or haematoma formation, and also runs the risk of peripheral nerve injury in the limb. This is particularly true of removal of forearm fracture plates.

Specific indications for removal of metalwork would include the following:

- Very specific local tenderness caused by prominence of the metalwork under the skin.
- Occasionally the removal of intramedullary nails in the lower limb long bone of high-class athletes because these can sometimes impair performance.
- At a similar elite end of the scale, metalwork in the hand and wrist of accomplished musicians, because some authorities have reported that even the small changes caused by metalwork can interfere with performance. However, it should be borne in mind that this is true only for elite performers.

By and large metalwork in adults should stay where it is put provided that it is not responsible for any specific problems.

OSCE COUNSELLING CASE 4.4 – 'Doctor, with this open fracture of my tibia, am I going to lose my leg?'

A direct question requires a direct answer but one that is couched properly in terms of relative risk.

Any fracture in the lower limb does have the potential to result in a loss of limb if its treatment or the fracture itself leads to complications. Open fractures are actually life-threatening injuries when considered on the global scale of health care.

Consider the likelihood of survival of someone sustaining an open tibial fracture as a result of the tsunami that struck Indonesia on Boxing Day 2004. By the time help arrived the casualty would almost certainly have died from either gangrene or tetanus. Such drastic infective complications are almost unheard of in fortunate countries with advanced medical care.

With appropriate management to convert the dirty traumatic wound into a clean surgical wound and the unstable displaced fracture into a reduced stable fracture followed by reconstruction, after a short interval of 48–72 h, of the soft tissue envelope, there is a considerable reduction in the risk of problems of non-union or infection and dramatic reduction in the risk of limb loss. Thus, although no guarantee can ever be given, the patient should be reassured that the chance of this happening is extremely low.

This question also presents an opportunity to challenge the patient about his or her concept of amputation. In the right circumstances amputation is an extremely good operation that can restore someone to independent mobility, free from pain, and to a pretty much normal level of activity from a position where he or she had been severely disabled as a result of the injuries or their complications. It is most commonly required for patients whose fractures are associated with very severe soft tissue injuries, particularly those with nerve injuries, arterial injuries requiring repair and troublesome post-traumatic muscle contractures. Thus amputation should be regarded as an enormous single step back towards normality from a bad situation.

BACK PROBLEMS

? Questions for each of the clinical case scenarios given

Q1: What is the likely differential diagnosis?
Q2: What issues in the given history support the diagnosis?
Q3: What additional features in the history would you seek to support a particular diagnosis?
Q4: What clinical examination would you perform and why?
Q5: What investigations would be most helpful and why?
Q6: What treatment options are appropriate?

Clinical cases

CASE 4.9 – The teenager with thoracic back pain.

A 13-year-old girl has complained of increasing back pain in the lower thoracic/interscapular spine. This is aggravated by her schoolwork, in particular when she is doing homework. She is able to do games at school and this only moderately aggravates her symptoms.

CASE 4.10 – The young adult with a trapped nerve.

A 32-year-old man had had minor twinges of back pain over the course of the past week. He was lifting his golf clubs out of the boot of his car when he experienced a searing pain and was unable to straighten up; he had severe pain radiating all the way from the back down to the foot of his right lower limb.

CASE 4.11 – The pathological fracture.

A 72-year-old otherwise healthy woman had a minor fall when she slipped on some spilt milk on her tiled kitchen floor. She experienced very severe lower back pain and has been brought in by ambulance from home because she is unable to weight bear. She mentions that for the last couple of weeks she has had a strange woolly feeling in the right leg.

CASE 4.12 – DIY gone wrong.

A 53-year-old man was attempting his own loft conversion and fell backwards through the loft hatch. He has severe lower back pain and has been brought in from home with spinal immobilization. Q3 is not applicable in this case.

OSCE Counselling Cases

OSCE COUNSELLING CASE 4.5 – 'Doctor I have terrible backache. The scan shows that I have a slipped disc. Don't I need an operation to take the slipped disc away?'

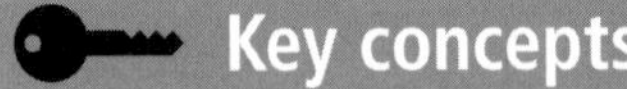

Key concepts

The surgical sieve

As mentioned before in the section 'The painful hip', the surgical sieve is helpful when approaching patients with back problems, especially in the light of features drawn from their history.

Children and teenagers are most likely to have problems of developmental or rarely, but very importantly, malignant origin. Young adults tend to experience spinal problems associated with early degenerative change, and elderly people have problems caused by either osteoporosis or malignancy.

Trauma, naturally, can affect any age group. Serious spinal injuries are very often seen after high-velocity or high-energy transfer road traffic accidents, or falls from heights by unskilled people inadvisedly attempting DIY.

Answers

CASE 4.9 – The teenager with thoracic back pain.

Q1: What is the likely differential diagnosis?

A1

During the adolescent growth spurt aches and pains can come and go; however, if they are persistent they must be investigated because failure to recognize problems such as a slipped capital femoral epiphysis can be catastrophic.

Q2: What issues in the given history support the diagnosis?

A2

Thoracic back pain is either postural in origin or may result from Scheuermann's disease, an osteochondritic process affecting the midthoracic vertebrae, which is often asymptomatic and only discovered in later life as an incidental radiological finding. The third and most unlikely, but most important, possibility is that of a malignant or infective process. Given that the youngster in question is otherwise well and able to take part in activities, the most likely diagnosis is that of poor posture or Scheuermann's disease.

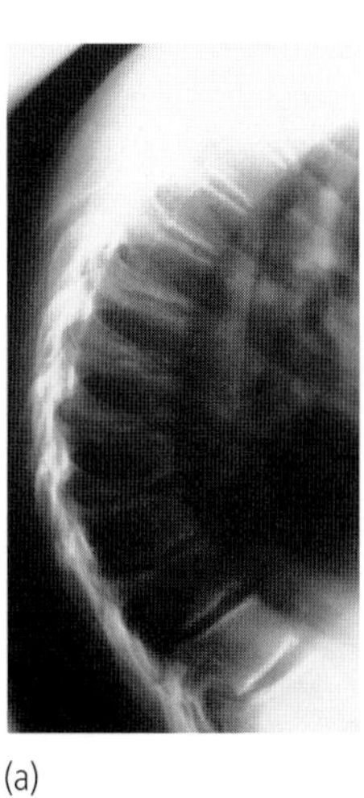

(a)

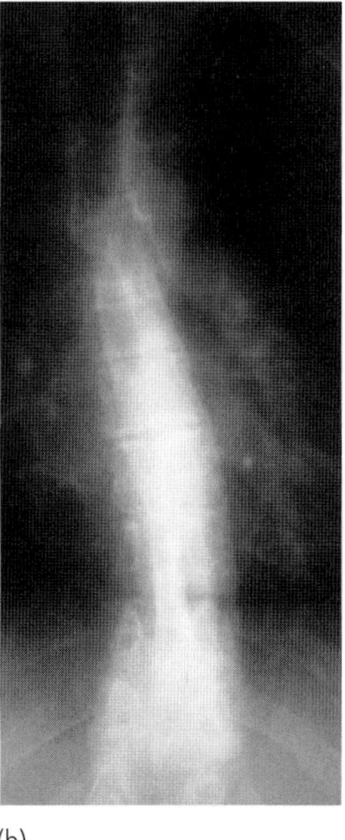

(b)

Figure 4.12 The teenager with thoracic back pain: Scheuermann's disease.

 Q3: What additional features in the history would you seek to support a particular diagnosis?

A3

Malignancy affecting the thoracic spine is usually secondary to a previously known problem; however, primary tumours do occur, originating in the bone marrow, or any of the musculoskeletal, vascular or neural elements of the spine. Rest pain and night pain support the diagnosis of infection or malignancy. The fact that posture, i.e. sitting at a desk and working, aggravates the symptoms strongly favours a purely mechanical origin. Other features indicating serious pathology are symptoms of nerve compression, altered sensation and altered power.

 Q4: What clinical examination would you perform and why?

A4

The spine specifically should be examined with the patient standing, seated and lying prone. Neurological examination of the limbs would exclude any evidence of spinal or spinal nerve root involvement. Inspection of the spine will give a clear indication of any kyphotic changes that are commonly associated with Scheuermann's disease or lateral curvature of the spine – scoliosis – which may have remained undetected through the youth's early childhood. Postural scoliosis, which is habitual rather than a structural problem with the spine, will correct when the patient forward flexes to try to touch the floor. A true structural scoliosis will actually be accentuated by this manoeuvre. Careful palpation of the spine will elicit any areas of tenderness.

 Q5: What investigations would be most helpful and why?

A5

Plain AP and lateral radiographs of the spine to include the whole spine should be taken if a structural scoliosis is defined. Magnetic resonance imaging (MRI) would be indicated to further define any suggestion of bony destruction. Scheuermann's disease, the most probable radiologically manifest problem, is recognized by simple anterior wedging of the thoracic vertebrae.

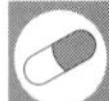 Q6: What treatment options are appropriate?

A6

For management of Scheuermann's disease and thoracic pain of a purely postural origin, physiotherapy is all that is needed. The prognosis is excellent.

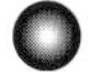

CASE 4.10 – The young adult with a trapped nerve.

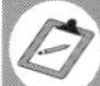

Q1: What is the likely differential diagnosis?

A1

The most likely differential diagnosis is that of a prolapsed intervertebral disc, which usually occurs at the level of L5/S1, trapping the S1 nerve root.

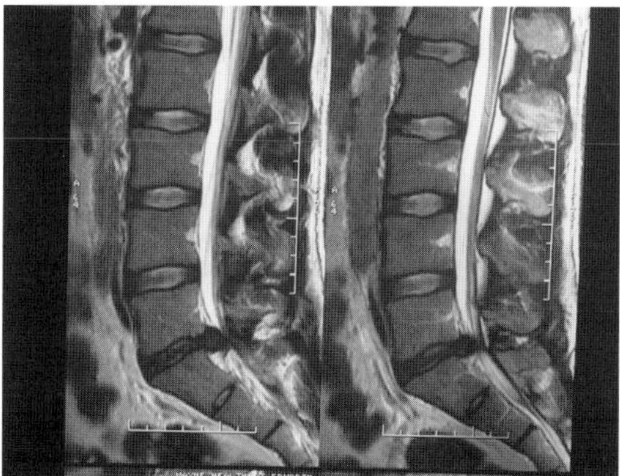

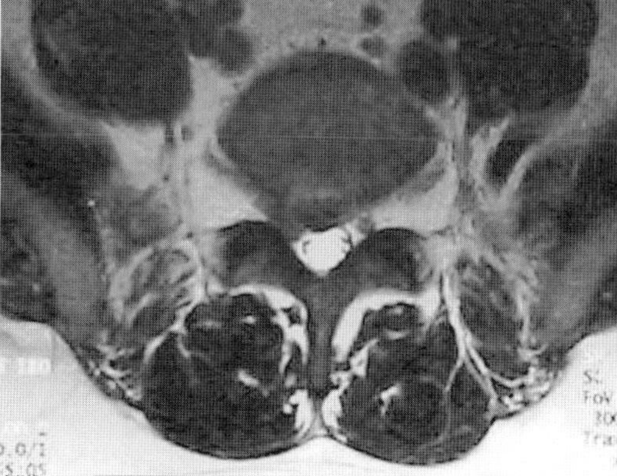

Figure 4.13 The young adult with a trapped nerve: a prolapsed intervertebral disc.

Q2: What issues in the given history support the diagnosis?

A2

A prolapsed intervertebral disc can occur against a long-standing history of mechanical back pain in young adults, with a simple event such as stooping to lift a comparatively light weight causing the degenerate disc to prolapse. This results in nerve root entrapment, inflammation and radicular pain as described.

Q3: What additional features in the history would you seek to support a particular diagnosis?

A3

Specific questions should be asked about previous episodes of lower back pain. In mechanical back pain, the lower back pain is a dominant symptom and such referred pain as the patient experiences is normally vague and referred into one or both thighs, usually anteriorly. The pain from a prolapsed disc resulting in nerve root entrapment is usually extreme. The resulting referred leg pain is worse than the back pain and may radiate all the way to the foot in the case of 'sciatica' or down to the knee in the front of thigh in the case of 'femoralgia'. Lower lumbar disc prolapses are much more common because the lower lumbar spine is subject to tremendous stresses in ordinary everyday life. Femoralgia occurs as a result of a prolapsed disc higher in the lumbar spine and, although less common, is readily recognizable if it is sought.

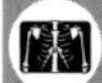 Q4: What clinical examination would you perform and why?

A4

Neurological examination is mandatory. The patient may not be able to stand but should be encouraged to do so if he can. If possible the patient should be asked to walk on tiptoes. This is the most reliable way of assessing plantar flexion (S1 nerve root-innervated muscular strength). Careful inspection of the back will show the lumbar spine to have a loss of lordosis as a result of paraspinal muscle spasm and there will often be a scoliosis concave to the side in which the nerve root is entrapped, resulting from greater muscle spasm on that side.

Further clinical examination requires a thorough neurological examination of the patient's lower limbs plus saddle (urogenital/perianal) area, including digital rectal examination.

Tests for sciatic nerve root tension or femoral nerve root tension should be left until the end of examination.

Power inhibition often occurs as a result of the extreme pain and so it is useful for the patient to be given a potent analgesic, possibly even a morphine injection, before power testing is carried out.

In an L5 nerve root entrapment there may be weakness in great toe dorsiflexion and foot inversion. In an S1 nerve root entrapment there may be weakness in plantar flexion and foot eversion. The ankle jerk may be lost in either of the above cases. With femoralgia the quadriceps may be weak and there may be loss of the patellar tendon jerk. Sensory blunting is usually in a characteristic dermatomal distribution.

Examination of the perianal area is crucial. If the disc prolapse is central rather than lateral, cauda equina syndrome may result. In this case the patient will have no desire to void if nerve root entrapment affects those nerves mediating sensation to the bladder. Painless retention results and, unless surgical decompression is carried out urgently, incontinence and loss of sexual function will be permanent. Such patients usually have bilateral lower leg sciatic pain and bilateral perianal numbness with loss of anal tone. Careful clinical examination will often demonstrate the presence of a full bladder in a patient in whom there is no desire to void. Passage of a catheter is usually easy and pain free, with little sensation of catheter insertion experienced by the patient. A large volume of urine is usually drained.

Lastly, sciatic nerve root tension signs can be identified by the straight-leg raise. Care must be taken to do this gently and it is often a good idea to start with the pain-free leg, and to watch the patient's face. Lift the pain-free leg into the air gently, while encouraging the patient to relax. When he experiences pain enquire whether it is in the back or the ipsilateral or contralateral leg. Pain in the ipsilateral leg is a cross-over sign when examining the pain-free leg, suggesting a central disc prolapse. Keep the foot in its current position and then flex the knee. This should relieve leg pain. Note whether the pain is experienced solely in the back because this goes against sciatic nerve root tension.

Repeat the process with the contralateral leg. Bow-string signs and dorsiflexion of the foot to elicit pain again can also be performed after relieving pain by flexing the knee. However, the simple straight-leg raise test is normally enough to confirm or refute the diagnosis.

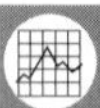 Q5: What investigations would be most helpful and why?

A5

A plain lateral radiograph of the lumbar spine is indicated to exclude any unexpected destructive malignant pathology. The gold standard investigation is MRI.

 Q6: What treatment options are appropriate?

A6

In spite of the catastrophic nature of presentation most cases of sciatica will respond to analgesia supported by a low regular dose of diazepam to help relieve muscle spasm and progressive physiotherapy. Long periods of bed rest are best avoided.

The patient should be encouraged to return to work as early as possible and to stop smoking. Interestingly, both of these are important features in long-term recovery.

In patients who fail these conservative measures a discectomy is indicated.

In cases of cauda equina syndrome emergency MRI should be performed with spinal decompression by an appropriately skilled orthopaedic or neurosurgical spinal surgeon as soon as possible.

 CASE 4.11 – The pathological fracture.

 Q1: What is the likely differential diagnosis?

A1

The differential diagnosis is restricted essentially to the diagnoses underlying pathological spinal fractures. The most common example would be an insufficiency fracture caused by osteoporosis.

Other origins of pathological weakness in the spinal bones include malignant deposits, which may be primary or secondary. The most common primary deposit would probably be myeloma. Secondary deposits usually originate in the breast, thyroid, lung, prostate or kidney.

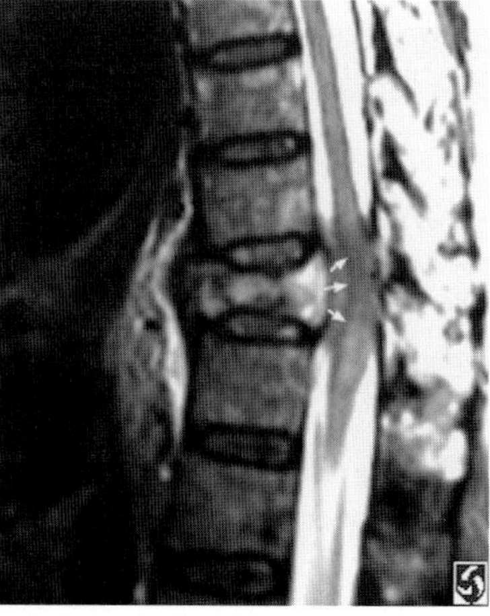

Figure 4.14 The pathological fracture: pathological spinal fractures.

 Q2: What issues in the given history support the diagnosis?

A2

A history of previous insufficiency fractures would strongly support a diagnosis of an osteoporotic fracture. Obviously a history of a known malignancy would indicate the possibility of a tumour deposit.

In the given history the feeling of abnormal sensation in one lower limb hints at involvement of spinal nerve roots, which is certainly not typical in osteoporotic fractures.

 Q3: What additional features in the history would you seek to support a particular diagnosis?

A3

Specific questions should be asked about the past medical history to elicit the problems outlined above, plus general questions about the patient's overall health, well-being, vitality, weight loss etc.

 Q4: What clinical examination would you perform and why?

A4

Clinical examination should be performed with the patient lying supine and carrying out the spinal immobilization precautions for the injured area. It must be presumed, in the presence of a fall, a history suggestive of a fracture and abnormal neurological symptoms, that the spinal injury is potentially unstable. Further movement without appropriate care could easily result in worsening neurological damage.

Otherwise neurological examination should be carried out exactly as for Case 4.10.

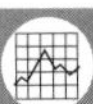 Q5: What investigations would be most helpful and why?

A5

Again plain radiographs are essential, and may demonstrate a simple wedge compression consistent with an osteoporotic insufficiency fracture. In the history presented, it is quite possible that the AP view of the lumbar spine would demonstrate loss of the pedicle at the level of the fracture – a radiological finding suggestive of malignant destruction.

Further investigations should include FBC, ESR, biochemistry screen including liver function tests, CRP, urine for Bence Jones proteins and protein electrophoresis of the serum.

Magnetic resonance imaging is mandatory to define the extent of any soft tissue mass associated with a pathological fracture and to assist in planning of surgery for decompression of such a mass and stabilization of the spine to allow for mobilization of the patient.

 Q6: What treatment options are appropriate?

A6

Should the woman's fracture be entirely attributable to osteoporotic change, she simply needs to be given analgesia and gently and progressively mobilized thereafter.

Care should be taken to ensure that she has appropriate treatment for her osteoporosis to help reduce the risks of further fractures. In the case of spinal cord or spinal nerve root compression with an associated fracture, caused by a malignant deposit, surgical decompression after preoperative treatment with steroids to reduce associated tumour-related swelling would have a reasonable chance of restoring lower limb function in this woman. The more severe the preoperative nerve impairment, the less the chance of complete resolution of symptoms with spinal decompression and operative stabilization of the spine – hence the importance of careful handling of the patient preoperatively.

 CASE 4.12 – DIY gone wrong.

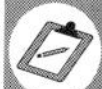 Q1: What is the likely differential diagnosis?

A1

The most likely differential diagnosis is a burst fracture – an unstable fracture of one of the lumbar vertebrae; less likely is a stable wedge compression fracture.

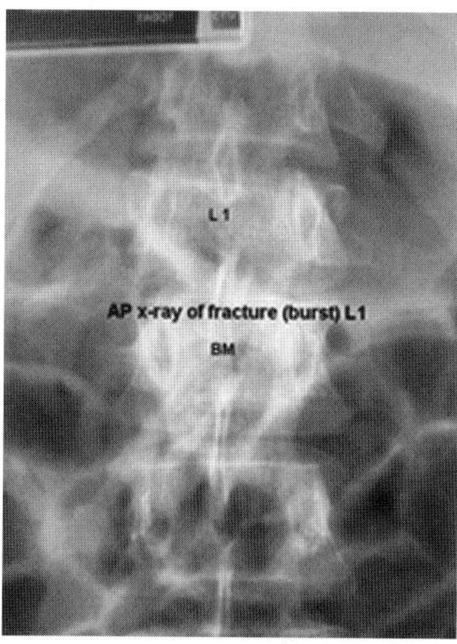

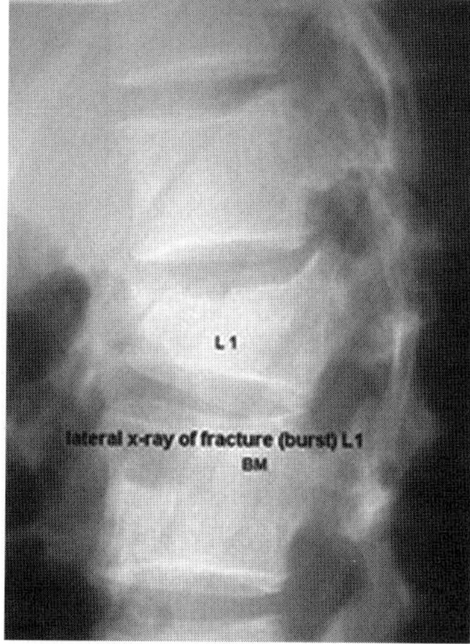

Figure 4.15 DIY gone wrong: a burst fracture.

 Q2: What issues in the given history support the diagnosis?

A2

It is impossible from the history to determine whether the fracture sustained is stable or unstable unless there is neurological injury. Neurological injury is a certain sign that the associated fracture is unstable.

 Q3: What additional features in the history would you seek to support a particular diagnosis?

A3

Not applicable.

 Q4: What clinical examination would you perform and why?

A4

Again full spinal precautions must be taken, including immobilization of the cervical spine. In a conscious patient, if the neck is pain free and non-tender to palpation, and the patient has good head control, cervical spinal immobilization can be dispensed with without a radiograph. In cases of doubt, immobilization and thorough radiological evaluation should be carried out.

The patient should be examined thoroughly in the supine position from the neurological point of view, paying particular attention to loss of sensation, reflexes and power in the lower limbs, and the urogenital triangle as described above.

In addition, specific examination of the feet, ankles, knees and hips should be carried out because in a fall from a height, typical associated injuries include fractures of the calcaneum, distal articular surface of the tibia (plafond), tibial plateau, femoral condyles, hips and pelvis.

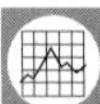 Q5: What investigations would be most helpful and why?

A5

Plain radiographs will help confirm the level of the spinal fracture and may give important information as to whether or not, in the patient who is neurologically intact, the fracture is stable.

It is important to understand that a fracture may be completely unstable but the patient neurologically completely normal.

Features suggesting instability include loss of the anterior vertebral body height: greater than 30 per cent of the posterior vertebral body height suggests posterior element injuries. Again this hints at the potential for unstable motion of this injured spinal segment.

On the AP radiograph, wedging in the lateral direction suggests a rotational rather than a true wedge compression mechanism, further indicating instability. Clear-cut signs of instability on the plain radiographs are those of a retropulsed fragment encroaching on the spinal canal and loss of posterior vertebral height; both of these features are visible on the lateral view; on the AP view, the signs are widening of the distance between the pedicles in comparison to the vertebrae above and below.

Computed tomography will define the precise architecture of the bones at this level and facilitate planning of spinal surgery if this is deemed necessary.

Further radiographs should be carried out of the feet, tibial plateaux, hips, pelvis etc. if areas of tenderness have been elicited.

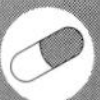

Q6: What treatment options are appropriate?

A6

In incomplete spinal nerve injuries steroids of varying doses have been tried. These are currently out of favour because the improvements in neural function were marginal and the risks of steroid administration appreciable.

Full spinal immobilization should be continued until the spine either is recognized as being stable or becomes stable through healing or surgical intervention.

OSCE Counselling Case – Answer

OSCE COUNSELLING CASE 4.5 – 'Doctor I have terrible backache. The scan shows that I have a slipped disc. Don't I need an operation to take the slipped disc away?'

Surgery for prolapsed discs does not cure back pain. The indication for surgery to remove a prolapsed disc, or rather that portion of the disc that has prolapsed, is chronic back pain that fails to settle with appropriate conservative measures including a very committed, specific physiotherapy programme.

In such cases discectomy is by and large successful in relieving leg pain but has little or no impact on back pain. Indeed long-term follow-up studies of patients undergoing surgical versus non-surgical management for sciatica in relation to prolapsed lumbar discs show that there is no overall difference in outcome.

There are specific risks associated with discectomy and these include nerve root injury at the time of surgery, chronic fibrosis as a consequence of surgical intervention and more immediate problems such as epidural haematoma, which can lead to paraplegia, although this is exceedingly rare.

A degenerate disc that leads to a disabled motion segment in the spine is occasionally a source of back pain, which can be managed with spinal fusion. The risks of spinal fusion surgery are similar to, but greater than, those of simple discectomy, and hence every effort should be made to optimize patients' conditions through non-surgical means; patients should be well informed about the risks of any surgery that they consider.

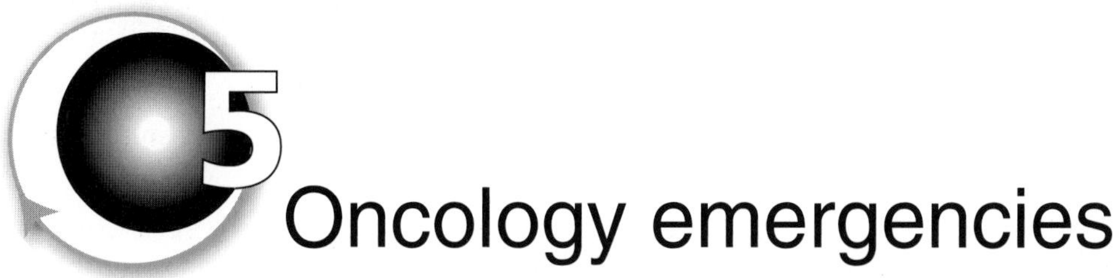

5 Oncology emergencies

Daniel Rea

? Questions for each of the clinical case scenarios given

Q1: What is the likely diagnosis?
Q2: What aspects of the physical examination are most relevant?
Q3: What investigations would be performed?
Q4: How would the diagnosis be confirmed?
Q5: What would be the initial management?
Q6: What issues need to be addressed following acute management?

Clinical cases

CASE 5.1 – A 66-year-old man complains of recent-onset bilateral leg weakness, polydipsia, constipation and difficulty passing urine.

A 66-year-old man has been sent to the accident and emergency department (A&E) with a 10-day history of progressive lower limb weakness. In addition he complains of low thoracic back pain. He complains of frequency and difficulty passing urine, constipation and excessive thirst. He was diagnosed with early prostate cancer 2 years ago and is being treated with goserelin (a luteinizing hormone-releasing hormone or LHRH agonist). In other respects he is in good health and he lives alone in a second-floor flat.

CASE 5.2 – A 48-year-old woman develops fever 10 days after adjuvant chemotherapy for early breast cancer.

A 48-year-old woman presents to A&E while visiting a relative. She complains of feeling unwell and has a temperature of 38°C. She underwent a mastectomy and reconstructive surgery 6 weeks earlier for a node-positive invasive breast cancer. Ten days ago she started her first cycle of a planned programme of chemotherapy at a hospital 200 miles away. She does not know what drugs she was given. She is normally fit and well with no other medical complaints. She has a respiratory rate of 24/min, pulse 120 beats/min and blood pressure 95/60 mmHg.

CASE 5.3 – A 59-year-old smoker has dyspnoea, and arm and facial swelling.

A 59-year-old man presents to his GP with a 1-week history of progressive facial swelling, swelling of both arms and shortness of breath on climbing a flight of stairs. He has smoked 20 cigarettes per day for 40 years and works as a garage foreman. He is sent down to A&E following a chest radiograph that shows a widened mediastinum and a right hilar mass. He had a previous chest radiograph 6 months earlier, which was normal apart from some patchy shadowing in the left midzone, which is no longer present.

 OSCE Counselling Cases

OSCE COUNSELLING CASE 5.1 – 'How will I cope at home if complete recovery is not achieved?'

The 66-year-old man with prostate cancer and leg weakness (described in Case 5.1) is now clinically stable and awaiting imaging investigations. He is aware of the likely cause of his symptoms and signs, and asks the above question 'How will I cope at home if compete recovery is not achieved?'.

OSCE COUNSELLING CASE 5.2 – 'How long have I got to live?'

He then goes on to ask how long he has to live.

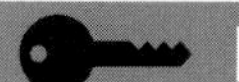 Key concepts

- Cytotoxic chemotherapy involves the use of drugs with a narrow therapeutic index so side effects are common and can be life threatening.
- Prompt intervention usually results in complete resolution of acute toxicity but late toxicities may be slow to resolve or irreversible.
- As acute toxicity is reversible, aggressive management of severe complications is appropriate even in cases of advanced incurable malignancy.
- Short-term neutropenia is very common after cytotoxic chemotherapy of common solid malignancies, but requires intervention only when accompanied by infection.
- Acute complications of malignancy require prompt assessment and, where invasive intervention is appropriate, this should be introduced as soon as possible to relieve symptoms and limit the extent of damage and disability. Supportive care and symptom relief should be introduced immediately. Acute complications of malignant disease rarely resolve completely and often mark a transition into a new 'phase' of the patient's illness. Careful assessment of the consequences of a new complication is required and may have implications for future prognosis, physical and psychological health. They usually indicate failure of current therapy and indicate a need to review this.

Answers

CASE 5.1 – A 66-year-old man complains of recent-onset bilateral leg weakness, polydipsia, constipation and difficulty passing urine.

Q1: What is the likely diagnosis?

A1

The likely diagnosis is spinal cord compression secondary to bone metastasis from prostate cancer that has become refractory to first-line endocrine therapy. This is complicated by hypercalcaemia as a result of widespread bone involvement.

Q2: What aspects of the physical examination are most relevant?

A2

- Hydration status
- Functional status (how well can he walk?)
- Presence of spinal tenderness
- Presence of a sensory level
- Degree and extent of lower limb weakness, muscle tone and reflexes
- Sacral sensation, anal tone and presence of palpable bladder.

Q3: What investigations would be performed?

A3

- Whole spine magnetic resonance imaging (MRI)
- Urea and electrolytes (U&Es)
- Creatinine, calcium, albumin and prostate-specific antigen (PSA)
- Full blood count (FBC) and international normalized ratio (INR).

Q4: How would the diagnosis be confirmed?

A4

Whole spine MRI will identify the presence and level of spinal cord compression; imaging of the whole spine will identify additional lesions that will affect decision-making and permit treatment planning. Corrected serum calcium will establish the presence of hypercalcaemia, which may be accompanied by biochemical evidence of dehydration and renal failure.

 Q5: What would be the initial management?

A5

- High-dose dexamethasone
- Intravenous rehydration, followed by intravenous bisphosphonate
- Catheterization if in retention
- Spinal decompression and stabilization as treatment of choice if technically achievable and multiple levels of compression excluded
- Urgent radiotherapy to the sites of compression if surgery is contraindicated.

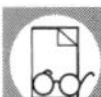 Q6: What issues need to be addressed following acute management?

A6

The prognosis after spinal cord compression is generally poor with a median survival of 12 months; however, functional status is superior for patients treated surgically. Postoperative radiation will be required and second-line options for treatment for advanced prostate cancer should be considered. Rehabilitation after treatment will depend on the degree of neurological recovery and may require extensive physiotherapy. Physiotherapy, occupational therapy and nursing assessment of the patient and home environment will be required to facilitate discharge planning. Home adjustments or relocation may be needed. Ongoing monitoring of hypercalcaemia is needed together with maintenance bisphosphonates. Long-term control may be achieved with oral bisphosphonates but, if unsuccessful, regular intravenous bisphosphonates are required.

 CASE 5.2 – A 48-year-old woman develops fever 10 days after adjuvant chemotherapy for early breast cancer.

 Q1: What is the likely diagnosis?

A1

This is neutropenic sepsis. Virtually all cytotoxic drugs cause myelosuppression and infection is a frequent complication of myelosuppression. Infection can progress rapidly and may be fatal if uncontrolled.

 Q2: What aspects of the physical examination are most relevant?

A2

Examination should focus on assessment of the severity of presumed infection and the potential source of infection. Vital signs should be confirmed. Surgical wounds should be examined, including donor sites for reconstruction. Respiratory and abdominal examinations are important. Examination of the oral cavity and perineal area should be performed, noting ulceration and the presence of candidiasis. The peripheral circulation should be assessed and any evidence of widespread bleeding noted.

 Q3: What investigations would be performed?

A3

- An FBC including differential white blood cell count (WCC)
- Arterial blood gases
- Blood cultures, including separate cultures from indwelling lines
- U&Es and creatinine
- Urine culture and swabs from any open wounds should be taken
- Chest radiograph
- Sputum culture if produced.

 Q4: How would the diagnosis be confirmed?

A4

Neutropenia will be confirmed by blood count; arbitrarily neutropenia is defined as an absolute neutrophil count $< 1.0 \times 10^9$/L. Associated thrombocytopenia may also be present; if detected, coagulation status should be assessed, including D-dimers because disseminated intravascular coagulation can complicate severe sepsis.

 Q5: What would be the initial management?

A5

Rapid intravenous fluids should be commenced initially using plasma expanders where hypotension is present. Broad-spectrum intravenous antibiotics should be administered using the regimen recommended by the local hospital neutropenic sepsis policy. Where a source of infection is suspected, such as a respiratory focus, secondary antibiotics should be added again following the local protocol. An allergy history should be obtained and a recent antibiotic history noted, which might influence drug choice. Pulse oximetry and blood gas evaluation may indicate the need for oxygen supplementation. The patient should be catheterized if not passing urine freely or if hypotension persists after fluid load. If hypotension does not respond adequately to fluid load, the patient should be managed in a high-dependency or intensive care environment. Inotropic support may be required to maintain adequate cardiac output. Severe metabolic acidosis may require correction and artificial ventilation may be needed. The use of granulocyte colony-stimulating factors (G-CSFs) in established neutropenic sepsis is controversial but is commonly given to patients with severe sepsis and marked neutropenia

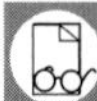 Q6: What issues need to be addressed following acute management?

A6

Neutropenic sepsis in solid tumours (non-leukaemic) usually responds promptly to simple treatment and most patients make a full, uncomplicated recovery after the return of normal neutrophil function. Intravenous antibiotics are generally administered for at least 24 h after resolution of fever, with appropriate oral antibiotics thereafter until all signs of infection have resolved. In cases where fever does not settle within 48 h full clinical review should take place. Repeat cultures should be taken, microbiological advice sought and change in antibiotics considered. The possibility of a viral or fungal infection should also be considered and treated if appropriate The treating oncologist should be notified of the details of the episode and will need to take all the patient's circumstances into account when deciding appropriate modification of the treatment programme. Consideration of dose reduction or prophylaxis against future neutropenic sepsis is an appropriate strategy if further chemotherapy is used.

 CASE 5.3 – A 59-year-old smoker has dyspnoea, and arm and facial swelling.

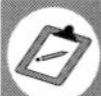 Q1: What is the likely diagnosis?

A1

This is superior vena caval obstruction (SVCO) secondary to malignancy. The patient's smoking history and the rapid appearance of the radiological abnormality make the most likely diagnosis small cell lung cancer, but it is not possible reliably to exclude a non-small cell lung cancer or a high-grade lymphoma. The symptoms could be caused by venous thrombosis although this does not explain the abnormal radiology. There may be associated thrombus.

 Q2: What aspects of the physical examination are most relevant?

A2

Full examination is required but should focus particularly on the respiratory and circulatory systems. The presence of clubbing should be noted and the chest and upper body should be examined for venous distension/diversion. The neck veins should be examined and the degree of facial swelling noted. Periorbital swelling may be present and the ability to close the eyes should be assessed. A paradoxical pulse and reduced-output state may indicate coexistent cardiac tamponade. Examination of the entire body for evidence of metastatic deposits is required. Lymph node masses and liver involvement may help with a source of histological confirmation and assist staging assessment.

 Q3: What investigations would be performed?

A3

Computed tomography will define the mediastinal abnormality more accurately than chest radiograph, and identify areas of external compression and associated thrombus. Computed tomography should include the abdomen to complete staging of the malignancy. Phlebography will establish patency of the superior vena cava and should be performed in conjunction with percutaneous stent insertion. Bronchcoscopy should be performed to obtain a tissue diagnosis and indication of the presence of a primary bronchogenic neoplasm. Full blood count, INR, U&Es, creatinine, calcium and liver function tests are useful ancillary investigations; low sodium could indicate syndrome of inappropriate antidiuretic hormone secretion (SIADH) which would favour a diagnosis of small cell lung cancer. High calcium would indicate a possible squamous cell carcinoma or bone involvement. Tumour markers are of modest value, a high carcinoembryonic antigen (CEA) level being indicative of a probable adenocarcinoma and a high lactate dehydrogenase (LDH) possibly indicating a lymphoid malignancy.

 Q4: How would the diagnosis be confirmed?

A4

Either phlebography or CT will confirm the clinical diagnosis of SVCO but both may be needed for complete evaluation. Histological diagnosis of the type of malignancy can usually be obtained at brochoscopy but, if no malignancy is seen, CT-guided biopsy or mediastinoscopy may be required to sample areas of suspected malignancy.

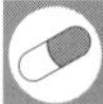 Q5: What would be the initial management?

A5

Radiologically guided stent placement provides the optimal means to palliate SVCO, resulting in rapid relief of symptoms. Anticoagulation should commence after stent placement. High-dose corticosteroids may provide temporary relief of symptoms but could make interpretation of lymphoma histology more difficult, and should therefore be avoided if possible until a tissue diagnosis has been obtained. The underlying disease should be treated correctly. A bulky high-grade lymphoma causing SVCO should be treated initially with chemotherapy, which may be curative. A small cell lung cancer has a high response rate to chemotherapy and localized disease will respond well to radiotherapy, but treatment is non-curative. Non-small cell lung cancer presenting with SVCO is very unlikely to be amenable to surgical resection, but can be usefully palliated by either chemotherapy or radiotherapy.

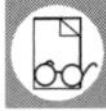 Q6: What issues need to be addressed following acute management?

A6

Assuming that this patient does indeed have small cell lung cancer, stenting successfully relieves the obstruction and he will start to respond to chemotherapy. The long-term outlook is bleak with a median survival of around 12 months. The patient may need psychological support and help adjusting to his fatal prognosis. He may need to retire on ill-health grounds and require help accessing appropriate financial support. Irrespective of his physical requirements, he and his family or close friends should be seen by a lung cancer support nurse or specialist palliative care nurse (Macmillan nurse), who can help explore all of the above issues and help access appropriate support as and when required. Close communication between hospital and community-based care is essential to the optimal future management of this patient.

OSCE Counselling Cases – Answers

OSCE COUNSELLING CASE 5.1 – 'How will I cope at home if complete recovery is not achieved?'

The reality is that complete recovery after spinal cord compression is unusual unless diagnosed very early when minimal cord damage has taken place. In the case described it is very difficult to predict the outcome. The patient is likely to be shocked and frightened by the diagnosis and needs time to adjust to the change in circumstances. It is reasonable to suggest that detailed discussion be deferred until the extent of residual deficit is known, so that there can be a realistic assessment of what the patient will be able to do and how independent he will be. In discussing treatment options the patient can expect to have the best- and worst-case scenarios described and an indication of how likely any of the possible outcomes are. Rather than guess at these it is entirely appropriate to request specialist assistance at this stage.

OSCE COUNSELLING CASE 5.2 – 'How long have I got to live?'

All doctors encountering patients with terminal malignant disease will be asked this question. The atmosphere and environment in which this issue is discussed are important. An explanation that the answer is complicated and will take time is acceptable, provided that you return soon; where possible anticipating the question that is going to be asked will allow you to control the circumstances.

You need to establish that the patient is ready to discuss this question and that you are sure that he or she wishes to hear an answer to the question. The patient may be expressing a whole series of anxieties about the terminal illness and not really wish to be confronted with a direct answer in weeks or months. Ensure that the patient has the appropriate support from relatives or friends. If this is not possible an additional member of staff should be present who knows the patient well and will be able to stay with him or her after you leave. It is important to find time to spend talking about the question and the reaction to your answers.

You should explain that estimating prognosis is inaccurate on an individual basis, with wide variations between patients. Ask the patient to tell you what he thinks the prognosis might be; you can guide him forwards or backwards in his estimate. Avoid being too specific about providing a median survival figure; instead a sensible range is a better way to illustrate the likely prognosis. You will need to gauge how the patient is reacting during the conversation, taking things more slowly when he displays unease. Always try to conclude the discussion on an optimistic aspect of the consultation.

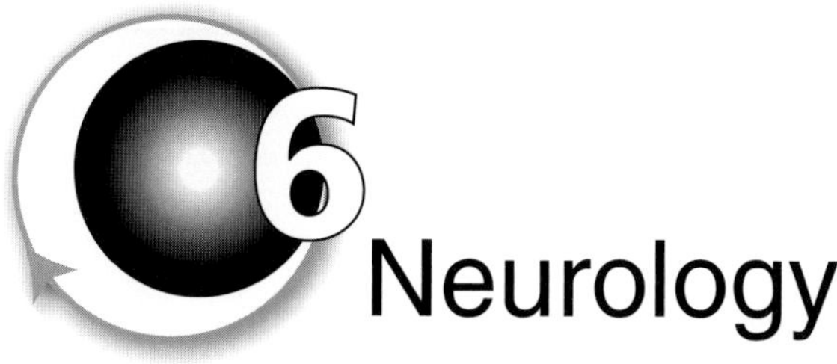

6 Neurology

Stuart Weatherby

DISORDERS OF CONSCIOUSNESS

? Questions for each of the clinical case scenarios given

Q1: What is the likely differential diagnosis?
Q2: What issues in the given history support/refute a particular diagnosis?
Q3: What additional features would you seek to support a particular diagnosis?
Q4: What clinical examination would you perform and why?
Q5: What investigations would be most helpful and why?
Q6: What treatment options are appropriate?

Clinical cases

CASE 6.1 – A 58-year-old previously well man suffers an episode of loss of consciousness just after leaving the golf club bar with his friends.

The patient smells of urine, seems a bit dazed, has a mild headache and feels achy, but otherwise is normal. He can't recall anything about the incident. He is a smoker.

CASE 6.2 – A 24-year-old woman who is known to have epilepsy started fitting after a family argument and an ambulance was called.

The ambulance team tell you that when they arrived in hospital she had been fitting for 30 min. She is still fitting when she arrives in hospital and appears non-responsive. Her body is thrashing violently on the bed. Her eyes are screwed tightly shut. Her oxygen saturation is 99 per cent air. Her pupils react to light and her plantar responses are downgoing. The rest of the examination is normal.

CASE 6.3 – A 21-year-old woman presents with a history of an episode of loss of consciousness 3 months ago.

She is otherwise well and plays hockey for the university's first team. Her friends witnessed it and have come to the clinic with her. The event occurred while she had been out socializing in a hot and busy pub. After standing for 25 min waiting to be served at the crowded bar she felt light-headed and became very pale and sweaty, her vision darkened and she crumpled down onto the floor. She was unrousable for a few seconds but then came round quickly with no confusion. While unrousable her limbs were observed to jerk two to three times. A medical student who was in the pub told her that she had had an epileptic 'fit'. Examination is normal and no postural blood pressure drop is noted.

OSCE Counselling Case

OSCE COUNSELLING CASE 6.1 – The patient with epilepsy.

Q1: What are the issues that need to be discussed with a patient newly diagnosed with epilepsy?

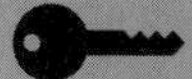

Key concepts

Seizure type can be described on the basis of the clinical phenotype, and also on the basis of the underlying aetiology. Below is a simplified classification to enable an understanding of the relevance of various terminologies. There are two main types: generalized and partial (see below for overview).

Partial (focal) seizures

Only part of the brain (the focus) is affected and consciousness is not lost, although it can be impaired. Partial seizures are sometimes termed 'localization-related seizures' because an underlying structural abnormality is implied.

Generalized seizures

The 'whole brain' is affected and the key clinical feature is loss of consciousness.

A generalized seizure can involve the whole brain at onset (primary generalized seizure – the whole brain has a predisposition to seizure) or may start as a partial (focal) seizure that then spreads to involve the whole brain (secondary generalized seizure).

In most adults epilepsy is partial either with or without secondary generalization. Structural lesions should be excluded (space-occupying lesions and cerebrovascular disease are more common in elderly people; minor structural lesions including scarring, focal areas of atrophy or cryptogenic foci are more common in younger adults).

Initial onset of primary generalized seizures is rare outside childhood and young adulthood. Although childhood and rare epilepsy syndromes are outside the scope of this text, it is, however, useful briefly to discuss juvenile myoclonic epilepsy. This is primary generalized epilepsy that usually starts in childhood or adolescence. It is associated with brief episodes of myoclonus (brief generalized, single body jerks). Juvenile myoclonic epilepsy is a condition that requires lifelong treatment.

The generalized seizures can be subdivided on phenotypic grounds rather than on the basis of underlying aetiology:

- Convulsive tonic–clonic (generalized convulsions): loss of consciousness and tonic and clonic phases of muscular contractions
- 'Absence type' (absence seizures) with sudden immediate and short-lived loss of consciousness with no loss of postural tone
- Other generalized seizure types, e.g. myoclonic (this may be brief generalized, single body jerks, often throwing the individual to the ground) and atonic (sudden loss of postural tone with a collapse to the ground – 'drop attack').

The partial seizures can also be subdivided on phenotypic grounds:

- Simple partial: only one part of one hemisphere of the cerebral cortex is affected, symptoms depending on the part affected, e.g. motor or sensory seizures. There is no impairment of consciousness but there can be post-ictal motor impairment, e.g. after a prolonged focal seizure affecting the right arm, it could be temporarily weak or paralysed; this is known as a post-ictal Todd's paralysis.

- Complex partial: only one part of one hemisphere of the cerebral cortex is affected initially but there is greater spread of the discharge to allow *impairment* of consciousness and often behavioural disturbances (e.g. automatisms). The seizure often starts as a focal seizure (if this affects *perception*, it is known as an aura).

Management of prolonged seizures/status epilepticus

Secure airway, give oxygen, assess cardiac and respiratory function, and give intravenous benzodiazepine. Carers in the community may be able to terminate serial seizures by giving rectal diazepam/lorazepam. In hospital, intravenous lorazepam 4 mg (or diazepam 10 mg) is more appropriate and should be given again after 10 min if there is no response. If there is a history of alcohol abuse thiamine should be administered intravenously. If there is any suspicion of hypoglycaemia, 50 mL 25 per cent glucose should be given intravenously. (Note that glucose given alone in someone with alcohol problems can precipitate Wernicke's encephalopathy.)

If fitting persists the patient should receive phenytoin 15 mg/kg i.v. at a rate not exceeding 50 mg/min, followed by maintenance doses of about 100 mg every 6–8 hours. An alternative is fosphenytoin, a pro-drug of phenytoin prescribed in terms of phenytoin equivalent (1.5 mg fosphenytoin ≡ 1 mg phenytoin). If fitting still persists (after 30 min) the patient should promptly be transferred to intensive care for more aggressive treatment to control seizures (e.g. phenobarbital). It is crucial to diagnose and treat the underlying cause of the seizures and also to recognize associated injuries or complications (e.g. aspiration pneumonia).

Answers

CASE 6.1 – A 58-year-old previously well man suffers an episode of loss of consciousness just after leaving the golf club bar with his friends.

 Q1: What is the likely differential diagnosis?

A1

Generalized seizure or syncope. In this situation there is very little history on which to base a diagnosis. However, it is a commonly occurring scenario. The differential diagnosis essentially breaks down into causes of seizure or causes of syncope. A number of causes for transient loss of consciousness are listed below.

- Epilepsy
- Cardiac:
  - arrhythmia
  - decreased cardiac output from mechanical causes, e.g. outflow obstruction
- Hypovolaemia
- Hypotension:
  - vasovagal attack
  - drugs
  - dysautonomia
- Vascular:
  - carotid sinus syncope
  - carotid disease
- Metabolic:
  - hypoglycaemia
  - anaemia
  - anoxia
- Multifactorial:
  - vasovagal
  - cardiac syncope
  - cough syncope
  - micturition syncope.

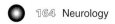

 Q2: What issues in the given history support/refute a particular diagnosis?

A2

The fact that the patient smells of urine, seems a bit dazed, has a mild headache and feels achy, and cannot recall anything about the incident are most consistent with a generalized convulsive seizure.

Seizures may be classified as generalized (consciousness lost) or partial (consciousness not lost). There is also a variant of partial seizures (complex–partial) in which consciousness is impaired. Epilepsy subtypes are briefly reviewed under 'Key concepts'.

 Q3: What additional features would you seek to support a particular diagnosis?

A3

The diagnosis of causes of loss of consciousness is fundamentally a clinical issue, and is based primarily on an accurate history. Insufficient history may be one reason that the misdiagnosis rate for epilepsy is so high (up to 26 per cent in one population-based study, the most common conditions mistaken for epilepsy being syncope and non-epileptic seizures). A corroborative history is essential.

Although the patient says that he cannot remember anything about the incident, he nevertheless should be questioned closely to try to find out how he felt just before he lost consciousness. Did the event truly begin abruptly (consistent with a seizure), or did he feel strange and/or have déja-vu or jamais-vu symptoms beforehand (these symptoms are suggestive of a complex–partial seizure that may have then become generalized). Did he develop a shaking in one side that progressed before he lost consciousness? (These symptoms suggest a partial motor seizure that became generalized.) Alcohol is known to provoke seizures and, as the patient had the event on leaving the golf club bar, he may have had alcohol. Medical problems such as hypoglycaemia in diabetes mellitus can also provoke seizures. A comprehensive past medical and drug history should be obtained. As he is a smoker it is important to question him for constitutional symptoms such as weight loss and cough with haemoptysis.

Witnesses should be interviewed (with the patient's permission) to get a description of the events.

WHAT WERE THE CIRCUMSTANCES?

In generalized seizures the event occurs abruptly, frequently without warning, and is not related to posture. The patient often appears normal before the event.

In syncope the patient often feels light-headed beforehand. Some types of syncope are related to circumstances, e.g. standing suddenly (postural hypotension), coughing (cough syncope), urination (micturition syncope – generally in men), in association with palpitations (syncope related to arrhythmia) or anxiety (e.g. in vasovagal syncope).

WHAT DID THE PATIENT LOOK LIKE?

Generalized seizures are usually of a tonic–clonic type and the patient tends to fall stiffly (tonic) and then start a coarse generalized limb shaking (clonic). This tends to go on for around 30 s, during which the patient is unresponsive to all stimuli. If examined during this period, the pupils are unreactive to light and the plantar responses are upgoing. The patient may bite his tongue and be incontinent of urine. When the patient regains consciousness he is often confused (post-ictal confusion) with aching muscles and a headache. In generalized seizures the patient can be cyanosed or look normal. It is

common for oxygen saturations to be low during a prolonged, generalized, tonic–clonic epileptic seizure. Often convulsive seizures of this type occur singly or in groups of two or three. Prolonged series of such seizures without regaining consciousness in between is called convulsive status epilepticus and requires urgent treatment (see later)

In syncope the patient often appears pale shortly before and during the event. The period of loss of consciousness tends to be very brief (seconds). There is no confusion afterwards

Q4: What clinical examination would you perform and why?

A4

- Look in the mouth for evidence of tongue biting (this can occur during a generalized seizure).
- Cardiovascular system: a common cause for seizures in this age group is cerebrovascular disease. Evidence of ischaemic heart disease should be sought. Postural hypotension, arrhythmia or cardiac murmurs can also be associated with syncopal events.
- Neurological examination should concentrate on looking for lateralizing signs. These may occur as a result of a focal cerebral lesion, e.g. from a stroke or a space-occupying lesion. Funduscopy, if it identifies papilloedema, suggests the presence of raised intracranial pressure from a space-occupying lesion.
- Respiratory examination: the patient smokes so the possibility of a cerebral metastasis from a bronchogenic carcinoma should be considered.
- Abdominal examination: if there is a history of alcohol excess it is important to assess for signs of chronic liver disease.

Q5: What investigations would be most helpful and why?

A5

- A BM stick allows rapid measurement of glucose.
- Electrocardiogram (ECG): should be done in all patients because epilepsy and cardiac causes of loss of consciousness can be difficult to distinguish. If arrhythmias are suspected a 24-hour ECG is helpful.
- Full blood count (FBC): anaemia or infection can provoke seizures.
- Urea and electrolytes (U&Es), calcium: hyponatraemia and hypocalcaemia in particular can provoke seizures.
- Blood glucose: hypoglycaemia can provoke seizures.
- Electroencephalogram (EEG): should be performed in all patients to support the diagnosis of epilepsy in patients with a suitable history and to help with seizure classification and localization. It is important to note that a 'normal' EEG does not exclude epilepsy, and a 'non-specifically abnormal' EEG does not necessarily imply an underlying significant neurological problem. Diagnosis of epilepsy is based primarily on a clear history. One reason for the high rates of misdiagnosis in epilepsy may be inappropriate interpretation of the EEG result. A single resting EEG shows abnormalities in only 50 per cent of patients with epilepsy. Sensitivity increases if the EEG is done within 24 h of a seizure, repeated or performed after sleep deprivation. Most useful of all is if the EEG can be performed during a seizure with video monitoring of the patient (video-telemetry). Conversely, normal phenomena, artefacts and non-specific abnormalities, occurring in about 20 per cent of the general population, are open to misinterpretation and may yield 'false-positive results'. Correct analysis of the EEG is dependent on the context in which it is performed. If an EEG

is requested as a 'screening tool' for a patient with, for example, 'funny turns', it may yield minor abnormalities and cause more diagnostic uncertainty than it solves.

- Brain imaging: computed tomography (CT) of the brain will exclude a space-occupying lesion and may identify evidence of cerebrovascular disease. It is often used for rapid assessment. Magnetic resonance imaging (MRI) of the brain is better at identifying small structural lesions and is the brain imaging modality recommended by many authorities.

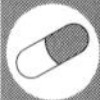

Q6: What treatment options are appropriate?

A6

This patient is likely to have suffered a secondary generalized seizure. However, a diagnosis of epilepsy cannot be made on the basis of a single seizure. Infection, drugs or metabolic problems can provoke seizures. Anti-epileptic drugs (AEDs) are therefore not usually started after a first seizure unless the risk of recurrence is thought to be high.

Epilepsy may be viewed as a chronic neurological condition characterized by recurrent unprovoked seizures. The nature of the seizures depends on which brain structures are affected.

Anti-epileptic drugs are usually started after the second seizure. Current indications and side-effect profiles for the various AEDs are readily available in the *British National Formulary*. The principles of treatment are addressed and commonly used 'first-line' monotherapy agents are discussed in brief.

A treatment should be effective, with minimal side effects for the patient. At present there is no clear consensus as to where the balance between efficacy and side effects lies. In circumstances where there is no urgency to start treatment, the decision should ideally be made jointly by the patient and a neurologist. Potentially 'acceptable' side effects will differ from patient to patient, and there are particular issues when prescribing for women, because drug interactions with the oral contraceptive pill, safety in pregnancy and breast-feeding need to be taken into account. The aim of treatment is to control seizures with a single agent (monotherapy), although a small proportion of patients may eventually require more than one AED.

There are now a large number of AEDs (including phenytoin, sodium valproate, carbamazepine, lamotrigine, levatiracetam, topiramate, oxcarbazepine, tiagabine, phenobarbital to name but a few). Some are licensed for use only as adjuncts (i.e. as an 'add on' treatment in patients with difficult to treat epilepsy), and should not therefore be initially used as monotherapy.

At present commonly prescribed first-line monotherapy AEDs in patients who do not require urgent treatment includes sodium valproate, lamotrigine and carbamazepine. Lamotrigine and sodium valproate are accepted as suitable for primary generalized seizures, partial/secondary generalized, and epileptic seizures of uncertain nature. Carbamazepine is not generally used for primary generalized seizures, because it may worsen this seizure type significantly.

CASE 6.2 – A 24-year-old woman who is known to have epilepsy started fitting after a family argument and an ambulance was called.

 Q1: What is the likely differential diagnosis?

A1

- Non-epileptic seizure disorder
- Status epilepticus.

Non-epileptic seizure disorder is overwhelmingly likely in this scenario. However, before making this diagnosis it is important to be confident that the other important diagnosis of prolonged generalized tonic–clonic seizure (status epilepticus) has been excluded. Status epilepticus is defined as continuous epileptic seizures for over 30 min or recurrent seizures over 30 min with failure to regain consciousness in between events. Untreated it carries a high mortality and occurs in 3–7 per cent of patients with epilepsy.

 Q2: What issues in the given history support/refute a particular diagnosis?

A2

Onset during a stressful event can be suggestive of a psychogenic factor. However, epileptic seizures can be triggered by stressful events so this feature is rather non-specific. The fact that the patient is known to have epilepsy does not help to support either an epileptic or a non-epileptic aetiology. A significant number of patients (30 per cent on average) have mixed epileptic and non-epileptic seizure disorders.

 Q3: What additional features would you seek to support a particular diagnosis?

A3

This case demonstrates the importance of making a diagnosis before starting potentially dangerous treatments. Non-epileptic seizure disorder is considered to have a psychogenic basis. Non-epileptic attacks are found to be most common in women between the ages of 20 and 50. Factors that may play a part in their onset often include a personal or family history of psychiatric disorder or depression, previous significant life events including bereavement, or a history of physical, sexual or emotional abuse.

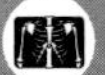 Q4: What clinical examination would you perform and why?

A4

The fact that the eyes are screwed tightly shut suggests a volitional component to the muscle activity. This would not be expected to occur in status epilepticus. Wild thrashing, hip thrusting, normal pupillary responses, normal oxygen saturations and normal plantar responses are suggestive of non-epileptic seizures. The patient may respond to deep pain stimuli during the seizure. In status epilepticus patients are completely unresponsive.

 Q5: What investigations would be most helpful and why?

A5

An EEG – although it seems rather self-evident, it is important to emphasize that non-epileptic seizures are NOT epileptic seizures.

Correct identification of non-epileptic seizures is particularly important to prevent inappropriate transfer to an intensive therapy unit (ITU) for epilepsy management (see later).

An EEG performed during the seizure will be normal in a non-epileptic seizure, but would be expected to show epileptiform discharges during generalized status epilepticus.

Serum prolactin is often elevated during and shortly after a prolonged generalized tonic–clonic seizure. It is not generally significantly elevated by a non-epileptic seizure. However, it should be remembered that prolactin levels can also be increased by drugs (e.g. phenothiazines). This can occasionally cause diagnostic confusion.

 Q6: What treatment options are appropriate?

A6

Patients with non-epileptic seizure disorder require a psychotherapeutic approach to help control their condition. The fits self-terminate.

Status epilepticus is a potential differential diagnosis in this situation, and the management of status epilepticus is outlined in Key concepts on p. 162.

 CASE 6.3 – A 21-year-old woman presents with a history of an episode of loss of consciousness 3 months ago.

 Q1: What is the likely differential diagnosis?

A1

- Syncope: simple faint (vasovagal syncope)
  - cardiac: cardiac arrhythmias
  - metabolic: hypoglycaemia, hyperventilation, drug related/provoked
- Epilepsy.

This history is highly suggestive of syncope and is most likely to be a vasovagal event.

 Q2: What issues in the given history support/refute a particular diagnosis?

A2

The symptoms related to posture, and the fact that she became pale and felt light-headed before losing consciousness (i.e. a relatively long premonitory period), suggest impairment of cerebral blood flow. The facts that she crumpled to the floor rather than falling stiffly, and that loss of consciousness was very short-lived with rapid recovery, are also highly suggestive of a syncopal event.

The circumstances of the events (a hot, crowded situation) are highly suggestive of vasovagal syncope. The fact that she is otherwise very active would suggest that a primary cardiac arrhythmogenic or structural lesion is less likely (although it does not entirely exclude it).

A few short-lived and transient limb-jerking movements are compatible with a syncopal event (and are NOT diagnostic of epilepsy), although longer-lasting jerking movements of the limbs are more suspicious of epileptic seizures.

 Q3: What additional features would you seek to support a particular diagnosis?

A3

- Is there is a past or family history of epilepsy or heart problems?
- Did she have palpitations before the event (more suggestive of an arrhythmia)?
- Was there any incontinence or tongue biting with the episode of loss of consciousness? This is common with epileptic seizures but not in syncope.

Remember that a patient may not volunteer aspects of a history that are potentially embarrassing, and 'direct' questioning may be needed to elicit this information.

Q4: What clinical examination would you perform and why?

A4

One would not usually expect to find any abnormalities in the general or neurological examination.

However, during examination, particular attention should be paid to excluding abnormalities in the cardiac system (e.g. arrhythmias, heart murmurs). A postural blood pressure drop may sometimes be found.

 Q5: What investigations would be most helpful and why?

A5

- ECG
- 24-h ECG
- Cardiac 'memo'

- Echocardiogram
- Tilt testing.

An ECG would help further to discount the (unlikely) possibility of a primary cardiac/arrythmogenic cause. Otherwise, no other investigations are necessary at present.

Importantly, an EEG is not indicated and if performed might complicate matters – a substantial proportion of 'normal' EEGs may show minor alterations in wave morphology that might confuse the unwary.

If she has further events, further investigation with a 24-h ECG may identify disorders of heart rhythm. If an arrhythmogenic cause is strongly suspected and the 24-h ECG is normal a cardiac 'memo' can be helpful. If a structural cause is strongly suspected an echocardiogram can identify evidence of outflow obstruction. Tilt-table testing is sometimes helpful in patients with severe and frequent episodes of syncope if cardiac abnormalities have been excluded.

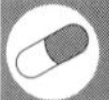

Q6: What treatment options are appropriate?

A6

This patient requires reassurance that the episode was a faint rather than an epileptic seizure, and to try to avoid precipitating activities.

OSCE Counselling Case – Answer

OSCE COUNSELLING CASE 6.1 – The patient with epilepsy.

Epilepsy is a long-term diagnosis and issues surrounding AED choice, seizure triggers (fatigue, alcohol and other drugs, stress and occasionally photosensitivity), issues for women, driving regulations, safety in the home, cognitive effects of epilepsy and AEDs all need to be discussed with the patient. It is important to document that this has been done in the notes for medicolegal reasons. A useful checklist is available from the Scottish Intercollegiate Guidelines (www.sign.ac.uk). Comprehensive guidelines from the National Institute for Health and Clinical Excellence (NICE) are also available from www.nice.org.uk.

The following issues need to be discussed:

- Explain what epilepsy is.
- Discuss the side effects of the various AED options.
- Discuss triggers to seizures, e.g. lack of sleep, infections, drugs, poor compliance with AED medication.
- SUDEP: SUDEP is the acronym for sudden unexplained death in epilepsy. There are around 500 cases in the UK every year, which, as a comparison, is more than the annual cases of cot deaths. The causes are not clear but SUDEP appears to be more frequent in those with poor seizure control who are non-compliant with treatment. It is considered that all patients with epilepsy should be informed of SUDEP, although clearly it is important to do this at an appropriate time, not necessarily at the time of diagnosis.

The following should also be discussed.

ISSUES FOR WOMEN

Oral contraception

Women taking one of the enzyme-inducing anticonvulsants (including carbamazepine, phenytoin and topiramate) may need to take a high-dose oral contraceptive because the low dose is likely to be less effective.

Pregnancy

The risk that children of parents with epilepsy will themselves develop epilepsy is only about 5 per cent, unless the parent has a clearly hereditary form of the disorder. Patients should be managed in an obstetric clinic with access to a physician specializing in epilepsy.

Use of the long-established AEDS (e.g. sodium valproate, carbamazepine and phenobarbital) during pregnancy appears to be associated with a two- or threefold increase in the risk of major congenital malformations in women with epilepsy. The risk of malformation appears to be dose related and a higher rate is seen in those women receiving two or more drugs. These risks may be minimized by taking folic acid supplements, so it is important for a patient to try to plan pregnancy in advance. Pre-pregnancy and post-delivery vitamin K is also recommended to prevent haemorrhagic disease of the newborn. There is less evidence of fetal problems with several of the more recently available AEDs (e.g. lamotrigine). However, at present no pharmaceutical company guarantees that their product is safe in pregnancy.

Patients usually elect to continue treatment in pregnancy because the risks of stopping are generally thought to be greater than the risks of continuing (e.g. injury during a fit or fetal hypoxia in prolonged generalized seizures).

LIFESTYLE

- Consider employment and relationship issues.
- Inform the patient about driving issues.

The doctor has a legal obligation to explain to the patient who has suffered an epileptic seizure that he or she must inform the Driver and Vehicle Licensing Agency (DVLA) and must not drive until the medical panel of the DVLA have considered the case. The patient is under a legal obligation to inform the DVLA.

After an unprovoked seizure the stipulation of the DVLA is that a patient with a group 1 licence (normal car licence) must not drive until he or she has been fit free for a year. DVLA guidelines on episodes of loss of consciousness are occasionally updated and vary depending on the type of licence, whether a seizure was provoked, and in episodes of 'unexplained' loss of consciousness (e.g. when the patient presents alone with no recall about the event) whether there is a high or low risk of recurrence. The DVLA website shows the current recommendations for driving after many types of illness (www.dvla.gov.uk/at_a_glance/content.htm).

No driving restrictions are currently required for a simple faint for a normal driving licence. If the faints are recurrent then the three 'Ps' should apply on each occasion (i.e. an identifiable provocation, a prodrome and a postural element).

After a syncope with a high risk of recurrence, if the cause is identified and treated the DVLA usually allow a patient to drive 4 weeks later. If the cause is not identified the stipulation is usually 6 months off driving (assuming that there are no further events).

STOPPING THE AED AFTER 2 YEARS OF SEIZURE FREEDOM

Between 70 and 80 per cent of fits will stop with a single AED. If fits stop, the risk of recurrence is 10 per cent after 5 fit-free years. After a period of seizure freedom it is appropriate to discuss the pros and cons of stopping treatment because the epilepsy may have remitted. After being fit free for 2 years the probability of remaining seizure free after stopping an AED is about 55–70 per cent if the patient continues on the AED. It is important to note that some primary epilepsy syndromes such as juvenile myoclonic epilepsy will not remit and the patient will require long-term treatment.

CEREBROVASCULAR DISEASE

? Questions for the clinical case scenario given

Q1: What is the likely differential diagnosis?
Q2: What issues in the given history support/refute a particular diagnosis?
Q3: What additional features would you seek to support a particular diagnosis?
Q4: What clinical examination would you perform and why?
Q5: What investigations would be most helpful and why?
Q6: What treatment options are appropriate?

Clinical case

CASE 6.4 – A previously well 39-year-old man attends A&E with a left-sided headache, neck pain and and slight word-finding difficulty after a mild whiplash injury 2 hours earlier.

He says his right arm doesn't 'feel right'. His wife has noticed a slight drooping of the eyelid on the left.

Answers

CASE 6.4 – A previously well 39-year-old man attends A&E with a left-sided headache and slight word-finding difficulty after a mild whiplash injury 2 hours earlier.

Q1: What is the likely differential diagnosis?

A1

- Dissection of the left carotid artery
- Migraine with aura
- Left-sided intracerebral haemorrhage
- Cerebrovascular disease causing a left-sided stroke in the middle cerebral artery territory

The most likely cause is a dissection of the left carotid artery.

Q2: What issues in the given history support/refute a particular diagnosis?

A2

Carotid artery dissection is a significant cause of stroke in patients younger than 40 years. Dissections are usually subadventitial (between the media and adventitia or within the media), creating a false lumen that can cause stenosis, occlusion or pseudoaneurysm of the vessel. Simultaneously, the dissection may cause the formation of a thrombus from which fragments embolize. Strokes resulting from carotid dissection may thus have a haemodynamic or an embolic origin. In this case a major clue to the cause of this patient's stroke is that he has a painful drooping left eyelid that suggests the possibility of Horner's syndrome. Horner's syndrome is caused by damage to the sympathetic supply to the eye. The sympathetic fibres travel with the carotid artery, and carotid dissection may damage these fibres. Horner's syndrome consists of ptosis, miosis, enophthalmos and sometimes loss of sweating on one half of the face. It is important to consider a carotid dissection in any case of painful Horner's syndrome.

As in this case, carotid artery dissections have non-specific presenting symptoms such as neurological deficits and headache. They often occur at a relatively young age and in previously healthy individuals, either spontaneously or after various degrees of trauma.

Neurologists manage stroke in all age groups. This patient is very young to have significant cerebrovascular disease. The other causes mentioned would not generally be expected to cause a Horner's syndrome but remain possibilities. Each aura symptom in migraine usually lasts only 20 minutes.

 Q3: What additional features would you seek to support a particular diagnosis?

A3

If the patient does not have a previous or family history of migraine this reduces the possibility of migrainous aetiology. Is there a history suggestive of a connective tissue disorder such as Marfan syndrome (a heritable condition that affects the connective tissue characteristics, including tall stature, lax joints, lens dislocation and cardiovascular abnormalities) or Ehlers–Danlos syndrome (heritable disorders of connective tissue, characterized by skin extensibility, joint hypermobility and tissue fragility caused by a defect in collagen)? These connective tissue disorders can predispose to arterial dissections.

 Q4: What clinical examination would you perform and why?

A4

Signs of an upper motor neuron pattern sensorimotor deficit in the right arm, and signs of Horner's syndrome (see above) should be found. It is also important to search for evidence of a head injury and, given the history of neck pain, to exclude evidence of spinal cord damage (bilateral limb weakness and sensory loss).

 Q5: What investigations would be most helpful and why?

A5

- CT/MRI of brain
- Non-invasive angiography of the carotid arteries
- Invasive contrast arteriography.

Computed tomography of the brain will in most circumstances be adequate to demonstrate ischaemic damage in the middle cerebral artery distribution, although MRI is more sensitive. Ultrasonography of carotid arteries is fast, convenient, non-invasive and highly sensitive, and may identify a dissection. Invasive contrast arteriography is more accurate but carries a greater risk. Non-invasive alternatives include CT and MR angiography (MRA). ECG and echocardiography may also be performed to rule out a cardiac source of cerebral emboli in many cases of 'young stroke'.

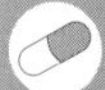 Q6: What treatment options are appropriate?

A6

- Aspirin
- Anticoagulation.

Formal anticoagulation for a period of months is usually favoured, although the evidence base for this is relatively poor. In practice the choice between anticoagulation agents and aspirin is made depending on various circumstances (e.g. how severe the stroke is, the length of time since the dissection).

DISEASES OF PERIPHERAL NERVES

? Questions for each of the clinical case scenarios given

Q1: What is the likely differential diagnosis?
Q2: What issues in the given history support/refute a particular diagnosis?
Q3: What additional features would you seek to support a particular diagnosis?
Q4: What clinical examination would you perform and why?
Q5: What investigations would be most helpful and why?
Q6: What treatment options are appropriate?

Clinical cases

CASE 6.5 – A 29-year-old man presents with a 10-day history of progressive, ascending leg weakness and numbness.

He suffered a 'stomach bug' while on holiday in Spain about 3 weeks ago. He was previously well.

CASE 6.6 – A 65-year-old man with type 2 diabetes (now requiring insulin for the last 5 years) presents with a progressive, ascending, symmetrical numbness and burning.

The symmetrical numbness and burning discomfort initially involved his feet (and more recently his ankles) over the last 8 years.

CASE 6.7 – A pregnant 35-year-old woman presents with a 4-month history of tingling in her left hand.

This is worse at night and often wakes her. She finds that hanging her left arm down outside the bed or shaking the left hand may help. She was previously well.

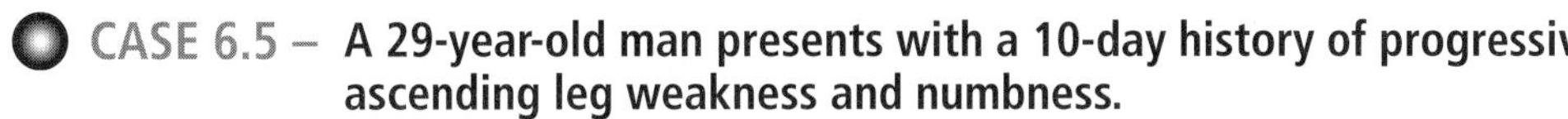

Answers

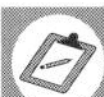

CASE 6.5 – A 29-year-old man presents with a 10-day history of progressive, ascending leg weakness and numbness.

Q1: What is the likely differential diagnosis?

A1

- Guillain–Barré syndrome (acute inflammatory demyelinating polyneuropathy or AIDP)
- Botulism
- Diphtheria
- Acute intermittent porphyria.

Q2: What issues in the given history support/refute a particular diagnosis?

A2

The story of ascending numbness and weakness about 10 days after an acute infection is typical of Guillain–Barré syndrome, which is an acute peripheral neuropathy causing weakness, paraesthesia and hyporeflexia. Progression generally stops 5 weeks after onset, and maximal weakness typically occurs at 2 weeks. The weakness is almost always symmetrical. Around 60 per cent of patients have a gastrointestinal or respiratory infection between 1 and 3 weeks before onset. Mortality of the disease ranges between 5 and 10 per cent, and the condition does not tend to recur. Cranial nerves may be involved in 45–75 per cent of cases and may be the dominant clinical feature, e.g. the Miller Fisher syndrome (a variant with ophthalmoplegia, ataxia and areflexia). A process similar to Guillain–Barré syndrome (termed 'chronic inflammatory demyelinating polyneuropathy' or CIDP) may occur over a period of months.

Botulism is often a food-borne disease (caused by the bacterium *Clostridium botulinum*), but wound botulism is increasingly recognized in injecting drug users. Although there can be an incubation period, the symptom progression is very rapid. Early oropharyngeal symptoms, ciliary paralysis (fixed pupils) and normal sensation distinguish it from Guillain–Barré syndrome.

Diphtheria is an acute infectious disease caused by *Corynebacterium diphtheriae*. There is often a high fever, and a tonsillar/pharyngeal membrane. The condition is now fortunately rare due to immunisation programmes.

Acute intermittent porphyria (an autosomal dominant metabolic problem with increased production and excretion of porphobilinogen) can also cause a rapidly advancing symmetrical peripheral neuropathy. However, it is rare and there are often accompanying features of abdominal pain.

 Q3: What additional features would you seek to support a particular diagnosis?

A3

The neuropathy may progress to involve the respiratory muscles and the patient may reach a critical state without any obvious prior clinical deterioration. The patient should be questioned if he suffers shortness of breath, particularly when lying flat (respiratory muscle weakness is more apparent in this position).

 Q4: What clinical examination would you perform and why?

A4

Guillain–Barré syndrome is an acute peripheral neuropathy. Examination should reveal a symmetrical global weakness of the legs and a reduction in sensation to all modalities in a stocking distribution. Reflexes become diminished and then absent as the disease progresses.

An important part of the clinical examination is to assess respiratory function. Forced vital capacity (FVC) measurements are essential. FVC is the volume of air expelled by a forced maximal expiration from a position of full inspiration. A peak expiratory flow rate, as used in assessing patients with asthma, is NOT appropriate and should not be used

Q5: What investigations would be most helpful and why?

A5

- Forced vital capacity: as the natural history of the condition is that it will continue to deteriorate over 5 weeks, regular FVC measurements are essential to detect incipient hypoventilatory respiratory failure.
- Lumbar puncture: an elevated cerebrospinal fluid (CSF) protein would be expected (but may remain normal in 10 per cent of cases). It may take 1–2 weeks after the onset of weakness for the elevation in CSF protein to become apparent. The CSF white cells should remain normal but, if they are significantly elevated (e.g. > 50), an associated HIV infection should be considered.
- Neurophysiology (nerve conduction studies): may be normal in the first 2–3 weeks but is then likely to demonstrate evidence of demyelination with conduction block, slowed distal latencies and decreased motor conduction velocities.
- Blood tests, U&Es, antibody tests, vitamin B_{12} and folate, serological studies for infection (e.g. *Mycoplasma* and *Campylobacter* species): blood investigations may identify low sodium (e.g. from syndrome of inappropriate antidiuretic hormone secretion or SIADH). Vitamin B_{12} deficiency would not really be expected to cause such a rapidly progressive neuropathy, but it is possible and is a treatable cause of neuropathy; if the lumbar puncture was normal, it should be considered further.

 Q6: What treatment options are appropriate?

A6

- Intravenous immunoglobulins
- Plasma exchange
- Deep vein thrombosis (DVT) prophylaxis.

Intravenous immunoglobulin (Ig) and plasma exchange therapy are comparable in terms of efficacy. Most patients generally receive intravenous Ig because this easier to administer, and may shorten recovery time by 50 per cent. As patients are likely to be relatively immobile prophylaxis with low-molecular-weight heparin should be considered.

Effective management also involves monitoring the patient closely to look for complications, in particular progressive respiratory failure, cardiac arrhythmias or autonomic instability. It is important to note that that a chronic form of Guillain–Barré syndrome – CIDP – exists and is characterized by a progressive or relapsing demyelinating polyneuropathy over 3 months. The findings on investigation are generally very similar to those of Guillain–Barré syndrome (AIDP), although patients with CIPD may also respond to corticosteroids.

 CASE 6.6 – A 65-year-old man with type 2 diabetes (now requiring insulin for the last 5 years) presents with a progressive, ascending, symmetrical numbness and burning.

 Q1: What is the likely differential diagnosis?

A1

Chronic sensory peripheral neuropathy caused by diabetes mellitus.

 Q2: What issues in the given history support/refute a particular diagnosis?

A2

The patient has had diabetes mellitus for long enough to develop complications. The slow progression, in a symmetrical fashion, affecting a 'stocking' distribution is typical of a peripheral neuropathy. The burning discomfort is consistent with neurogenic pain.

 Q3: What additional features would you seek to support a particular diagnosis?

A3

Although the likely cause is a chronic peripheral neuropathy caused by diabetes mellitus, one should take care before making such assumptions. The problem could be multifactorial. Other causes of a peripheral neuropathy should be excluded.

A history of chronic excess alcohol intake, vitamin B_{12} and folate deficiency, thyroid disease, renal failure, autoimmune diseases (which may cause a vasculitic neuropathy) or paraproteinaemia (e.g. multiple myeloma) should be sought.

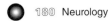

 Q4: What clinical examination would you perform and why?

A4

Examination should reveal a stocking sensory loss with loss of ankle jerk reflexes. Often dorsal column sensation (vibration sense, joint position sense and light touch) is preferentially affected. Look for other complications of diabetes mellitus (e.g. retinopathy, cerebrovascular disease, ischaemic heart disease, peripheral vascular disease, renal failure).

 Q5: What investigations would be most helpful and why?

A5

- Blood tests:
  - glucose
  - glycated haemoglobin (HbA1c)
  - urea and electrolytes
  - vitamin B_{12} and folate
  - thyroid function tests
  - immunoglobulins and electrophoresis
- Neurophysiology.

The blood tests are to identify other causes of a peripheral neuropathy and also to assess longer-term diabetic control (HbA1c).

Neurophysiological studies of nerve conduction are often useful in classifying whether the neuropathy is predominantly demyelinating (loss of the myelin insulation around the nerves, causing slow conduction velocity) or axonal (thinning of the nerve fibres themselves, causing small amplitude responses). Demyelinating peripheral neuropathies are more frequently the result of 'acquired' causes and may be aggressive, but are more often treatable. A cause should be identifiable in almost all cases. Axonal neuropathies are generally more indolent and slowly progressive.

In this case the cause is likely to be a diabetic peripheral neuropathy. However, in many cases of slowly progressive axonal peripheral neuropathy, investigations do not always reveal an identifiable cause. The neuropathy is then termed an 'idiopathic' axonal peripheral neuropathy.

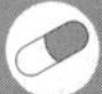 Q6: What treatment options are appropriate?

A6

Treatment is symptomatic treatment of the pain with drugs such as amitriptyline and gabapentin. Treatment of the cause, in this case optimizing diabetic control, will slow progression of the neuropathy.

CASE 6.7 – A pregnant 35-year-old woman presents with a 4-month history of tingling in her left hand.

 Q1: What is the likely differential diagnosis?

A1

- Left carpal tunnel syndrome
- Left ulnar neuropathy
- Left cervical root lesions.

The main sensory supply to the hand is from median and ulnar nerves (and a minimal contribution in the anatomical snuffbox from the radial nerve).

Carpal tunnel syndrome is a compressive problem affecting the median nerve.

 Q2: What issues in the given history support/refute a particular diagnosis?

A2

The most likely diagnosis is carpal tunnel syndrome. Carpal tunnel syndrome is more common in conditions where the carpal tunnel becomes narrowed, e.g. during pregnancy, trauma, rheumatoid arthritis, hypothyroidism. Worsening of symptoms at night, and relief on shaking the affected hand, are typical of carpal tunnel syndrome. The sensory disturbance in median/ulnar lesions affects only the hand. The sensory disturbance associated with cervical root lesions is more extensive and extends above the hand. It should be emphasized that cervical root lesions in this age group are very uncommon (although they occur with greater frequency in elderly people).

 Q3: What additional features would you seek to support a particular diagnosis?

A3

In carpal tunnel syndrome, although there may be weakness in the median nerve muscles, it is the sensory symptoms that predominate. An ulnar neuropathy typically causes a more pronounced functional deficit than median nerve compression.

Q4: What clinical examination would you perform and why?

A4

- Carpal tunnel syndrome: the sensory symptoms are confined to the anterior aspect of the lateral three and a half fingers. Thenar atrophy may be noted. Weakness of thumb abduction is a useful clinical sign for the motor component of carpal tunnel syndrome. Hyperflexion of the wrist for 60 s may elicit paraesthesia (Phalen's sign) and tapping the volar wrist over the median nerve (i.e. Tinel's sign) may produce paraesthesia in the median distribution of the hand.

- Ulnar nerve palsy: complete ulnar nerve paralysis causes a claw hand; wasting of the small hand muscles results in hyperextension of the fingers at the metacarpophalangeal joints and flexion at the interphalangeal joints. The sensory disturbance of ulnar neuropathy affects the medial one and a half fingers.
- Cervical root lesions: C6, C7 or C8 root damage can cause sensory loss in the hand, although this will extend into the forearm. Muscle weakness will be in the affected myotome and the relevant reflex arcs may be affected.

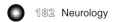

 Q5: What investigations would be most helpful and why?

A5

- Nerve conduction/electromyography (EMG) studies are helpful in confirming the clinical diagnosis.

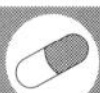 Q6: What treatment options are appropriate?

A6

- For carpal tunnel syndrome: reduction of pressure on the median nerve will provide relief. In this case fluid retention and oedema are likely to reduce after pregnancy and the symptoms may then remit. Placing the hand in a splint may be of symptomatic benefit. Injecting the carpal tunnel with corticosteroid could provide relief. Often surgical release of the carpal tunnel is necessary.
- For ulnar nerve palsy: surgical release at the site of compression may be needed.
- For cervical root lesions: surgical decompression at the site of the cervical root lesion may be needed. As mentioned earlier, cervical root lesions in this age group are very uncommon.

HEADACHE

? Questions for each of the clinical case scenarios given

Q1: What is the likely differential diagnosis?
Q2: What issues in the given history support/refute a particular diagnosis?
Q3: What additional features would you seek to support a particular diagnosis?
Q4: What clinical examination would you perform and why?
Q5: What investigations would be most helpful and why?
Q6: What treatment options are appropriate?

Clinical cases

CASE 6.8 – A 40-year-old woman attends the accident and emergency department (A&E) with her worst-ever headache.

It started suddenly in the occipital area 5 h ago and was associated with nausea and vomiting and some photophobia. Her neck became stiff after around 2 h.

CASE 6.9 – A 25-year-old woman presents to A&E with a severe gradual-onset headache.

It is right sided, throbbing and periorbital, and there is associated nausea. She has had similar episodic headaches over the last 5 years and they generally last 10 h before settling.

CASE 6.10 – A 70-year-old woman presents with sharp shooting pains in the region of the left cheek.

The pains last a few seconds and occur several times a day. She finds that yawning or touching the left cheek provokes attacks of the pain.

CASE 6.11 – A 70-year-old woman presents with a gradual-onset diffuse headache, which is more severe in the left temporal region.

She comments that wearing her spectacles has become uncomfortable and combing her hair exacerbates the pain.

CASE 6.12 – A 22-year-old woman presents with a 2-week history of headache of gradual onset.

It is generalized, worse in the morning and exacerbated by coughing and straining. There is associated nausea. She started the combined oral contraceptive pill 6 weeks ago.

CASE 6.13 – A 40-year-old man (previously well) presents with a 6-day history of gradual-onset worsening headache, lethargy, myalgia and fever, and (by the sixth day) altered behaviour.

He is brought to hospital after his wife called an ambulance because he had a generalized seizure.

Answers

 CASE 6.8 – A 40-year-old woman attends A&E with her worst-ever headache.

 Q1: What is the likely differential diagnosis?

A1

- Subarachnoid haemorrhage
- Thunderclap headache
- Bacterial meningitis
- Viral meningitis
- Cerebral venous sinus thrombosis
- Migraine.

 Q2: What issues in the given history support/refute a particular diagnosis?

A2

The history is typical of subarachnoid haemorrhage. This classically presents with sudden-onset, worst-ever headache with nausea, vomiting, photophobia and neck stiffness (although this can take a few hours to develop).

The 'textbook' description of subarachnoid haemorrhage is of a sudden-onset, worst-ever headache similar to a blow to the back of the head. If patients present in this way subarachnoid haemorrhage should be at the top of the differential diagnosis. In practice patients do not always follow the textbook description. A useful operational definition is of sudden-onset, first or worst headache, usually occipital and maximal within moments, that may develop over minutes and lasts at least 1 h. Subarachnoid haemorrhage may occur outside these parameters but is rare. A thunderclap headache may present in exactly the same manner as a subarachnoid haemorrhage, but does not tend to last longer than an hour.

 Q3: What additional features would you seek to support a particular diagnosis?

A3

Temperature may be mildly elevated by subarachnoid haemorrhage or cerebral venous sinus thrombosis. Bacterial and viral meningitis may cause a high fever. Thunderclap headache is not associated with a fever.

Approximately 1 per cent of all headaches seen in A&E are subarachnoid haemorrhage. The most common differential diagnosis for acute headache admitted to hospital is migraine. However, the symptoms of migraine tend to evolve and the headache is not usually of sudden onset. The headache is often frontal and may be unilateral. Thunderclap headaches may be recurrent. A history of previous normal investigations for a recurrent headache of this type may preclude the need to exclude subarachnoid haemorrhage on each occasion.

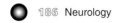

Sudden-onset headache can also occur in other conditions such as cerebral venous sinus thrombosis (although this mode of presentation is rare), which tends to be more common in females. Bacterial meningitis may very rarely present in this fashion, although in fact the patient usually has a more gradual-onset headache and may have a purpuric rash. Viral meningitis is unlikely because the patient often has a prodromal illness and a sudden-onset headache would be exceptional.

Q4: What clinical examination would you perform and why?

A4

If the patient has had a subarachnoid haemorrhage they may have focal neurological signs that give a clue as to the cause of the bleed, e.g. a nerve III palsy suggests a posterior communicating artery aneurysm. If there is elevated intracerebral pressure funduscopy may reveal papilloedema. In bacterial meningitis a purpuric rash may be identified and the patient may also have signs of septicaemia.

Patients with subarachnoid haemorrhage, bacterial meningitis, cerebral venous sinus thrombosis or migraine may have focal neurological abnormalities. Viral meningitis and thunderclap headache are not associated with focal neurological deficits.

Q5: What investigations would be most helpful and why?

A5

- FBC: an FBC will show elevated white cells in a bacterial (neutrophilia) or viral (lymphocytosis) meningitis. It will be normal in migraine, thunderclap headache and cerebral venous sinus thrombosis. The FBC would be expected to be normal in subarachnoid haemorrhage.
- Uncontrasted CT of the brain: this will show the presence of blood in about 98 per cent of cases of subarachnoid haemorrhage when done within 12 h.
- Lumbar puncture after 12 h: a lumbar puncture should be carried out in cases where the CT brain scan does not show blood. It is 100 per cent accurate for the presence/absence of subarachnoid haemorrhage if carried out appropriately within 12 h to 2 weeks of symptom onset. It will also identify elevated white cells (as occur in meningitis). The accurate diagnosis of a subarachnoid haemorrhage is dependent on identifying blood breakdown products in the CSF, rather than the identification of red blood cells (as red cells in the CSF can be due to a subarachnoid haemorrhage or a 'traumatic tap'). Blood within the CSF is broken down into bilirubin and is measurable after 12 h.

Therefore, in a subarachnoid haemorrhage bilirubin will be identified in the CSF when performed after 12 h, whereas bilirubin breakdown products are not identified in a 'traumatic tap'.

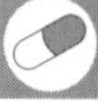

Q6: What treatment options are appropriate?

A6

If investigations reveal subarachnoid haemorrhage calcium antagonists (e.g. nimodipine) should be given. They reduce the mortality and morbidity from cerebral artery vasospasm provoked by the presence of subarachnoid blood and need to be given to all patients. Non-invasive or invasive angiography should be performed to identify the presence of an aneurysm which can then be ablated by either neuroradiological or neurosurgical techniques.

If investigations reveal an elevated CSF pressure but are otherwise normal, MRI of the brain with venogram sequences will identify/exclude the presence of a cerebral venous sinus thrombosis. The more typical presentation and management of cerebral venous sinus thrombosis are addressed in Case 6.12.

If investigations are normal the differential diagnosis lies between thunderclap headache and migraine. A thunderclap headache is of sudden onset, whereas migraine headaches are generally of more gradual onset (it is good practice in this situation to retake the initial history). Migraine lasts longer than a thunderclap headache, and features of nausea, vomiting, photophobia and phonophobia are often more pronounced than in thunderclap headache. Furthermore, migraine may be associated with focal neurological symptoms and signs.

Although the history would be unusual for meningitis it is appropriate to briefly discuss this important condition here. Patients in whom bacterial meningitis is suspected generally have a gradual-onset headache, rash, neck stiffness, nausea, vomiting, photophobia and confusion (although not necessarily all of them). A purpuric rash indicates a more generalized sepsis. In bacterial meningitis the lumbar puncture results typically show raised protein, low glucose and raised white cells (neutrophils). If the lumbar puncture has been performed after the patient has been on antibiotics (i.e. a partly treated bacterial meningitis) the white cells are often lymphocytes. In viral meningitis the findings are normal (or very slightly raised) protein, normal glucose and raised white cells (lymphocytes). In tuberculous meningitis the findings are raised protein, low glucose and raised white cells (lymphocytes).

In suspected bacterial meningitis it is important to start appropriate antibiotics on an empirical basis as soon as possible (i.e. before doing a lumbar puncture). Instituting antibiotic therapy 1–2 h before lumbar puncture will not significantly decrease the diagnostic sensitivity if the culture of the CSF is done together with testing for bacterial antigens and with blood cultures. In most patients, initial empirical therapy with a broad-spectrum cephalosporin (cefotaxime or ceftriaxone), supplemented with ampicillin in young infants and older adults, is appropriate. In patients with suspected bacterial meningitis it is currently considered appropriate to start corticosteroids at the same time as initiating antibiotics (and to continue steroids for the first 4 days). Most regions have their own local policies and these should be consulted because the situation regarding antimicrobial treatment may be subject to variation. Bacterial meningitis should be notified to public health physicians who will contact trace and give prophylactic antibiotics as necessary. In immunocompromised patients, patients in whom tuberculous meningitis is suspected or in cases of recent foreign travel, other treatment regimens are necessary.

CASE 6.9 – A 25-year-old woman presents to A&E with a severe gradual-onset headache.

Q1: What is the likely differential diagnosis?

A1

Migraine.

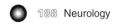

 Q2: What issues in the given history support/refute a particular diagnosis?

A2

Episodic gradual-onset severe headaches in young women are almost always migraine.

 Q3: What additional features would you seek to support a particular diagnosis?

A3

She should be questioned for other features of migraine. Some patients find that various foodstuffs may precipitate their headaches (e.g. cheese, chocolate, red wine, citrus fruit, crisps). There may be a hormonal component to the symptoms and the headaches may be worse around the time of periods. Some hours before the onset of headache, patients may suffer premonitory symptoms, e.g. of hunger, or anxiety. An aura may precede the headache. Often there is a family history of migraine.

 Q4: What clinical examination would you perform and why?

A4

Examination is normal.

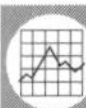 Q5: What investigations would be most helpful and why?

A5

The diagnosis of migraine is based on history. No investigations are necessary.

Migraine is the most common primary headache, affecting between 10 and 20 per cent of the population of the USA, and occurs more commonly in women. The International Headache Society (www.i-h-s.org) has carefully classified all headache types. There are two main types of migraine: migraine with and migraine without aura. The cardinal feature of migraine aura is that it evolves slowly; most aura symptoms develop over 5–20 min and usually last less than 60 min. The headache generally follows soon after the aura. Auras vary in type and complexity. Visual auras are the most common and include scotomata ('blind spots' in the visual field), fortification spectra and geometric visual patterns, whereas progressive sensory disturbance is the second most common migraine aura. The typical migraine headache is of gradual onset, throbbing and unilateral, although it may be bilateral in a substantial minority. Nausea, vomiting, photophobia and phonophobia are often accompanying features.

 Q6: What treatment options are appropriate?

A6

Many patients will respond to simple analgesics, especially non-steroidal anti-inflammatory drugs, which are often given with an anti-emetic, e.g. metoclopramide. Diclofenac and domperidone suppositories may also be helpful. If these measures do not work, the triptan class of anti-migraine drugs (selective serotonin agonists) may be used. These drugs significantly reduce the severity and duration of the migraine headache, but are not effective if given during the aura. They should be taken at the onset of the headache. Several guidelines are available for the diagnosis and management of migraine. The guidelines of the British Association for the Study of Headache are available from www.bash.org.uk. In cases of frequent migraine prophylactic agents are often considered. β Blockers and amitriptyline are examples of commonly used prophylactic agents.

A number of other issues are also worthy of note:

- The combined oral contraceptive pill is currently contraindicated in women with migraine with aura as a result of concerns about increased stroke risk.
- If patients have frequent migraines, they sometimes respond by taking frequent doses of analgesics. This can lead to increased chronicity of the headache and a rebound medication overuse headache. Codeine and other opiates are particularly problematic in this respect.

CASE 6.10 – A 70-year-old woman presents with sharp shooting pains in the region of the left cheek.

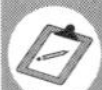 Q1: What is the likely differential diagnosis?

A1

Trigeminal neuralgia.

 Q2: What issues in the given history support/refute a particular diagnosis?

A2

Trigeminal neuralgia tends to occur in the over-60s and is more common in women. It is characterized by brief paroxysms of pain localized in the maxillary or mandibular divisions of the trigeminal nerve.

 Q3: What additional features would you seek to support a particular diagnosis?

A3

Attacks may be triggered by yawning, or touching the area of skin innervated by the mandibular branch of the trigeminal nerve. It is important to note that involvement of the ophthalmic branch is very rare.

Q4: What clinical examination would you perform and why?

A4

Examination is usually normal but may reveal altered sensation in the area of skin innervated by the mandibular branch of the trigeminal nerve.

 Q5: What investigations would be most helpful and why?

A5

Magnetic resonance imaging is generally used to exclude a vascular or other compressive lesion of the relevant divisions of the trigeminal nerve.

 Q6: What treatment options are appropriate?

A6

- Medical treatments:
  - carbamazepine
  - gabapentin
  - amitriptyline.
- Operative intervention: if the pain is refractory to medical treatments, neurosurgical procedures including microvascular decompression (to separate the trigeminal nerve from a compressing blood vessel) and percutaneous glycerol rhizolysis (injecting glycerol to damage the trigeminal fibres causing the pain) may be considered.

CASE 6.11 – A 70-year-old woman presents with a gradual-onset diffuse headache, which is more severe in the left temporal region.

 Q1: What is the likely differential diagnosis?

A1

- Temporal arteritis
- Space-occupying lesion.

 Q2: What issues in the given history support/refute a particular diagnosis?

A2

In a patient of this age it is always worth bearing in mind the possibility of a space-occupying lesion. This history is, however, typical of temporal arteritis.

Temporal arteritis is more common in the over-70s, especially in women. It is a medium-/large-vessel vasculitis. Affected vessels are infiltrated by lymphocytes, plasma cells and multinucleated giant cells, often in a patchy fashion. Temporal arteritis is closely linked to polymyalgia rheumatica (a clinical syndrome characterized by severe aching and stiffness in the neck, shoulder girdle and pelvic girdle). Temporal pain and tenderness are characteristic and thus the patient may complain of pain when wearing spectacles and combing her hair.

 Q3: What additional features would you seek to support a particular diagnosis?

A3

Patients may have constitutional symptoms such as malaise, lethargy, weight loss and night sweats. They may notice increasing discomfort in the jaw on talking or chewing (jaw claudication).

The inflammatory process in the blood vessels may occur throughout various areas of the body and cause ischaemia. Visual loss, stroke, angina and arterial aneurysms may all be associated.

 Q4: What clinical examination would you perform and why?

A4

There is likely to be tenderness over the temporal arteries, which may have diminished or absent pulses.

 Q5: What investigations would be most helpful and why?

A5

- ESR
- FBC
- LFT
- CT of brain
- Temporal artery biopsy.

An ESR is usually (but not always) elevated and gives additional support to the clinical diagnosis. Abnormal liver function tests may occur, and the FBC may show an anaemia, leukocytosis or thrombocytosis. If the patient has typical symptoms brain imaging is not necessary.

However, as this condition occurs in elderly people, and the headache phenotype can be rather variable, CT of the brain may be helpful to exclude a space-occupying lesion if there is clinical uncertainty as to the diagnosis. Furthermore, a raised ESR can be associated with other conditions (e.g. myeloma, infections and cancers). In cases of diagnostic uncertainty these conditions may need to be excluded.

Definitive diagnosis is achieved by temporal artery biopsy to identify the inflammatory lesions described above. The inflammation tends to be patchy and may not always appear in a single biopsy.

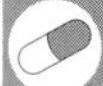 Q6: What treatment options are appropriate?

A6

Corticosteroids should be started immediately after clinical diagnosis. It is not necessary to perform a temporal artery biopsy first, because the inflammatory changes generally persist for 2 weeks. Treatment is usually with high-dose prednisolone orally, although if vision is threatened high-dose intravenous methylprednisolone infusions may be used initially. The response to treatment is typically rapid, within 48 h. In most cases it is usual to start the patient on 60 mg prednisolone and slowly to wean the dose down over several months once the symptoms are under control. If the ESR was initially raised it can be used to guide treatment. When a patient gets to a dose of around 10 mg prednisolone the dose reduction process is much slower (e.g. 1 mg/month). Often a dose threshold is found, below which the symptoms return, and patients may therefore require long-term corticosteroids. When a patient is placed on long-term steroids it is necessary to consider monitoring of bone density (using a DEXA scan) and instituting 'bone protection' with drugs such as bisphonates to reduce the likelihood of steroid-induced osteoporosis.

CASE 6.12 – A 22-year-old woman presents with a 2-week history of headache of gradual onset.

Q1: What is the likely differential diagnosis?

A1

- Cerebral venous sinus thrombosis
- Idiopathic intracranial hypertension
- Brain tumour.

Q2: What issues in the given history support/refute a particular diagnosis?

A2

This history is typical of both cerebral venous sinus thrombosis and idiopathic intracranial hypertension. The phenotype of the headache is of raised pressure (headache worse in the morning and exacerbated by coughing and straining) and other causes of raised pressure (e.g. brain tumour) are possible and need to be excluded. Prothrombotic states (e.g. the combined oral contraceptive pill [COC]) predispose to cerebral venous sinus thrombosis. Cerebral venous sinus thrombosis and idiopathic intracranial hypertension are more common in women.

Q3: What additional features would you seek to support a particular diagnosis?

A3

Ask for symptoms of lateralizing weakness or sensory disturbance. This suggests underlying structural lesions and would be consistent with a brain tumour or possibly cerebral venous sinus thrombosis. Idiopathic intracranial hypertension does not cause limb weakness. Disturbance of visual function (particularly enlargement of the blind spots) may occur in both idiopathic intracranial hypertension and cerebral venous sinus thrombosis. Impairment of consciousness can occur in brain tumours with oedema, or in cerebral venous sinus thrombosis. It does not occur in idiopathic intracranial hypertension.

 Q4: What clinical examination would you perform and why?

A4

Patients with idiopathic intracranial hypertension are almost always female and overweight. Examination of visual function is important. Visual fields may be affected in both conditions (enlarged blind spots and constricted visual fields). Funduscopy may reveal papilloedema. General neurological examination may reveal lateralizing signs.

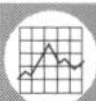 Q5: What investigations would be most helpful and why?

A5

- MRI of the brain with venogram sequences (MRV)
- Clotting studies
- D-Dimers
- Formal charting of visual fields, including measurement of blind spots
- Lumbar puncture with CSF pressure measurement (if imaging is normal).

Although CT of the brain is useful to exclude a tumour, the most appropriate imaging investigation is MRI of the brain with venogram sequences. This is more sensitive in identifying a cerebral venous sinus thrombosis. Recent evidence suggests that D-dimers are also often elevated in patients with acute and subacute cerebral venous sinus thrombosis, but their measurement is not sensitive enough to confirm/exclude the condition definitively. It is important to monitor vision carefully, because visual loss can occur rapidly in both cerebral venous sinus thrombosis and idiopathic intracranial hypertension. An early sign is development of enlargement of the blind spots, which can be detected by clinical examination of the visual fields (but much more sensitively by formal charting of the visual fields).

If imaging studies are normal then the likely diagnosis (if the patient is overweight and has papilloedema) is idiopathic intracranial hypertension. A lumbar puncture with CSF measurement will confirm the diagnosis by identifying raised intracranial pressure (considered as pressure > 25 cmH_2O).

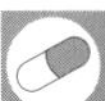 Q6: What treatment options are appropriate?

A6

If investigations identify a brain tumour oncological and neurosurgical opinions should be sought.

If investigations identify cerebral venous sinus thrombosis, the generally accepted treatment is formal anticoagulation, initially with heparin and then with warfarin for 3–6 months. Medications (such as COCs) associated with hypercoagulable states should be discontinued.

If investigations identify idiopathic intracranial hypertension, it is important to stop any medication that may precipitate the condition (e.g. COC and tetracycline antibiotics). Idiopathic intracranial hypertension occurs almost exclusively in overweight individuals and weight loss is the mainstay of treatment. Medications such as carbonic anhydrase inhibitors (e.g. acetazolamide) and/or diuretics (e.g. furosemide) are also used to reduce the CSF pressure.

It is important to realize that progressive visual field loss in idiopathic intracranial hypertension and cerebral venous sinus thrombosis is often asymptomatic. By the time the patient notices an impairment of visual acuity (a late-stage symptom in raised intracranial pressure), a significant degree of permanent visual loss may already have occurred. Regular monitoring of visual fields, both clinically and with formal perimetry, as part of the assessment of optic nerve function (together with visual acuity, colour vision and funduscopy) is vital. Idiopathic intracranial hypertension is a more chronic condition than cerebral venous sinus thrombosis and requires longer-term monitoring of visual function.

If a patient with either of these two conditions develops progressive visual loss that does not respond to medication, neurosurgical procedures to protect optic nerve function should be considered (CSF diversion, e.g. lumboperitoneal shunt, or optic nerve sheath fenestration). Although lumbar puncture can acutely reduce CSF pressure, the effect is transient. Repeated lumbar punctures do not help with longer-term management.

CASE 6.13 – A 40-year-old man (previously well) presents with a 6-day history of gradual-onset worsening headache, lethargy, myalgia and fever, and (by the sixth day) altered behaviour and confusion.

Q1: What is the likely differential diagnosis?

A1

- Encephalitis
- Brain abscess
- Brain tumour.

Q2: What issues in the given history support/refute a particular diagnosis?

A2

A brain tumour or abscess could present in this fashion. However, the prodrome of a viral-type illness is suggestive of encephalitis, as is the progressive evolution of symptoms. The altered behaviour and subsequent fit suggest involvement of the substance of the brain – as occurs in encephalitis. In meningitis behaviour change does not occur unless there is more extensive involvement (i.e. a meningoencephalitis) or the patient has systemic infection.

Q3: What additional features would you seek to support a particular diagnosis?

A3

Encephalitis: a history of close contacts with infectious diseases, travel abroad or tick/insect bites, or predisposition would increase the probability of an infectious cause

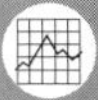 Q4: What clinical examination would you perform and why?

A4

Lateralizing neurological signs suggest a structural lesion within the brain but will not distinguish a cause. Similarly papilloedema will suggest raised intracranial pressure but may occur in all of the above causes. If the patient had a brain tumour that was metastatic general examination might reveal evidence of the primary. Fever, however, is not generally a feature of a brain tumour.

Q5: What investigations would be most helpful and why?

A5

- MRI of the brain
- EEG
- Lumbar puncture.

Computed tomography of the brain will essentially exclude an intracerebral mass lesion and may be done rapidly (can be useful particularly if the patient is confused), but the imaging modality of choice is MRI. This will better identify the nature of a space-occupying lesion and is much more sensitive at picking up the changes that occur in encephalitis. Herpes simplex virus (HSV) encephalitis is the most common and treatable encephalitis in the UK and abnormalities are frequently noted in the temporal lobes on MRI.

An EEG is helpful if further consideration is being given to a potential diagnosis of encephalitis. It will generally be abnormal, showing increased slow-wave activity and possibly epileptiform discharges. In HSV encephalitis, characteristic EEG changes of lateralized periodic complexes at regular 2–3 s intervals are seen.

A lumbar puncture is not generally helpful in investigating brain tumours. It is contraindicated in brain abscesses. If imaging excludes a mass lesion and significant oedema, a lumbar puncture can be helpful to investigate encephalitis. In HSV encephalitis the CSF is often under increased pressure with raised white cells (lymphocytes), elevated protein and modestly reduced glucose (i.e. the lumbar puncture results may be similar to those in tuberculous or fungal meningitis). Polymerase chain reaction (PCR) of the CSF is likely to detect the presence of HSV-1 or -2. General blood investigations (including FBC and U&Es) should of course also be performed in all patients – syndrome of inappropriate ADH secretion (SIADH) occurs reasonably frequently in encephalitis.

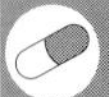 Q6: What treatment options are appropriate?

A6

In this patient the mostly likely diagnosis is encephalitis. The treatment options are:

- aciclovir
- corticosteroids
- anticonvulsants
- (antibiotics).

The aetiology of encephalitis is usually infectious and is most commonly the result of HSV-1 or -2, although varicella-zoster virus (VZV), Epstein–Barr virus (EBV), cytomegalovirus (CMV), measles, mumps, rubella, tick-borne disease and rickettsiae may also cause encephalitis. Outside the UK other infective agents such as West Nile and Japanese B viruses should be considered. In the immunocompromised individual fungal and parasitic agents should be considered. With the exception of HSV and VZV encephalitis, the viral forms of encephalitis are not currently treatable. Symptomatic treatment is necessary in all patients. The antiviral agent aciclovir given intravenously for 10–14 days reduces both mortality and morbidity in HSV and VZV encephalitis. It is given in all patients, because clinically it is not possible to distinguish between the various forms of encephalitis. If there is significant cerebral oedema treatment with the osmotic diuretic mannitol and/or corticosteroids needs to be considered (e.g. dexamethasone). If therapy is started early, the survival rate is > 90 per cent, although neuropsychiatric sequelae are common. If seizures are present, anticonvulsants should be started, and continued for some months once the condition has resolved.

In practice antibiotics (as used for empirical bacterial meningitis therapy) are often started on admission (because bacterial meningitis is sometimes initially considered). If the investigations suggest a brain tumour, the imaging characteristics may suggest that this is either primary or secondary (i.e. metastatic). Further investigation to identify the site of the primary tumour, and liaison with neurosurgeons and oncologists are indicated. If investigations suggest a brain abscess, investigation as to the source and whether there are predisposing factors (e.g. an immunodeficiency) must be carried out. Liaison with neurosurgical colleagues is necessary because drainage/excision is often used. Non-surgical management (e.g. with a prolonged course of brain-penetrating antibiotics) is usually reserved for those with an abscess in a difficult site for surgery.

CNS DEMYELINATION

? Questions for the clinical case scenario given

Q1: What is the likely differential diagnosis?
Q2: What issues in the given history support/refute a particular diagnosis?
Q3: What additional features would you seek to support a particular diagnosis?
Q4: What clinical examination would you perform and why?
Q5: What investigations would be most helpful and why?
Q6: What treatment options are appropriate?

Clinical case

CASE 6.14 – A 35-year-old white woman presents with a 3-day history of progressive numbness below the umbilicus, with mild weakness of the lower limbs and urinary frequency.

Five years previously she suffered a subacute episode of uncomfortable visual loss in the right eye with full recovery over a week.

Answers

CASE 6.14 – A 35-year-old white woman presents with a 3-day history of progressive numbness below the umbilicus, with mild weakness of the lower limbs and urinary frequency.

Q1: What is the likely differential diagnosis?

A1

- Inflammation of spinal cord (transverse myelitis)
- Spinal cord compression.

Q2: What issues in the given history support/refute a particular diagnosis?

A2

The most likely cause is inflammation of the spinal cord (transverse myelitis).

The symptoms of lower limb weakness, a sensory level at the umbilicus and urinary dysfunction localize the problem to the thoracic cord. In this age group the gradual-onset history is suggestive of transverse myelitis, although a gradual onset may also occur in certain causes of spinal cord compression (e.g. tumour and epidural abscess). The previous history of visual disturbance suggests a previous inflammatory lesion in the optic nerve (optic neuritis) and that this event is also the result of CNS inflammation (i.e. transverse myelitis). (A spinal cord infarction would be of sudden onset but would cause the same examination findings.)

Q3: What additional features would you seek to support a particular diagnosis?

A3

A preceding viral illness is suggestive of an inflammatory cause. Back pain is often a feature of spinal cord compression (trauma, tumour and epidural abscess), although mild back discomfort can occur in transverse myelitis. In cases of spinal cord compression caused by epidural abscess, patients may be systemically unwell with a fever.

Q4: What clinical examination would you perform and why?

A4

First, localize the lesion. In a thoracic spinal cord lesion the patient should have increased tone in the legs, a pyramidal pattern of weakness and a sensory level on the trunk. Lower limb reflexes will be brisk and plantar responses upgoing. A fever may occur in an epidural abscess. Mild pyrexia is compatible with a transverse myelitis.

Vertebral tenderness occurs in an epidural abscess, and may occur in spinal cord tumour. Although she has made a full symptomatic recovery from her previous visual problem, examination may reveal impaired colour vision and a pale optic disc in the affected eye (both signs of optic nerve damage).

 Q5: What investigations would be most helpful and why?

A5

- MRI of the brain and spinal cord
- Blood investigations, including inflammatory indices, autoimmune screen, vitamin B_{12} and folate
- Lumbar puncture for microbiological, biochemical studies and oligoclonal bands (this last test requires a serum sample too)
- Visual evoked potentials.

The subacute progressive onset after a viral infection in a previously well young woman is typical of transverse myelitis. Spinal cord compression, e.g. from a tumour, can present in a similar manner, but is rare. Compression from an intervertebral disc would be unlikely in this age group, and compression from an epidural abscess or spinal abscess is often, but not exclusively, associated with fever and localized spinal tenderness. Transverse myelitis is inflammation of the spinal cord. It may occur in isolation or in the setting of another illness. It may be associated with infections (viral or bacterial, e.g. *Mycoplasma pneumoniae*, *Borrelia* spp., syphilis or TB), autoimmune disease (e.g. systemic lupus erythematosus, Sjögren's syndrome or sarcoidosis). Occasionally vitamin B_{12} deficiency can produce a spinal cord syndrome that may mimic transverse myelitis. In the western world transverse myelitis, in this age group, is most frequently associated with multiple sclerosis (MS). It is likely that this patient has MS because she has had a previous event consistent with an inflammation in another part of the CNS (the optic nerves).

Magnetic resonance imaging at this level will help to distinguish between an inflammatory and a compressive lesion in the thoracic spinal cord. However, it is important to image the whole spinal cord because occasionally lesions higher up can produce a similar clinical picture. Imaging of the brain and cervical spine is necessary because MS causes a characteristic pattern of inflammation in the brain, and inflammatory changes may also be identified within the cervical spine.

A lumbar puncture may be helpful to look for further evidence of CNS inflammation. Oligoclonal bands unique to the CSF are consistent with the underlying cause of the symptoms being MS. Visual evoked potentials examine the integrity of the visual pathways by showing the patient a flashing chessboard pattern on a monitor and attaching electrical 'pick-ups' over the visual cortices. These may also provide paraclinical evidence of more widespread inflammatory problems within the CNS (as found in MS).

Multiple sclerosis is an idiopathic autoimmune inflammatory disease of the CNS characterized by inflammation and demyelination of the white matter in the brain and spinal cord. It is the most common neurological disease to affect young adults. The aetiology is uncertain, although both genetic and environmental factors are known to be important. In common with various autoimmune diseases, the condition occurs more frequently in women. Onset is usually between the ages of 30 and 40. Typically patients initially suffer relapsing episodes of neurological dysfunction, with full or partial remissions (relapsing–remitting MS). The relapses may be provoked by infection.

After about 10 years patients tend to slowly become more disabled even between relapses (secondary progressive phase MS).

Common forms of neurological disturbance in MS include transverse myelitis, optic neuritis (a subacute, usually unilateral, visual loss with pain on eye movement and a relative afferent pupillary defect, i.e. the pupil of the affected eye does not respond to light but the consensual reflex is maintained – there is usually a full clinical recovery), and brain-stem or cerebellar disturbances

A definite diagnosis of MS is given when a patient has had at least two attacks of demyelination (hence multiple) at two different sites in the CNS at different time points. Visual evoked potentials may provide paraclinical evidence of demyelination within the clinically unaffected visual system and provide some evidence of lesions disseminated in the site. MRI provides similar information and is more useful. Multiple sclerosis produces high-signal inflammatory lesions in the brain in a periventricular distribution, and inflammatory changes may also be found in the cervical spinal cord. Other autoimmune or connective tissue disorders may cause changes in the brain and spinal cord that can be identified on MRI, but the periventricular pattern is fairly specific to MS.

If a patient presents with an episode of transverse myelitis without a significant past history, he or she has a 'clinically isolated syndrome'. It is uncertain whether this could be a 'one-off' event, or the first symptom of MS. The presence of periventricular lesions on brain MRI, or oligoclonal bands in the CSF, is highly suggestive that such a patient will have further neurological events affecting the CNS and thus be diagnosed with MS.

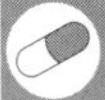

Q6: What treatment options are appropriate?

A6

Intravenous corticosteroids, usually given as 1 g prednisolone i.v. every day for 3 days, are the treatment of choice for all relapses in MS.

Corticosteroids speed up the rate of recovery but do not modulate the disease process itself. If there are frequent and problematic relapses, disease-modifying therapies (interferon-β or copolymer) can reduce the relapse rate.

DISORDERS OF CRANIAL NERVES

? Questions for each of the clinical case scenarios given

Q1: What is the likely differential diagnosis?
Q2: What issues in the given history support/refute a particular diagnosis?
Q3: What additional features would you seek to support a particular diagnosis?
Q4: What clinical examination would you perform and why?
Q5: What investigations would be most helpful and why?
Q6: What treatment options are appropriate? (Case 6.15 only)

Clinical cases

CASE 6.15 – A 35-year-old man who has recently had a viral infection presents with a 48-h history of progressive-onset drooping of the left side of his face.

He has noticed that his sense of taste is worse and noises seem louder.

CASE 6.16 – A 55-year-old man with diabetes presents with a 4-day history of progressive painful right periorbital pain, drooping of the right eyelid and double vision.

When he lifted his eyelid he noted that his right eye seemed to be deviated 'down and out' and he is unable to move it.

Answers

CASE 6.15 – A 35-year-old man who has recently had a viral infection presents with a 48-h history of progressive-onset drooping of the left side of his face.

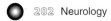

 Q1: What is the likely differential diagnosis?

A1

- Bell's palsy
- Tumour of the parotid gland.

The most likely diagnosis is Bell's palsy – an acute inflammatory lower motor neuron lesion of the facial nerve. It may be associated with a viral infection and may occur in all age groups and in both sexes. Maximum facial paralysis generally occurs in 48 h and in almost all cases within 5 days.

The facial nerve runs through the parotid gland, so parotid tumours may cause a facial nerve palsy. In this situation the onset may be more insidious.

There are a number of other causes of lower motor neuron facial palsies: Guillain–Barré, myasthenia gravis, sarcoidosis (a multisystem granulomatous inflammatory disease) and Lyme disease (caused by the tick *Borrelia burgdorferi*) can cause lower motor facial paralysis but are rare and usually bilateral. Moreover one would expect additional signs and symptoms.

 Q2: What issues in the given history support/refute a particular diagnosis?

A2

As mentioned in the answer above, Bell's palsy may be associated with a viral infection (particularly herpes simplex virus). It is important to remember that the facial nerve runs through the parotid gland and parotid tumours may cause facial nerve palsy. However, the onset would be expected to be insidious.

Hyperacusis (painful sensitivity to noise) occurs because of involvement of a branch of the facial nerve supplying the stapedius muscle (which acts to damp the ossicular chain). Taste sensation to the anterior two-thirds of the tongue is affected because the trigeminal nerve fibres that run in the chorda tympani nerve and supply the tongue join and travel with the facial nerve.

An upper motor neuron facial weakness is unlikely with this history, partly because other associated symptoms of sensory motor disturbance would be expected.

 Q3: What additional features would you seek to support a particular diagnosis?

A3

Bell's palsy affects only the facial nerve, and more extensive symptoms would therefore be unlikely. In cases of parotid tumour the patient may have noted swelling of the cheek.

 Q4: What clinical examination would you perform and why?

A4

Examination should confirm features of a left lower motor neuron facial lesion: left-sided facial weakness, difficulty in closing the left eye and an inability to furrow the left side of the forehead.

The forehead is bilaterally innervated by the facial nerve. In an upper motor neuron lesion causing unilateral facial paralysis the forehead is therefore spared.

It is important to examine the patient for signs of a viral herpes-zoster skin rash in the external auditory canal and mucous membranes of the oropharynx (this combination of Bell's palsy and herpes zoster is termed Ramsay Hunt syndrome).

 Q5: What investigations would be most helpful and why?

A5

Bell's palsy is a clinical diagnosis. In practice, if examination reveals only a lower motor neuron facial nerve palsy, no other investigations would be needed at this stage.

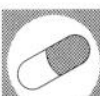 Q6: What treatment options are appropriate?

A6

If the eyelid does not close properly the cornea can be damaged. The eye must be protected in such cases, particularly during sleep, and can be taped shut to protect it.

Around 80 per cent of patients with Bell's palsy recover within a month. Early recovery of some motor function in the first 5 days is a favourable prognostic sign. A short course of oral corticosteroids combined with an antiviral agent is associated with improved recovery.

If the patient does not recover it is worth re-considering the cause, e.g. ultrasonography of the parotid gland will identify a tumour that may be causing compression of the facial nerve. Brain imaging will help identify tumours that invade the temporal bone and may cause facial palsy. A lumbar puncture will help in identifying evidence of Lyme disease or other infective agents.

 CASE 6.16 – A 55-year-old man with diabetes presents with a 4-day history of progressive painful right periorbital pain, drooping of the right eyelid and double vision.

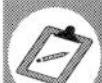 Q1: What is the likely differential diagnosis?

A1

- Compressive right nerve III palsy
- Infarction of the right nerve III.

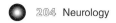

 Q2: What issues in the given history support/refute a particular diagnosis?

A2

The hallmarks of a nerve III palsy are unilateral ptosis and ophthalmoplegia, the eye being deviated down and out.

 Q3: What additional features would you seek to support a particular diagnosis?

A3

If the cause of nerve III palsy is compression the pupil of the affected eye will be fixed and dilated (i.e. a pupil-involving nerve III palsy).

If the cause of nerve III palsy is infarction of the nerve, the pupil of the affected eye is unaffected (i.e. a pupil-'sparing' nerve III palsy). Enlargement of the pupil is a sign of compression because the pupilloconstrictor fibres are peripherally located in the nerve. Infarction of nerve III characteristically involves the central portion of the nerve but spares the peripheral fibres.

Pain can be a feature of both compression or infarction of cranial nerve III. Nerve III infarction is common in people with diabetes and hypertension. It is important not to assume that this patient has a nerve III infarct just because he has a vascular risk factor.

 Q4: What clinical examination would you perform and why?

A4

Pupillary examination is important to help distinguish between a compressive nerve III palsy and a vascular cause, for the reasons outlined above. In a nerve III palsy the ptosis is often quite profound. The eye should be deviated 'down and out'.

As a rule of thumb all cases of painful pupil involving nerve III palsies suggest a compressive cause.

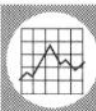 Q5: What investigations would be most helpful and why?

A5

If the patient has a painful pupil-involving nerve III palsy an urgent CT of the brain and a CT angiogram are needed.

The acute onset of a painful pupil-involving nerve III palsy suggests a rapidly expanding lesion such as an aneurysm, most commonly of the posterior communicating artery (PCA). It is vital not to miss this. There is a significant risk of the aneurysm bursting and causing a subarachnoid haemorrhage. CT and a CT angiogram are likely to identify an aneurysm, and if one is identified it is important to liaise with neurosurgical and neuroradiological colleagues to consider either clipping the aneurysm or endovascular ablation.

If no aneurysm is identified other causes of compressive nerve III palsy should be considered (e.g. tumours, carcinomatous lesions of the skull base or cavernous sinus, inflammatory lesions of the nerve or orbit, giant cell arteritis). However, these are often accompanied by other symptoms or signs. An ESR and MRI of the brain (with contrast and/or with venogram sequences) are helpful in identifying these other causes.

In a pupil-sparing nerve III palsy imaging may show evidence of cardiovascular disease and vascular risk factors should be explored.

MOVEMENT DISORDERS

? Questions for each of the clinical case scenarios given

Q1: What is the likely differential diagnosis?
Q2: What issues in the given history support/refute a particular diagnosis?
Q3: What additional features would you seek to support a particular diagnosis?
Q4: What clinical examination would you perform and why?
Q5: What investigations would be most helpful and why?
Q6: What treatment options are appropriate?

Clinical cases

CASE 6.17 – A 60-year-old woman attends with gradual-onset, very slowly progressive tremor in both hands over 10 years.

The tremor is not present at rest. She finds it difficult to drink or to use cutlery. She comments that her grandfather, mother and brother had or have similar symptoms. She finds that a small tot of whisky helps ease the tremor.

CASE 6.18 – A 25-year-old man with 'psychiatric problems' presents with a progressive 2-year history of 'movement problems' (both at rest and on intention) and slurring of speech.

His cousin died in his teens of a 'liver problem'.

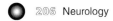

Answers

CASE 6.17 – A 60-year-old woman attends with gradual-onset, very slowly progressive tremor in both hands over 10 years.

 Q1: What is the likely differential diagnosis?

A1

Benign essential tremor.

 Q2: What issues in the given history support/refute a particular diagnosis?

A2

Benign essential tremor is familial in 50 per cent of cases (autosomal dominant) and there may be a striking improvement with alcohol. It tends to affect both hands. It is slowly progressive.

 Q3: What additional features would you seek to support a particular diagnosis?

A3

The tremor is characteristically coarse, affects the upper limbs distally and is exacerbated by sustained postures. Cerebellar tremor is different because it is particularly evoked when attempting fine coordinated movements.

 Q4: What clinical examination would you perform and why?

A4

Other than the coarse symmetrical tremor, more prominent when she holds her hands outstretched, no other abnormalities are identified.

 Q5: What investigations would be most helpful and why?

A5

Benign essential tremor is a clinical diagnosis and investigations are not generally necessary. Occasionally, in the early stages benign essential tremor can be confused with Parkinson's disease.

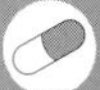 Q6: What treatment options are appropriate?

A6

Propranolol or primidone.

Not all patients require treatment and often treatment response is poor.

 CASE 6.18 – A 25-year-old man with 'psychiatric problems' presents with a progressive 2-year history of 'movement problems' (both at rest and on intention) and slurring of speech.

 Q1: What is the likely differential diagnosis?

A1

- An organic movement disorder – Wilson's disease
- A drug-related movement disorder
- A psychogenic movement disorder.

 Q2: What issues in the given history support/refute a particular diagnosis?

A2

Progressive onset tremor in a patient with a psychiatric problem might be a drug-related tremor caused by antipsychotic medication. It is possible that he has a dyskinesia from antipsychotic medication (which can also cause parkinsonian-type symptoms). An alternative is that he has a psychogenic movement disorder.

However, in any young patient with a movement disorder, it is important to consider and exclude the diagnosis of Wilson's disease. Wilson's disease is an autosomal recessive inherited condition caused by mutation in the *ATP7B* gene on chromosome 13q. The gene is expressed predominantly in liver, kidney and placenta and, to a lesser extent, in heart, brain, lung, muscle and pancreas; the result is an excess of tissue copper deposition. Liver disease is the most common presenting problem in children. Neurological features are a more common mode of presentation in adults. About 35–50 per cent of patients present with neurological or psychiatric symptoms. It is important because it is treatable. If left untreated it is fatal. As this young man has a psychiatric history and a family history of liver disease it is highly likely that the diagnosis is Wilson's disease.

Q3: What additional features would you seek to support a particular diagnosis?

A3

It would be important to find out his psychiatric medication and the doses. Antipsychotics can cause dyskinesia. Even if he is on high doses of antipsychotic medication, Wilson's disease must be excluded.

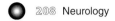

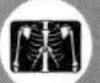 Q4: What clinical examination would you perform and why?

A4

Typical findings in Wilson's disease are irregular, random, brief, abrupt movements of the arms (chorea). A brown crescentic deposit in the periphery of the iris, known as the Kayser–Fleischer ring, is often found, particularly in those with significant neurological involvement. It is a granular deposit of copper. If the patient has brown eyes it may not always be easy to visualize. Signs of liver disease may also be present.

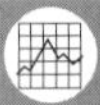 Q5: What investigations would be most helpful and why?

A5

- Slit-lamp microscope examination to identify the Kayser–Fleischer ring
- Low serum copper level
- Low serum caeruloplasmin level
- Increased 24-hour urinary copper level
- An MRI of the brain often shows changes in the basal ganglia.

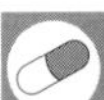 Q6: What treatment options are appropriate?

A6

Copper-chelating agents such as penicillamine, with monitoring of serum copper to guide treatment.

MISCELLANEOUS

? Questions for each of the clinical case scenarios given

Q1: What is the likely differential diagnosis?
Q2: What issues in the given history support/refute a particular diagnosis?
Q3: What additional features would you seek to support a particular diagnosis?
Q4: What clinical examination would you perform and why?
Q5: What investigations would be most helpful and why?
Q6: What treatment options are appropriate?

Clinical cases

CASE 6.19 – A 30-year-old woman presents with a 3-month history of feeling generally lethargic, intermittent drooping of her left eye and intermittent double vision.

She feels that her muscles are generally weaker. These symptoms are worse towards the end of the day. She has also noticed that her voice is weaker, also worse at the end of the day.

CASE 6.20 – A 50-year-old, previously well man presents with a 5-month history of progressive weakness in his upper and lower limbs.

The symptoms initially affected the hands, the right more than the left. He comments that the muscles in his hands have got 'thinner' and he has noticed some 'flickering' of the muscles in his arms. There are no sensory symptoms.

CASE 6.21 – A 50-year-old man presents with a 12-month history of gradual-onset tremor in his right hand.

It is present at rest and he feels that it is aggravated by stress. His handwriting is deteriorating and getting smaller and he feels that his movements are generally slower. Otherwise his health is good.

OSCE Counselling Case

OSCE COUNSELLING CASE 6.2 – How would you explain a diagnosis of multiple sclerosis (MS) to a patient?

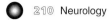

Answers

CASE 6.19 – A 30-year-old woman presents with a 3-month history of feeling generally lethargic, intermittent drooping of her left eye and intermittent double vision.

 Q1: What is the likely differential diagnosis?

A1

- Myasthenia gravis
- Lambert–Eaton myasthenic syndrome (LEMS).

 Q2: What issues in the given history support/refute a particular diagnosis?

A2

The history is typical of myasthenia gravis, caused by antibodies against acetylcholine (ACh) nicotinic postsynaptic receptors at the neuromuscular junction. Myasthenia gravis has a bimodal age distribution and predominantly affects young adults (aged about 20s to 30s) and the over-50s. It is characterized by fluctuating weakness worsened by exertion. Weakness increases during the day and improves with rest. The hallmark of the history and examination is significant fatiguing of the muscles with use.

It can be difficult in practice to distinguish LEMS from myasthenia. Both conditions present with increasing weakness after exertion, and there are also some clinical differences. It is rare for LEMS to present with double vision or dysphagia. In LEMS the muscles of the trunk, shoulder and pelvic girdle are most frequently involved. It is caused by an autoimmune attack directed against the voltage-gated calcium channels on the presynaptic motor nerve terminal. Fifty per cent of LEMS cases are associated with an underlying neoplasm, particularly small cell carcinoma of the lung.

In this particular situation the patient is young. LEMS tends to affect older age groups and occurrence at the age of 30 would be very unusual.

 Q3: What additional features would you seek to support a particular diagnosis?

A3

The patient should be questioned to determine whether she has fatiguing weakness in other muscle groups. In around 25 per cent of patients myasthenia can be confined to the eye muscles and the clinical features are therefore limited to ptosis and diplopia (ocular myasthenia). However, it may spread to other areas over years (generalized myasthenia). In generalized myasthenia the weakness tends to involve predominantly ocular, facial and bulbar muscles (weakness of speech and swallowing), as well as axial muscles (especially weakness of head flexion).

A history of particular drug usage should be sought. A number of drugs, including aminoglycosides, tetracyclines, penicillamine, β blockers, lithium and corticosteroids can worsen myasthenic symptoms and may therefore provoke symptom onset.

Myasthenia can be associated with autoimmune diseases, and symptoms of thyroid dysfunction should be sought.

 Q4: What clinical examination would you perform and why?

A4

On examination she has a mild ptosis of the left eye. Eye movements appear normal but after you have finished testing them she complains that the double vision seems to be starting again. There is mild proximal muscle weakness. Sensory and reflex examinations are normal.

If the diagnosis of myasthenia gravis is suspected, it is important actively to assess the patient for fatiguability of muscle power. This is an 'add-on' to the general neurological examination, and so will be found only if it is specifically considered. One method is continually or repeatedly test power in a particular muscle group (e.g. upgaze of the eyes to demonstrate a fatiguable ptosis). Sensory examination and deep tendon reflexes are normal. In LEMS reflexes are often depressed. It is very important to remember that respiratory muscle weakness may occur and forced vital capacity (FVC) measurements should be made. Testing for signs of thyroid disease or an enlarged thymus should be carried out.

 Q5: What investigations would be most helpful and why?

A5

MYASTHENIA GRAVIS

- Anti-ACh receptor antibodies
- Thyroid function tests and anti-thyroid antibodies
- Anti-striated muscle (anti-SM) antibodies
- CT of the chest
- Neurophysiological studies
- FVC
- Tensilon test.

Anti-ACh receptor antibodies are present in around 85 per cent of patients with generalized myasthenia and 50 per cent of patients with pure ocular myasthenia. Thyroid abnormalities are associated in around 4 per cent. Computed tomography of the chest is needed because a proportion of patients with myasthenia gravis have a thymoma. Anti-SM antibodies are present in about 84 per cent of patients with thymoma who are younger than 40 years.

Tensilon (edrophonium) is a short-acting ACh esterase inhibitor. It potentiates neuromuscular transmission by reducing breakdown of ACh at the neuromuscular junction. A positive Tensilon test is one that shows a significant improvement in muscle power after administration. The test is usually carried out in a double-blind fashion. It is not now used so frequently because of concerns about cardiac side effects. A therapeutic trial of pyridostigmine may provide the same information.

In myasthenia gravis, neurophysiological studies show a decremental response to repetitive stimulation.

As fatiguability of respiratory muscles may result in hypoventilatory failure, forced vital capacity measurements may be needed to monitor respiratory function.

LAMBERT–EATON MYASTHENIC SYNDROME (LEMS)

The anti-voltage-gated calcium channel antibodies can be identified with a blood test. Neurophysiological tests often show a marked and progressive increment in the amplitude of response (often termed 'incremental response').

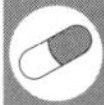

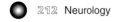

Q6: What treatment options are appropriate?

A6

MYASTHENIA GRAVIS

- Pyridostigmine
- Corticosteroids
- 'Steroid-sparing' immunosuppressive agents
- Immunoglobulins
- Plasma exchange
- Thymectomy.

Pyridostigmine is a longer-acting ACh esterase inhibitor and is helpful for symptomatic control. It may be sufficient in patients with mild ocular symptoms only. Patients with generalized myasthenia also need disease-modifying therapy. Immunosuppression with corticosteroids followed by steroid-sparing agents (e.g. azathioprine) is the standard oral medication of choice. As a short-term 'dip' in myasthenic control can occur when steroids are started, it is common practice to start treatment in hospital and to increase the steroid doses very slowly. Intravenous Ig (IVIG) or plasma exchange can be useful in producing improvement more rapidly. If the patient is found to have a thymoma, it should be surgically removed. In young patients with thymic hyperplasia and high anti-ACh receptor antibodies, thymectomy appears to induce remission in a proportion of patients (although there is no comprehensive evidence base for this).

LAMBERT–EATON MYASTHENIC SYNDROME

An underlying malignancy clearly would require treatment. For the neurological condition, treatment with 3,4-diaminopyridine may be effective. Plasma exchange and IVIG are also helpful.

CASE 6.20 – A 50-year-old, previously well man presents with a 5-month history of progressive weakness in his upper and lower limbs.

Q1: What is the likely differential diagnosis?

A1

- Motor neuron disease (MND)
- Progressive cervical myeloradiculopathy (progressive compression of the cervical cord and cervical nerve roots)

- Multifocal motor neuropathy
- Myasthenia gravis.

 Q2: What issues in the given history support/refute a particular diagnosis?

A2

The most likely diagnosis in this case is MND. Motor neuron disease is a progressive degenerative disorder of motor neurons. As the motor neuron pathway starts within the central nervous system (in the Betz cells), and travels peripherally, the clinical features of MND may be predominantly upper motor neuron, lower motor neuron or both. Motor neuron disease usually starts in the fourth to seventh decades of life. It is universally fatal, with a mean disease duration of 3 years. It begins insidiously with weakness (which may be asymmetrical), muscle atrophy or fasciculations in one or more limbs. As the disease progresses the weakness becomes more symmetrical. It is likely that the 'thinning' of the muscles described by the patient represents atrophy and that the flickering is fasciculations. There are no abnormalities of sensation in MND. No loss of anal sphincter tone occurs, because smooth muscles are not involved.

 Q3: What additional features would you seek to support a particular diagnosis?

A3

The most common form of MND involves a combination of upper and lower motor neuron features. Lower motor neuron signs include atrophy and fasciculations and upper motor neuron (i.e. corticospinal tract) signs include upgoing plantar response, spasticity and brisk tendon reflexes. More rarely the disease may predominantly affect the motor nuclei of the lower brain stem and cause weakness of the muscles of the jaw, tongue and pharynx (this is termed 'progressive bulbar palsy'). If lower motor neuron features predominate the appearances may be similar to myasthenia gravis or LEMS (helpful distinguishing features include the fact that eye signs are common in myasthenia but do not occur in MND, and wasting and fasciculations do not occur in myasthenia/LEMS). If the features are of a dominant lower motor neuron problem of the limbs, a rare form of motor peripheral neuropathy called multifocal motor neuropathy is a possible differential diagnosis (helpful distinguishing features include the fact that in multifocal motor neuropathy there is often little wasting of the muscles). High cervical cord compression (involving exiting nerve roots, i.e. cervical myeloradiculopathy) can mimic the more typical cases of MND where there are mixed upper and lower motor neuron signs. However, with a spinal cord lesion sphincter function is often affected, whereas sphincter function is preserved in MND.

 Q4: What clinical examination would you perform and why?

A4

Examination will normally show mixed upper and lower motor neuron features, as noted above.

 Q5: What investigations would be most helpful and why?

A5

- Serum creatine phosphokinase (CPK)
- Neurophysiological studies (EMG and nerve conduction tests)
- MRI of the cervical spine.

Serum CPK is often elevated in MND, but this is non-specific. MRI of the cervical spine will exclude a cervical cord lesion. In MND neurophysiological studies will show denervation in the muscle groups of at least three different segments of the body (because MND is a diffuse process) and no sensory abnormalities. In multifocal motor neuropathy, neurophysiological studies identify conduction block. The neurophsiological features of myasthenia gravis or LEMS are discussed in Case 6.17.

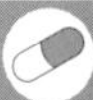 Q6: What treatment options are appropriate?

A6

- Symptomatic support
- Riluzole.

Treatment is symptomatic support, although symptomatic treatments for complications (cramps, spasticity, drooling, dysphagia, ventilatory failure) are the mainstay of managing this disease. As the disease progresses speech and swallowing may become so weak that vocal communication and oral feeding become impossible. A communication board may help with communication and a percutaneous gastrostomy feeding tube may be necessary to maintain adequate nutrition.

Ventilatory failure as a result of progressive muscle weakness develops in the later stages of the disease. Nocturnal hypoventilation may cause early-morning headache and lethargy. Non-invasive respiratory support (e.g. noctural ventilatory support using a tight-fitting mask) can help alleviate these symptoms.

The use of invasive ventilation (e.g. ventilation via tracheostomy) is a complex issue. It will prolong life but may well prolong suffering. It may also result in an altered mode of death (e.g. pneumonia). To try to accommodate patients' wishes it is important to discuss these issues at an appropriate, but relatively early, stage in the disease.

Riluzole is a disease-modifying therapy that has a modest effect. It results in a modest decrease in risk of tracheostomy or death by about 20 per cent over 12 months of treatment. However, it does not cause symptomatic improvement and does not prevent death. Side effects such as fatigue, nausea and worsening liver function may necessitate discontinuing treatment.

 CASE 6.21 – A 50-year-old man presents with a 12-month history of gradual-onset tremor in his right hand.

 Q1: What is the likely differential diagnosis?

A1

Parkinson's disease.

 Q2: What issues in the given history support/refute a particular diagnosis?

A2

Although other conditions (e.g. benign essential tremor, vascular parkinsonism or Parkinson 'plus' syndromes) can cause diagnostic confusion, this history is particularly suggestive of Parkinson's disease.

 Q3: What additional features would you seek to support a particular diagnosis?

A3

The cardinal features of Parkinson's disease are tremor, bradykinesia and rigidity. Patients are often noted to have an 'expressionless' face and their handwriting becomes smaller (micrographia). They have poor arm swing and may have stooped posture (particularly later on). Frequent falls, shuffling gait, difficulty in initiating movements and 'freezing up' occur later on in the disease course.

Some patients with cerebrovascular disease may have a parkinsonian appearance. This tends to manifest in a slow, stiff, rigid-type gait and tremor is not a major feature.

 Q4: What clinical examination would you perform and why?

A4

The tremor is 'pill rolling' (imagine rolling a pill between the index finger and thumb), which occurs at rest and NOT by intention. This is an important difference from cerebellar tremor, which is typically brought out by testing limb coordination (e.g. when attempting to touch the tip of the examiner's moving finger).

The tone will appear generally increased (rigidity) and movements (especially rapid alternating movements) slower (bradykinesia).

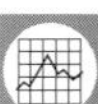 Q5: What investigations would be most helpful and why?

A5

None. In typical cases the diagnosis is made on clinical grounds alone.

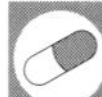 Q6: What treatment options are appropriate?

A6

- None
- Dopamine agonist
- L-Dopa with a peripheral decarboxylase inhibitor
- Catechol-*O*-methyltransferase (COMT) inhibitors

- Apomorphine
- Neurosurgery.

Treatment is symptomatic and does not alter the disease course. If the patient does not have functional limitation treatment can be deferred. In this particular case the patient appears to be limited and it would be appropriate to begin treatment.

There is an argument for trying to delay drug treatment in Parkinson's disease for as long as possible. The earlier treatment is started, the earlier the patient starts to develop difficult side effects such as unwanted movements (dyskinesias). These issues should be discussed with the patient. The 'gold standard' for treatment is L-dopa, which must be combined with a peripheral decarboxylase inhibitor to minimize peripheral side effects such as nausea and vomiting (examples include Madopar and Sinemet). This is the most efficacious treatment. However, there is evidence that treatment with this class of agent may be associated with an earlier onset of limiting dyskinesia, relative to the newer (but less efficacious) dopamine agonists that boost in vivo dopamine production. Currently it is usual practice to delay the use of L-dopa and to begin treatment with a dopamine agonist. Treatment response in the early years of the disease is very good. L-Dopa is added in when the effects of the dopamine agonists are no longer sufficient. In later disease the disease itself and the effects of treatment become more unpredictable. Patients may experience episodes when they abruptly 'freeze'. Higher doses of medication may be required to control symptoms and these may cause limiting dyskinesias. Catechol-*O*-methyltransferase inhibitors are used as treatment adjuncts, e.g. to prolong the duration of action of L-dopa or to minimize its dose. Apomorphine given subcutaneously is used in the late stage, when patients are poorly responsive to oral treatment; this reduces the duration of the 'off' periods when patients are unable to move. Neurosurgery (deep brain stimulation) may benefit carefully selected patients who have symptoms that cannot be controlled with medication.

OSCE Counselling Case – Answer

OSCE COUNSELLING CASE 6.2 – How would you explain a diagnosis of MS to a patient?

Patients need to be informed by a senior doctor and given time to ask any questions that they may have. They should be given the opportunity to have family members with them if they wish. Offering a follow-up consultation soon afterwards is also useful to address any issues that may subsequently occur to the patient. Specialist nurses play a particularly valuable role in this follow-up.

It should be explained that patients with MS have a tendency to inflammation within the brain and spinal cord, and that they may therefore experience episodes (termed 'relapses') of weakness, sensory problems or visual disturbance.

Patients are often they are very frightened that they may quickly become disabled. At diagnosis it is important to try to help the patient be positive about the condition. It can be helpful to explain that a significant proportion of patients do not suffer significant fixed deficit for many years, and that there is even a category of 'benign' MS. It is also helpful to explain that there are effective symptomatic treatments for MS. In addition, if a relapse causes a significant functional deficit, corticosteroid pulses speed recovery. If there are frequent and problematic relapses, disease-modifying therapies (interferon-β or copolymer/copaxone) can reduce the relapse rate.

It should be explained that the cause of MS is unknown but that there is a genetic susceptibility and infections can trigger relapses. Pregnancy is not a problem in MS, and in fact there is often a slight improvement during pregnancy. The risk of MS occurring in the offspring of patients with MS is about 3–5 per cent. The patient should be offered the contact details of the MS Society, who are also able to offer support and advice. As MS is a chronic neurological disease all patients receive regular follow-up. Many regions also have specialist nurse support for this condition.

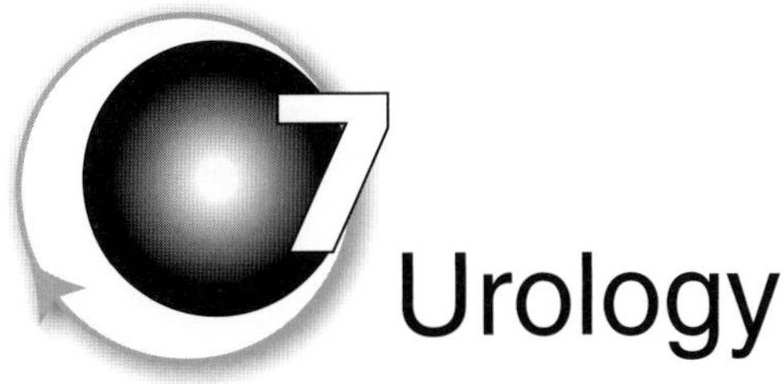

7 Urology

Suresh Ganta and Alan P. Doherty

HAEMATURIA

? Questions for each of the clinical case scenarios given

Q1: What is the likely differential diagnosis?
Q2: What issues in the given history support/refute a particular diagnosis?
Q3: What additional features would you seek to support a particular diagnosis?
Q4: What clinical examination would you perform and why?
Q5: What investigations would be most helpful and why?
Q6: What treatment options are appropriate?

Clinical cases

CASE 7.1 – 'I can see blood in my urine.'

A 65-year-old man presents to his GP with painless total haematuria with some clots. He has no associated urinary symptoms. He has been a moderate smoker for the last 40 years and worked in a chemical factory for 25 years. He has noticed a half-stone weight loss (about 3 kg) over the last 4 months.

CASE 7.2 – 'I have to go quite frequently and also have blood in my urine.'

A 35-year-old woman presents with dysuria and hourly urinary frequency. She has significant urgency and terminal haematuria. She has suprapubic discomfort and a feeling of incomplete emptying of her bladder. She has also had flu-like symptoms over the last 2 days. She has two children and is a smoker.

CASE 7.3 – 'There is blood on testing my urine.'

A 37-year-old businessman has an insurance medical health check and is found to have blood in his urine with a dipstick test. He is completely asymptomatic. He does not smoke and has had no urinary symptoms.

OSCE Counselling Case

OSCE COUNSELLING CASE 7.1 – 'How do I prevent recurrent urine infections?'

A 45-year-old woman presents with recurrent urinary infections. She has had three vaginal deliveries and required a forceps delivery for the last child who is now aged 18 years. She has noticed some stress leakage of urine and has a mild vaginal prolapse.

Key concepts

Haematuria

This is the presence of blood in the urine and is confirmed by the presence of >10–20 red blood cells (RBCs)/mL in the urine. Macroscopic (frank, visible) haematuria is more serious because it is more often associated with pathology than microscopic (on testing, i.e. urinalysis) haematuria. It may be either associated with symptoms of bladder irritability and pain, or painless. Painless haematuria may be the only symptom of an underlying cancer. Surprisingly, < 50 per cent of patients presenting with macroscopic haematuria are found to have a serious underlying disease.

Bladder cancer

This commonly presents with painless macroscopic haematuria (90 per cent). In 10 per cent of cases presenting with bladder cancer, microscopic haematuria is the only presenting symptom. Transitional cell carcinoma is the most common type of bladder cancer in Europe and the USA.

Bladder tumours are graded according to cytological and nuclear factors into a well-differentiated G1, intermediate differentiation of G2 and poorly differentiated G3.

Tumours are staged according to the depth of invasion into the muscle wall:

- pTa: non-invasive papillary carcinoma confined to the lamina propria
- pT1: tumour invades the subepithelial connective tissue known as the lamina propria
- pT2: tumour invades muscle (called the detrusor muscle)
- pT3: tumour invades perivesical tissue
- pT4: tumour invades prostate, uterus, vagina, or pelvic or abdominal wall.

Treatment depends on the stage and grade of the tumour as well as the general condition of the patient. Main options for muscle invasive tumours are surgery and radiotherapy with or without chemotherapy.

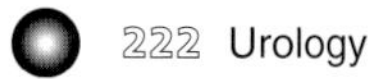

Answers

CASE 7.1 – 'I can see blood in my urine.'

Q1: What is the likely differential diagnosis?

A1

- Bladder cancer
- Bleeding from the prostate
- Renal carcinoma
- Bladder stone and
- Cystitis.

Q2: What issues in the given history support/refute a particular diagnosis?

A2

Frank haematuria has a 20 per cent probability of detecting an underlying urological malignancy. Ninety per cent of bladder cancers present with haematuria. Pain may be absent with malignancy and is usually associated with an inflammatory process causing haematuria. Smoking and occupational exposure to chemicals such as aromatic amines in the leather/textile/rubber/paint industry are known risk factors for bladder cancer.

Q3: What additional features would you seek to support a particular diagnosis?

A3

Duration of bleeding and degree of bleeding would indicate the severity of the condition and determine the need to resuscitate. A history of previous operations to the urinary tract should also be sought.

Q4: What clinical examination would you perform and why?

A4

Clinical examination is performed to determine blood loss, e.g. pallor, plus complete physical examination to identify abdominal masses and digital rectal examination (DRE) to examine the prostate.

Q5: What investigations would be most helpful and why?

A5

- Urine microscopy: to rule out infection
- Urine cytology: overall sensitivity < 75 per cent, higher for high-grade tumours
- Intravenous urogram (IVU): identifies anatomy and function of the upper tracts
- Ultrasonography: identifies abnormality of renal parenchyma
- Cystoscopy: 'gold standard' for assessment of the bladder – flexible cystoscopy under local anaesthetic or a rigid cystoscopy under general anaesthetic. This identifies the site of bleeding and whether biopsy/resection is possible.

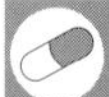

Q6: What treatment options are appropriate?

A6

Bladder tumours are diagnosed and staged after transurethral resection of the tumour (TURBT) and complete removal. Computed tomography (CT) may be appropriate in certain cases with larger tumours, to assess the extent of invasion into the bladder muscle wall and the distant spread.

Superficial bladder tumours are prone to recurrence after endoscopic treatment and ablation of the tumour, because there is often a urothelial field change. The rate of developing further recurrences depends on the size of largest tumour, number of tumours, T category, grade of tumour at diagnosis, and whether a recurrence was noted at 3 months after the primary resection.

A bladder tumour is more likely to progress and affect survival if it is poorly differentiated and higher stage, and has a high recurrence rate.

MANAGEMENT

Superficial bladder cancer (Tis, Ta, T1)

Small, solitary, low-grade mucosal diploid tumours (Ta)

- Low risk or recurrence
- TURBT
- Surveillance for recurrence by cystoscopy.

Multifocal, high-grade aneuploid tumours (Tis or T1)

- TURBT followed by a single dose of intravesical chemotherapy
- Intravesical immunotherapy/chemotherapy (single postoperative dose or every week for 6 weeks):
  - Bacille Calmette–Guérin (BCG)
  - intravesical course of chemotherapy, e.g. mitomycin.

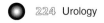

Invasive bladder cancer (T1–T4)

Radical cystectomy with pelvic lymphadenectomy and urinary diversion

External beam bladder irradiation

Systemic chemotherapy using M-VAC (methotrexate/vinblastine sulfate/doxorubicin [adriamycin]/*cis*-platinum).

Metastatic bladder cancer

Chemotherapy

- M-VAC/paclitaxel-based chemotherapy
- Gemcitabine/*cis*-platinum.

Untreated metastatic bladder cancer has a 2-year survival rate of < 5 per cent.

Box 7.1 Additional considerations for haematuria

Haematuria is a symptom of underlying cancer in the genitourinary tract in 20 per cent of patients with frank haematuria and 5 per cent of patients with microscopic haematuria. Microscopic haematuria in those aged over 50 years and macroscopic haematuria at any age are suspicious of an underlying urological malignancy and must be referred urgently. These patients should be seen within 2 weeks of referral.

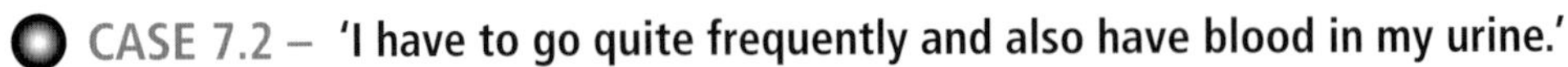

CASE 7.2 – 'I have to go quite frequently and also have blood in my urine.'

Q1: What is the likely differential diagnosis?

A1

- Urinary tract infection (UTI)
- Carcinoma *in situ* of the bladder
- Interstitial cystitis
- Bladder stones or lower ureteric stone.

Q2: What issues in the given history support/refute a particular diagnosis?

A2

- Dysuria and frequency
- Suprapubic pain or discomfort, common to patients with cystitis
- Feeling an incomplete emptying of bladder, with flu-like symptoms.

 Q3: What additional features would you seek to support a particular diagnosis?

A3

Recurrent infections often have an underlying predisposing cause. They are common in sexually active women but also occur in older postmenopausal women prone to constipation and immobility. Bladder outflow obstruction typically presents with a reduced urine flow, frequency and incomplete bladder emptying, with a high post-micturition residual volume. A history of diabetes, uterine prolapse, recent urethral instrumentation, indwelling long-term urethral catheters or stents and urinary stone disease is relevant.

Ureteric reflux of urine is another cause of re-infection and may be associated with an ascending infection (pyelonephritis), which typically presents with loin pain, fever and being systemically unwell.

 Q4: What clinical examination would you perform and why?

A4

- General examination to assess sepsis and dehydration
- Abdominal examination for masses or palpable bladder
- Vaginal examination for prolapse (in men a rectal examination to assess the prostate).

Q5: What investigations would be most helpful and why?

A5

- Dipstick:
  - leukocyte esterase test: detects pus cells in the urine
  - nitrate reductase test: detects bacteria that reduce nitrate to nitrite
- Urine microscopy and culture: identify organism and antimicrobial sensitivity
- Urine cytology: to rule out transitional cell carcinoma (TCC)
- Plain radiograph of the abdomen: identifies renal tract calcification
- Ultrasonography of renal tract: assesses renal cortex thickness and scarring (common after recurrent ascending infections) and measures post-micturition residual
- IVU: anatomy of renal tract
- Cystoscopy: if haematuria is present or there are significant symptoms
- Micturating cystourethrogram: indicated only if renal scarring is noted and clinical features suggest ureteric reflux.

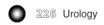

 Q6: What treatment options are appropriate?

A6

It is important to classify UTIs into simple and complicated or recurrent ones. A simple UTI is often treated empirically with broad-spectrum antibiotics followed by appropriate treatment based on urine cultures, which often take 2–3 days. Further investigations are needed if there are three episodes of cystitis in women and a single episode of infection in men.

A complicated urine infection or recurrent infection is often due to resistant organisms and requires a modified approach, often with advice from a microbiologist.

Treat predisposing causes: obstruction (urethral dilatation if the urethra is stenosed), correction of uncontrolled diabetes, treatment of stone disease and prolapse.

 CASE 7.3 – 'There is blood on testing my urine.'

 Q1: What is the likely differential diagnosis?

A1

Causes of asymptomatic microscopic haematuria by incidence:

- Benign essential haematuria (37 per cent)
- Benign prostatic hyperplasia (BPH) (24 per cent)
- UTI (27 per cent)
- Urinary stone disease (6 per cent)
- Bladder tumour (2 per cent)
- Renal cyst (1.5 per cent)
- Renal tumour (0.5 per cent).

 Q2: What issues in the given history support/refute a particular diagnosis?

A2

A nephrological cause for microscopic haematuria is common in those aged under 40 years and may be associated with hypertension and proteinuria.

 Q3: What additional features would you seek to support a particular diagnosis?

A3

- Benign causes:
  - infection
  - trauma, vigorous exercise-induced haematuria, menstruation and sexual activity
- Nephrological cause:
  - is there young-onset hypertension?
  - is there proteinuria?
  - renal insufficiency
  - red cell casts or dysmorphic red cells in urine.

Risk factors for significant disease with microscopic haematuria include:

- Smoking
- Occupational exposure to chemicals or dyes (benzenes or aromatic amines)
- History of urological disorder or disease, irritative voiding symptoms and UTI
- Analgesic abuse
- History of pelvic irradiation.

Q4: What clinical examination would you perform and why?

A4

Examine for abdominal masses and any pelvic masses, including assessment of prostate.

 Q5: What investigations would be most helpful and why?

A5

- Urine microscopy: rules out infection
- Urine phase contrast microscopy: for dysmorphic erythrocytes indicating glomerular source of bleeding
- Urine cytology: identifies transitional cell carcinoma
- IVU and ultrasonography: assess the anatomy of the renal tract and collecting system
- Renal biopsy: rarely indicated and usually supervised by a nephrologist
- Cystoscopy: the 'gold standard' investigation for the bladder.

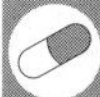

Q6: What treatment options are appropriate?

A6

The incidence of underlying urological malignancy in those presenting with microscopic haematuria is 5–7 per cent; it is therefore important to investigate all patients with microscopic haematuria.

A patient with asymptomatic microscopic haematuria, proteinuria and hypertension who is aged under 40 years is likely to have a glomerular cause for the microscopic haematuria. Immunoglobulin IgA nephropathy is the most common cause found on renal biopsy when no urological cause is noted.

Glomerular causes

- Age < 50 years
  - IgA nephropathy
  - thin basement membrane disease
  - Alport's disease (hereditary nephritis)
  - mild focal glomerulonephritis (GN)
- Age > 50 years
  - IgA nephropathy
  - Alport's disease (hereditary nephritis)
  - mild focal GN.

Referral to a nephrologist is recommended if risk factors for underlying nephrological cause are present.

Investigation of asymptomatic microscopic haematuria may also reveal an underlying urological pathology such as urinary stone disease, infections, BPH or urological cancer that is treated appropriately.

OSCE Counselling Case – Answer

OSCE COUNSELLING CASE 7.1 – 'How do I prevent recurrent urinary infections?'

Re-infection with the same strain of the organism is more common than persistence of the urinary pathogen. Colonic or perineal flora are the reservoir for these re-infecting strains. A relapse within 7 days of treatment usually indicates failure to eradicate the infection. In contrast, if bacteriuria is absent 14 days after infection and followed by a recurrence of infection, this is likely to be a re-infection. It is therefore essential to treat every infection with the appropriate antibiotic for an adequate length of time to prevent relapse.

General measures to prevent infections include adequate fluid intake, appropriate frequent voiding and postcoital micturition. It is good to achieve a short voiding interval and high flow rate, drinking large amounts of fluid to dilute the bacteria.

Regular intake of cranberry juice has been shown to be helpful in reducing recurrent infections.

Although not proven, excessive scrubbing and cleaning may damage genital skin and vaginal mucous membranes by excessive douching and reduce the normal barrier to infection.

Wiping the anus from front to back after passing stool is commonly advised.

Investigation and treatment of the predisposing factors such as stones, urethral diverticulum and diabetes.

STONE DISEASE

? Questions for each of the clinical case scenarios given

Q1: What is the likely differential diagnosis?
Q2: What issues in the given history support/refute a particular diagnosis?
Q3: What additional features would you seek to support a particular diagnosis?
Q4: What clinical examination would you perform and why?
Q5: What investigations would be most helpful and why?
Q6: What treatment options are appropriate?

Clinical cases

CASE 7.4 – 'I have pain in my loin.'

A 45-year-old woman presents to her GP with significant loin pain associated with nausea and vomiting. She has had a similar episode before and has required an operation to remove a stone in her ureter.

CASE 7.5 – 'I have recurrent infection and a dull ache in my loin.'

A 35-year-old woman presents with dysuria and passing stones/debris in her urine. She also has a dull loin ache. She has had recurrent UTIs that her GP has been treating with antibiotics for the last 2 years. She has two children and is a smoker.

CASE 7.6 – 'I have a fever and quite severe pain in my loin.'

A 37-year-old businessman had quite severe pain in his loin with a high temperature and feeling unwell.

OSCE Counselling Cases

OSCE COUNSELLING CASE 7.2 – 'How do I prevent recurrent stone formation?'

A 45-year-old woman presents with a 4-year history of recurrent urine infections. She has had two normal deliveries and has a normal menstrual cycle. Clinical examination and investigations are unremarkable.

Q1: What general measures would you recommend to reduce urine infections?

OSCE COUNSELLING CASE 7.3 – 'How do I counsel for extracorporeal shock wave lithotripsy?'

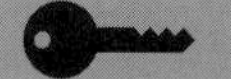

Key concepts

Presentation

- Renal pain is usually felt in the loin, sometimes spreading to the umbilicus and testis.
- Obstruction of the lower ureter may lead to bladder irritability or pain in the scrotum, penile tip or labia majora. Stones can also cause a recurrent painful desire to micturate, with only a little urine passed each time (strangury).

Predisposing factors for stone formation

- Low urine volume.
- Metabolic disorders of calcium: absorptive hypercalciuria is the most common abnormality detected in patients with calcium oxalate stones and is present in about 60 per cent of such patients. It is caused by an altered intestinal response to vitamin D, leading to increased absorption of calcium and hypercalcaemia, and decreased parathyroid hormone (PTH) secretion.
- Elevated urinary excretion/concentration of oxalate, calcium or uric acid; decreased excretion of inhibitors of stone growth; increase in urinary pH.

Basic advice and treatment for recurrent stone formers

Most important risk factor is urine volume: if the volume is doubled, the risk of forming further stones is reduced by a factor of four.

Crystalline composition of renal calculi

- Calcium oxalate (40 per cent)
- Calcium phosphate (15 per cent)
- Mixed oxalate/phosphate (20 per cent)
- Struvite (15 per cent)
- Uric acid (10 per cent)
- Miscellaneous stones 15 per cent (cystine, rare metabolites, drugs etc.).

Analysis of stone to determine composition can be useful in the management of patients with renal stones.

Answers

CASE 7.4 – 'I have pain in my loin.'

Q1: What is the likely differential diagnosis?

A1

- Ureteric colic
- Acute appendicitis
- Diverticulitis
- Ruptured aortic aneurysm
- Salpingitis
- Pyelonephritis.

Q2: What issues in the given history support/refute a particular diagnosis?

A2

- History consistent with ureteric colic, e.g. loin pain radiating to groin
- Haematuria on urinalysis and persistent pain.

Q3: What additional features would you seek to support a particular diagnosis?

A3

Duration of bleeding and degree of bleeding would indicate the severity of the condition and determine the need to resuscitate. Obtain history of previous operations to the urinary tract.

CRITERIA FOR ADMISSION

- Pain not adequately controlled
- Temperature > 37.5°C and signs of sepsis/obstructed kidney/unstable patient
- Unable to tolerate diet and fluids
- Deranged urea and electrolytes (U&Es) and raised white blood cell count (WCC).

 Q4: What clinical examination would you perform and why?

A4

Clinical examination to determine blood loss, e.g. pallor, complete physical examination to identify abdominal masses and DRE to examine the prostate.

 Q5: What investigations would be most helpful and why?

A5

- Urine microscopy: to rule out infection.
- Urine cytology: to identify TCC in the urinary tract.
- IVU: 90 per cent of stones are radio-opaque and are seen on an IVU; it is useful to assess the anatomy and function of the urinary tract and also identify the size of stone and the degree and level of obstruction.
- CT (helical/spiral CT) is the current 'gold standard' for imaging abdominal pain and can identify ureteric calculi and other causes of abdominal pain. It has a sensitivity and specificity of 96 per cent and 100 per cent, respectively.

 Q6: What treatment options are appropriate?

A6

Urgent intervention is indicated in a patient with an obstructed, infected upper urinary tract, impending renal deterioration, intractable pain or vomiting, anuria, or high-grade obstruction of a solitary or transplanted kidney.

Box 7.2 Additional considerations for abdominal pain and haematuria

An older patient with a ruptured abdominal aortic aneurysm may also present with severe abdominal pain and microscopic haematuria. This is a fatal condition and needs urgent surgical attention.

 CASE 7.5 – 'I have recurrent infection and a dull ache in my loin.'

 Q1: What is the likely differential diagnosis?

A1

- Pelviureteric junction (PUJ) obstruction
- Urinary stone disease
- Ureteric reflux disease
- Xanthogranulomatous pyelonephritis (XGPN)
- Renal tract tuberculosis (TB).

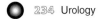

 Q2: What issues in the given history support/refute a particular diagnosis?

A2

Recurrent UTIs, fever, passing grit and stones.

 Q3: What additional features would you seek to support a particular diagnosis?

A3

A history of loin pain after increased fluid intake and alcohol would suggest obstruction of the PUJ.

Xanthogranulomatous pyelonephritis represents an unusual suppurative granulomatous reaction to chronic infection, often in the presence of chronic obstruction from a calculus, stricture or tumour, and may present with symptoms of long-standing inflammation and loin pain in patients with urinary stone disease. CT and ultrasonography show areas of pus and necrotic debris within the kidney.

Renal tract TB, although uncommon in the UK, should be considered. Pulmonary TB precedes the development of genitourinary TB.

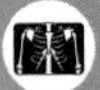 Q4: What clinical examination would you perform and why?

A4

Look for nephromegaly and complications of infections with perirenal collections.

 Q5: What investigations would be most helpful and why?

A5

- Radiograph of the abdomen: identifies renal tract calcifications
- Ultrasonography: hydronephrosis and dilatation of renal pelvis
- IVU: function and anatomy of the renal tract
- Dimethylsuccinic acid (DMSA) scan: identifies the split function of the kidney, and also useful to identify cortical scars for defining chronic infection
- Technetium-99m-labelled mercaptoacetyl triglycine (MAG-3): identifies the presence of underlying obstruction to the kidney.

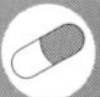 Q6: What treatment options are appropriate?

A6

Staghorn calculi require a multimodal approach to their treatment and often need more than one procedure to ensure complete removal, which is necessary because residual stone fragments quite rapidly form a nidus for further stone formation.

Struvite stones are invariably associated with urinary infections – specifically, the presence of urease-producing bacteria, including *Ureaplasma urealyticum* and *Proteus* spp. (most common); they lead to the hydrolysis of urea into ammonium and hydroxyl ions, resulting in an alkaline urine. The resultant increase in ammonium and phosphate concentrations combined with the alkaline urine (pH > 7.2) is necessary for struvite and carbonate apatite crystallization.

Treatment includes antimicrobials to reduce infection, and urinary acidifying agents to reduce stone formation.

A combination of extracorporeal shock wave lithotripsy (ESWL) and percutaneous nephrolithotomy (PCNL) is used to treat staghorn calculi.

Chemolytic therapy may be used either as a local irrigation via a nephrostomy or as oral agents. The latter have a role in patients who are not candidates for surgical removal of calculi and are also used as adjunctive therapy to dissolve residual apatite or struvite calculi and fragments after surgery, or to achieve partial dissolution of renal calculi to facilitated surgical removal.

Rarely open surgical treatment becomes necessary for the removal of large, complex renal calculi – either anatrophic nephrolithotomy (bivalving the kidney on the lateral aspect) or pyelolithotomy (opening the renal pelvis).

 CASE 7.6 – 'I have a fever and quite severe pain in my loin.'

 Q1: What is the likely differential diagnosis?

A1

Upper UTI: pyelonephritis is commonly associated with loin pain, fever and rigors. High-grade obstruction with infection in an obstructed renal system is commonly associated with severe pain and rapid septicaemia. In this case the patient will be very sick with hypotension, poor peripheral perfusion and circulatory collapse.

 Q2: What issues in the given history support/refute a particular diagnosis?

A2

Stone disease and being unwell with fever would suggest infection and possible obstruction of the ureter.

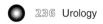

 Q3: What additional features would you seek to support a particular diagnosis?

A3

History of diabetes or immunosuppression is important as a predisposing factor.

Infection with a gas-forming organism is not uncommon in patients with diabetes – 'emphysematous pyelonephritis'. This has a high mortality rate.

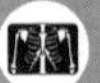 Q4: What clinical examination would you perform and why?

A4

Circulatory collapse is common with overwhelming sepsis and needs to be identified to institute appropriate resuscitation.

Complications of pyonephrosis and a perinephric abscess occur in an obstructed system that is infected. Very rarely an abscess will form and can even burst in the loin, or a psoas abscess can form in the femoral triangle.

 Q5: What investigations would be most helpful and why?

A5

- Full blood count (FBC), renal function and electrolytes
- Urine and blood cultures: most common organisms are coliforms (*Escherichia coli*, enterococci, *Proteus* spp., *Klebsiella* spp.)
- Ultrasonography: hydronephrosis, perinephric abscess
- Radiograph of the kidney, ureter and bladder: underlying stone
- Non-contrasted CT: renal tract calcification and obstructing stones in the ureter.

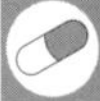 Q6: What treatment options are appropriate?

A6

Impaired glomerular filtration inhibits the entry of antibiotics into the collecting system and requires emergency decompression by means of either percutaneous nephrostomy or ureteral stenting. The best course is treatment of sepsis and resuscitation as appropriate and urgent drainage of the kidney, and treat pyonephrosis with a nephrostomy. Identify the cause of the obstruction.

The most common pathogen is *Escherichia coli*. Intravenous ampicillin and aminoglycoside provide broad antibiotic coverage, although oral fluoroquinolones may be a reasonable alternative; the type of antibiotic should be adjusted once the culture results are known.

OSCE Counselling Cases – Answers

OSCE COUNSELLING CASE 7.2 – 'How do I prevent recurrent stone formation?'

- By increasing fluid intake (e.g. cranberry juice) and frequency of bladder emptying, and pelvic floor relaxation to allow for complete bladder emptying
- Replacement of oestrogens in postmenopausal women
- Voiding after intercourse (in women). Postcoital antibiotics (if infections are noted particularly after intercourse)
- Prophylactic low-dose antibiotics (may be necessary to break the cycle of re-infection of urine).

OSCE COUNSELLING CASE 7.3 – 'How do I counsel for ESWL?'

Extracorporeal shock wave lithotripsy is a non-invasive form of stone fragmentation achieved by directing shock waves onto the stone. Shock waves are generated by electrohydraulic, piezoelectric, electromagnetic sources, which are focused on to the ureteric or renal calculus, resulting in stone fragmentation. Stones are localized using radiographs or ultrasonography. A water-filled cushion in a silicone membrane provides the interface between the patient and the shock wave generator to minimize energy dissipation.

Acute UTIs, uncorrected bleeding disorders, pregnancy, sepsis and uncorrected obstruction distal to the stone are all considered absolute contraindications. Patients with cardiac and pulmonary problems are treated with caution. Dysrhythmias are common during lithotripsy and are controlled by cardiac gating. In this setting, the shock wave is discharged by the R wave in the cardiac cycle, which prevents most tachyrhythmias. Stone sizes > 2 cm in diameter may require insertion of a JJ stent into the ureter to aid passage of stone fragments, and prevent the distal obstruction of the ureter from impacted stone fragments in the ureter – described as '*steinstrasse*' (stone street).

The stone fragmentation rate depends on the stone composition, stone size and position; calculi composed of calcium oxalate dihydrate, magnesium ammonium phosphate and uric acid fragment readily with ESWL. Calcium oxalate monohydrate and certain forms of calcium phosphate stones (e.g. brushite) are more difficult to fragment with ESWL and cystine stones are often resistant to such fragmentation. Stones within the lower pole calyx with an acute infundibulopelvic angle often do not clear, and this needs to be taken into consideration when offering advice.

The overall success rates are around 40–70 per cent.

The side effects of ESWL include pain, haematuria and loin bruising. Subcapsular haematomas in the perinephric region may be associated with severe loin pain and bruising, and may require parenteral opiates. Haematuria associated with stone fragmentation may present with clots.

The cardiac dsyrhythmias may occur with previous cardiac abnormalities.

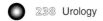

BLADDER OUTFLOW OBSTRUCTION

? Questions for each of the clinical case scenarios given

Q1: What is the likely differential diagnosis?
Q2: What issues in the given history support/refute a particular diagnosis?
Q3: What additional features would you seek to support a particular diagnosis?
Q4: What clinical examination would you perform and why?
Q5: What investigations would be most helpful and why?
Q6: What treatment options are appropriate?

Clinical cases

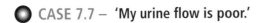

CASE 7.7 – 'My urine flow is poor.'

A 64-year-old painter presents with a reduced urinary stream and incomplete emptying of the bladder with nocturia of two to three times a night. He is a smoker and has ischaemic heart disease.

CASE 7.8 – 'I am unable to pass urine.'

CASE 7.9 – 'My husband is confused and wet.'

OSCE Counselling Case

OSCE COUNSELLING CASE 7.4 – What are the effects of surgery on the prostate?

Key concepts

Lower urinary tract symptoms:

- Bladder outflow obstruction
- Benign prostatic enlargement
- BPH
- Acute urinary retention
- Acute or chronic urinary retention
- Chronic urinary retention
- Detrusor failure.

Answers

CASE 7.7 – 'My urine flow is poor.'

Q1: What is the likely differential diagnosis?

A1

- BPH
- Diabetes mellitus
- Cystitis
- Prostatitis
- Prostate cancer.

Q2: What issues in the given history support/refute a particular diagnosis?

A2

Obstructive symptoms: namely hesitancy, reduced stream or interrupted stream, nocturia, frequency, terminal dribbling, incomplete emptying of the bladder.

Q3: What additional features would you seek to support a particular diagnosis?

A3

- Aetiology: previous endoscopic procedures or infections, stone disease, family history of prostate cancer
- General fitness and quality of life: co-morbidity with ischaemic heart disease, hypertension, diabetes etc.
- Scoring systems exist that would quantify the lower urinary tract dysfunction and the effect on the quality of life, i.e. international prostate symptom score (IPSS).

Q4: What clinical examination would you perform and why?

A4

Examination of the abdomen for a palpable bladder or masses and DRE to assess the size and consistency of the prostate.

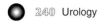

 Q5: What investigations would be most helpful and why?

A5

Urine dipstick, midstream urine (MSU) for culture and sensitivity, blood for serum creatinine, serum prostate-specific antigen (PSA) (if aged between 45 and 70 years and/or clinical examination suggests malignancy), urine flow rate and post-void residual volume of bladder by ultrasonography.

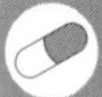 Q6: What treatment options are appropriate?

A6

Conservative treatment: advice to all patients should be appropriate fluid intake; avoid caffeine or bladder stimulants and reduce intake of fluid after 8.00pm.

 CASE 7.8 – 'I am unable to pass urine.'

 Q1: What is the likely differential diagnosis?

A1

- Obstruction to the urine outflow: prostatic enlargement
- Stress
- Neurological conditions: common in patients with multiple sclerosis and spinal cord compression (cauda equina lesion); consider this diagnosis in patients with associated abnormal neurology and in younger patients.

 Q2: What issues in the given history support/refute a particular diagnosis?

A2

History of previous obstructive lower urinary tract symptoms.

 Q3: What additional features would you seek to support a particular diagnosis?

A3

Trigger for acute urinary retention may be:

- Urine infection
- Alcohol intake
- Exacerbation of chronic obstructive airway and use of inhaled β-receptor agonists, or any drug with anticholinergic effects or α-adrenergic effects, such as antihistamines and ephedrine sulfate, which may precipitate retention

- Postoperative (major pelvic or orthopaedic surgery)
- Constipation
- Other conditions that may cause urinary retention are genital herpes, urethral stone, prostatitis and haematuria with clot retention.

Medical history of co-morbidity: diabetes, renal impairment.

Assess suitability for surgery and for α blockers (would cause postural hypotension, and judicious use is needed in elderly patients with a compromised cardiovascular system).

Q4: What clinical examination would you perform and why?

A4

- Confirm palpable bladder and abdominal examination to identify masses
- DRE to identify masses in rectum and prostate assessment
- Focused neurological examination including power and tendon reflexes in the legs and feet, examination for loss of sensation in the legs, feet and perineum. Testing for anal tone, contraction of pelvic floor muscles and the presence of the bulbocavernosus reflex (tests the integrity of the sacral cord reflex, i.e. pudendal afferents, sacral segments S2–4 and pudendal efferents. This is seen as a reflex contraction of the pelvic floor on stimulation of the glans or clitoris. This may also be elicited by gently pulling the urethral catheter).

Q5: What investigations would be most helpful and why?

A5

- Catheter specimen of urine for microscopy and culture: UTI
- Serum creatinine: renal dysfunction caused by back pressure into the renal collecting system
- Ultrasonography of renal tract: assessment of kidneys.

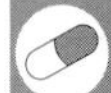

Q6: What treatment options are appropriate?

A6

- Initial treatment: symptomatic pain control, relief of retention with a urinary catheter
- Medical treatment: there is a role for α blockers in acute urinary retention. This can be started and a trial without catheter may be given within 48 h of starting the treatment. If this fails the options are either to proceed to surgery or to give another trial without a catheter in 2 weeks
- Surgical treatment: the 'gold standard' procedure is a transurethral resection of the prostate (TURP); however, there are several other modalities of treatment including laser treatment and microwave ablation that are being developed to achieve the same effect.

CASE 7.9 – 'My husband is confused and wet.'

Q1: What is the likely differential diagnosis?

A1

Acute confusional state with incontinence:

- Diabetic acidosis, electrolyte abnormalities
- Infections and dehydration
- Cerebral metastasis
- Intracranial haemorrhage/cerebrovascular accident (CVA).

Q2: What issues in the given history support/refute a particular diagnosis?

A2

Gradually increasing confusion and urinary incontinence may be caused by urinary retention, with back pressure on the renal collecting system causing uraemia. UTIs or sepsis may lead to general deterioration of health and confusion with loss of control of bodily functions. CVA or intracranial haemorrhage is associated with a neurological deficit.

Q3: What additional features would you seek to support a particular diagnosis?

A3

Urinary flow may be preserved with overflow urinary incontinence but continue to hold a significant residual volume – as much as 3–4 L. Overflow occurs with a palpable bladder when filling continues in an over-distended bladder; this is commonly painless. Precipitating factors such as constipation or a recent change of medication may be useful.

Q4: What clinical examination would you perform and why?

A4

Clinical examination to identify palpable bladder, DRE for constipation, rectal lesions and assessment of prostate; focused neurological examination.

Q5: What investigations would be most helpful and why?

A5

- Urine dipstick and microscopy: to rule out infection
- U&Es: uraemia

- Ultrasonography identifies hydronephrosis and renal cortical thickness (long-standing hydronephrosis is associated with a thinning of the renal cortex).

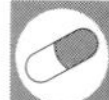 Q6: What treatment options are appropriate?

A6

Catheterization in chronic retention has the risk of inducing sepsis, and decompression of urine and pressure in the renal collecting system are associated with haematuria and a postobstructive diuresis. The haematuria may need to be treated with bladder washouts. It is important to correct the volume depleted as a result of diuresis to prevent a dehydration-induced/hypovolaemic acute tubular necrosis, in addition to the existing renal dysfunction.

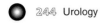

OSCE Counselling Case – Answer

OSCE COUNSELLING CASE 7.4 – What are the effects of surgery on the prostate?

Transurethral resection of the prostate is performed using a resectoscope through the urethra. It is commonly associated with postoperative bleeding, which is controlled with continuous bladder irrigation. The use of anticoagulants before the procedure increases the risk of bleeding.

Irrigating fluid (glycine) may be absorbed into the circulation, causing a transurethral resection syndrome with hypervolaemia and 1–3 per cent hyponatraemia. Mental confusion, nausea, vomiting and visual disturbance are noted, which are the result of fluid absorption and hyperammonaemia (glycine breaking down into ammonia and glycolic acid).

Surgery is associated with retrograde ejaculation in around 65–80 per cent. The subsequent urine sample shows spermatozoa on microscopy.

Erectile function: there is conflicting evidence, with either no change or some reduction in erectile function.

Failure to void after a TURP is present in up to 20 per cent of cases as a result of either insufficient resection of the prostate or detrusor failure.

Incontinence is rare (3 per cent) with urge and stress incontinence. Pre-existing detrusor overactivity caused by obstruction may manifest as urge incontinence and can be very distressing. Appropriate patient selection and counselling will reduce this risk. Resection close to the striated sphincter near the apex of the prostate may lead to sphincteric weakness, which manifests as stress incontinence or total incontinence. Conservative treatment with pelvic floor exercises may be helpful. An additional surgical procedure may be required to correct incontinence.

The alternatives, such as microwave and laser ablation of the prostate, are still not as effective as TURP.

PROSTATE CANCER AND PSA

? Questions for each of the clinical case scenarios given

Q1: What is the likely differential diagnosis?
Q2: What issues in the given history support/refute a particular diagnosis?
Q3: What additional features would you seek to support a particular diagnosis?
Q4: What clinical examination would you perform and why?
Q5: What investigations would be most helpful and why?
Q6: What treatment options are appropriate?

Clinical cases

CASE 7.10 – 'I have a raised PSA of 4 ng/mL.'

A 45-year-old businessman presents with a raised PSA after routine testing as part of his insurance screen. He is fit and well, and has no urinary symptoms.

CASE 7.11 – 'I have difficulty in passing urine.'

A 73-year-old man presents with haematuria on and off, passed clots about 3 weeks ago which settled, and has difficulty passing urine, with hesitancy, nocturia and terminal dribbling.

CASE 7.12 – 'I have severe back pain and am "off my legs".'

An 82-year-old man from a nursing home was noted to be 'off his legs' and has been complaining of back pain for about 3 weeks. He has been losing weight over the last 3 months and has a reduced appetite.

OSCE Counselling Cases

OSCE COUNSELLING CASE 7.5 – 'Do I need a blood test to check for prostate cancer?'

OSCE COUNSELLING CASE 7.6 – 'Will I be incontinent after my prostate operation?'

Q1: What are the main complications of radical retropubic prostatectomy and will I be incontinent after a prostate operation?

Key concepts

The incidence of prostate cancer is about 10 000 new cases in the UK per year, and postmortem findings show a higher incidence with increasing age. Over 50 per cent of patients aged over 90 have prostate cancer, but few of these are clinically significant. It is therefore said that 'you are more likely to die with prostate cancer than from prostate cancer'. Prostate cancer is androgen dependent, which is useful in its treatment.

The higher the PSA level the more likely is the presence of prostate cancer. Large cancers can cause symptoms of bladder outflow obstruction. Prostate cancer may present with metastasis, and cord compression caused by spinal metastases is a surgical emergency.

The Gleason grade for prostate cancer utilizes the architecture of the gland to describe the level of differentiation. Scores range from 1 to 5, with 1 being the least aggressive and 5 being the most aggressive. To represent the heterogeneity of prostate cancer the most predominant grade and the second most predominant grade are added to make up the Gleason score, e.g. 3 + 2 = 5.

Treatment depends on the stage and grade of the tumour, and the co-morbidity of the patient.

Localized prostate cancer is often treated with an intention to cure. Options include radical prostatectomy or radical radiotherapy. Low-grade, low-volume prostate cancer and localized cancer in elderly men may be treated with active surveillance.

Locally advanced prostate cancer may be treated with radiotherapy or hormone treatment, with androgen withdrawal by castration, either surgically or using drugs (anti-androgens or gonadotrophin-releasing hormone or GnRH analogue).

Answers

 CASE 7.10 – 'I have a raised PSA of 4 ng/mL.'

 Q1: What is the likely differential diagnosis?

A1

- BPH
- Prostate cancer
- Prostatitis
- UTI
- Prostatic calculi
- Instrumentation of the urethra and prostate.

A raised PSA is not specific for prostate cancer but can occur with a range of conditions. PSA levels in serum are related to the size of the prostate. PSA may also increase with age and the age-specific PSA range in a man younger than 50 years is < 2.5 ng/mL, whereas in a man > 70 years PSA levels of up to 6.5 ng/mL are acceptable.

 Q2: What issues in the given history support/refute a particular diagnosis?

A2

There is no history of a previous UTI and urethral instrumentation or symptoms to suggest prostatitis. Prostate cancer needs to be excluded.

 Q3: What additional features would you seek to support a particular diagnosis?

A3

Urinary symptoms suggest a urinary infection and symptoms of prostatitis. Risk factors of prostate cancer include family history, age and race (more common in black men and less common in Asian men). Radical treatment of prostate cancer would require an estimated lifespan of at least 10 years to benefit from the treatment.

Q4: What clinical examination would you perform and why?

A4

Clinical examination should include a DRE to assess the prostate. A tender prostate would suggest prostatitis. The presence of a nodule or hard lobe of the prostate suggests a cancer. Digital rectal examination is also useful to assess local spread to the seminal vesicles and laterally beyond the prostate in advanced disease.

Q5: What investigations would be most helpful and why?

A5

- Urine microscopy: isolates urine infection.
- Repeat PSA is more useful in borderline elevations and also in the presence of urine infection, prostatitis or recent instrumentation.
- Transrectal ultrasonography is useful to identify abnormal anatomy of the prostate and also to target prostate biopsies.
- Prostate biopsy: the gold standard for making a diagnosis.
- Bone scan: if the PSA is > 10 ng/mL, a bone scan would be useful to identify bony metastases.

Q6: What treatment options are appropriate?

A6

LOCALIZED PROSTATE CANCER

Treatment options are radical prostatectomy, radical radiotherapy, brachytherapy and active surveillance.

REASONS FOR A RADICAL PROSTATECTOMY

- Removes a potential source of metastatic and locally advanced disease.
- Other treatments may be as good (yet to be proven) but not likely to be better.
- Early prostate cancers allow for a nerve-sparing prostatectomy with preservation of potency.
- Removes a gland that grows with age and may eventually cause lower urinary tract symptoms.
- Early assessment of cure with PSA measurements (which should be zero).
- Use of salvage radiotherapy is effective, safe and well established in cases of failure. Surgery after radiotherapy is possible although far less well established.
- No risk of second malignancy.
- Keyhole (laparoscopic) approach is minimally invasive.

REASONS FOR RADICAL RADIOTHERAPY/BRACHYTHERAPY

It has comparable results to radical surgery, although surgery may be better for poorly differentiated disease. There is no need for invasive treatment.

REASONS FOR CHOOSING ACTIVE MONITORING

In lower-grade tumours with small-volume disease it may be reasonable to monitor them closely with frequent PSA measurements and to treat aggressively if evidence of disease or grade progression is noted.

- High-grade prostatic intraepithelial neoplasia (PIN): this may be a pre-neoplastic condition and also suggests that there is adjacent prostate cancer; a repeat biopsy is recommended. Close observation is prudent.
- Normal biopsy: PSA needs to be monitored because there is a risk of a false-negative biopsy as a result of a sampling error; a rising PSA would necessitate further investigation (repeat prostate biopsies).

CASE 7.11 – 'I have difficulty in passing urine.'

Q1: What is the likely differential diagnosis?

A1

- BPH
- Prostate cancer
- Urethral stricture
- Urinary stones.

Q2: What issues in the given history support/refute a particular diagnosis?

A2

Presents with local symptoms of urinary outflow obstruction. Family history of prostate cancer is a known risk factor for prostate cancer.

Q3: What additional features would you seek to support a particular diagnosis?

A3

Prostate cancer may be locally advanced with urinary obstruction and may present with haematuria. Locally advanced prostate cancer may also involve the trigone of the bladder and obstruct one or both ureters, causing hydronephrosis and uraemia. Metastatic prostate cancer spreads to bones and lymph nodes. The presence of bony pain and nodal enlargement is elicited.

Q4: What clinical examination would you perform and why?

A4

Clinical examination to identify the presence of a palpable bladder and DRE to identify the stage of the prostate cancer.

 Q5: What investigations would be most helpful and why?

A5

- Urine microscopy: rule out infection or prostatitis
- PSA: > 10 ng/mL is associated with an increased risk of metastatic prostatic cancer
- U&Es: uraemia
- Transrectal ultrasonography and prostate biopsy: confirm diagnosis of prostate cancer
- Ultrasonography of renal tract: hydronephrosis and renal cortex thickness
- Bone scan: metastatic screen.

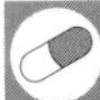 Q6: What treatment options are appropriate?

A6

Symptomatic prostate cancer is treated on the basis of being clinically localized or metastatic. Clinically localized disease is treated with radical treatment, i.e. surgery, radiotherapy or active surveillance. Brachytherapy is not suitable for patients with lower urinary tract symptoms because subsequent transurethral surgery has a high risk of incontinence.

Locally advanced prostate cancer may be treated symptomatically. Bladder outflow obstruction may be treated with hormones if there are no signs of urinary retention. Hormone treatment is known to reduce the size of the prostate and will improve the urinary symptoms. Hormone treatment may be followed by surgery or radiotherapy in selected patients.

Intermittent hormone treatment is being considered and has the advantage of a 'treatment holiday' to improve the quality of life of patients on hormone therapy/androgen withdrawal without affecting survival.

CASE 7.12 – 'I have severe back pain and am "off my legs".'

 Q1: What is the likely differential diagnosis?

A1

- Spinal cord compression from tumour or osteoporotic collapse
- Subdural or epidural abscess or haematoma
- Transverse myelitis
- Multiple sclerosis (MS)
- Acute postviral – Guillain–Barré disease.

 Q2: What issues in the given history support/refute a particular diagnosis?

A2

- Pain in the back or radiating from the back – can be exacerbated by coughing or movement
- Loss of sensation in lower part of the body
- Retention of urine
- Bowel and bladder dysfunction, incontinence.

 Q3: What additional features would you seek to support a particular diagnosis?

A3

Sequence of events with pain, loss of function and loss of sensation should be sought. The pain and mild weakness may last hours to days, but the transition to total loss of function distal to the lesion may take only minutes.

Patients who are started on hormone treatment with androgen withdrawal (GnRH analogues) have a 'testosterone flare' resulting from the initial stimulation of the testosterone release by the GnRH release; this must be monitored carefully because it may induce an enlargement of the spinal metastasis and precipitate cord compression. Therefore, it is important to use an anti-androgen for 2 weeks before the GnRH injection.

Q4: What clinical examination would you perform and why?

A4

- Examination of the abdomen and DRE
- Focused neurological examination necessary to identify cord compression
- Spine tenderness (percussion tenderness is especially prominent with metastatic carcinoma, vertebral infection, or spinal or epidural abscess), paraparesis, sensory deficits of the limbs or trunk, and corticospinal reflex changes.

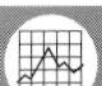 Q5: What investigations would be most helpful and why?

A5

- PSA
- Transrectal ultrasonography and prostate biopsy: diagnose prostate cancer
- Plain spinal radiograph: identifies sclerosis, osteoporosis and crush fractures
- CT or magnetic resonance imaging (MRI): tumours in spine with cord compression and nerve root involvement.

 Q6: What treatment options are appropriate?

A6

Any patient with suspected spinal cord compression should be admitted as an emergency for investigation and treatment. Once paralysed, only 5 per cent walk again; 30 per cent of patients survive to 1 year.

Best results are obtained when treatment is instituted early:

- Medical treatment: dexamethasone to relieve the oedema, analgesia
- Radiotherapy: useful to reduce the compression urgently
- Surgery: surgical decompression, urgent referral to a neurosurgeon.

OSCE Counselling Case – Answer

OSCE COUNSELLING CASE 7.5 – 'Do I need a blood test to check for prostate cancer?'

If the PSA is elevated the risk of having prostate cancer depends on the value:

- PSA 4–10: risk of underlying prostate cancer is 25 per cent
- PSA > 10: risk of underlying prostate cancer is 50 per cent

The probability (percentage) of prostate cancer depends on age and DRE (Table 7.1).

Table 7.1 PSA score and DRE result

Age (years)	< 50		51–60		61–70		71–80	
PSA (ng/mL)	DRE –	DRE +	DRE –	DRE +	DRE –	DRE +	DRE –	DRE +
< 2.5	9	37	12	39	15	42	20	44
2.6–4.0	9	41	12	42	16	44	20	47
4.1–6.0	10	41	14	44	17	47	22	48
6.1–10.0	11	–	15	48	19	50	25	42
10.1–20.0	13	55	19	54	25	58	31	60
> 20.0	22	82	45	74	43	81	59	84

DRE = digital rectal examination; PSA = prostate-specific antigen.
DRE – = normal DRE; DRE + = abnormal DRE.
Data from Potter et al. (2001) Age, prostate-specific antigen, and digital rectal examination as determinants of the probability of having prostate cancer. *Urology* **57**, 1100–4.

A prostate biopsy has a 1–3 per cent risk of complications of bleeding, infection and urinary retention.

BENEFITS OF PSA TESTING

1. It may provide reassurance if the test result is normal.
2. It may find cancer before symptoms develop.
3. It may detect cancer at an early stage when treatments could be beneficial.
4. If treatment is successful, the consequences of more advanced cancer are avoided.
5. Screening might detect the cancer at an earlier stage. Tumours detected by PSA testing are now thought to be significant tumours that should be treated.

DOWNSIDE OF PSA TESTING

1. It can miss cancer and provide false reassurance.

2. It may lead to unnecessary anxiety and medical tests when no cancer is present.
3. It might detect slow-growing cancer that may never cause any symptoms or shorten lifespan.
4. The main treatments of prostate cancer have significant side effects, and there is no certainty that the treatment of tumours discovered by screening makes any difference to the overall survival of the patients treated.

Routine PSA screening is not currently recommended in the UK for asymptomatic individuals; however, the PSA test may be performed in patients aged over 50 years who present with lower urinary tract symptoms or who request it.

Those with a family history of prostate cancer and from an African–Caribbean origin should be advised to be tested from the age of 40 years or may even have PSA testing earlier.

OSCE COUNSELLING CASE 7.6 – 'Will I be incontinent after my prostate operation?'

Q1: What are the main complications of RRP and will I be incontinent after a prostate operation?

Surgery is commonly offered to patients with an expected survival of over 10 years and localized prostate cancer.

Surgery may be performed by an open or laparoscopic route: the open approach may be retropubic or perineal. A bilateral nerve-sparing approach may be considered if suitable; this is more likely to preserve erectile function. A laparoscopic route has the advantage of minimum morbidity with acceptable oncological outcomes.

Inpatient stay varies with approach used: open operations require a stay of 4–7 days and the laparoscopic route requires 2–4 days.

The following are the common complications:

- Impotence: where bilateral nerve sparing is performed the return of erectile function is between 50 and 70 per cent. Bilateral nerve sparing is only safely offered to patients with early disease, i.e. screen detected. Taking all types of radical prostatectomy together, i.e. nerve and non-nerve-sparing, recent studies suggest that over 56 per cent of men will be completely impotent and a further 29 per cent will have a reduced erection.
- Incontinence: severe incontinence is noted in 1–3 per cent, and occasional loss of control in 10–20 per cent of patients.
- Mortality: the mortality rate is 0.7 per cent.

INCONTINENCE

? Questions for each of the clinical case scenarios given

Q1: What is the likely differential diagnosis?
Q2: What issues in the given history support/refute a particular diagnosis?
Q3: What additional features would you seek to support a particular diagnosis?
Q4: What clinical examination would you perform and why?
Q5: What investigations would be most helpful and why?
Q6: What treatment options are appropriate?

Clinical cases

CASE 7.13 – 'I have a urinary leak every time I cough or strain.'

A 48-year-old woman is postmenopausal and has a minor leak of urine every time she coughs and sneezes. She has three children, the last one needing a forceps delivery.

CASE 7.14 – 'I have recurrent infections and can't get to the toilet in time.'

A 24-year-old teacher with frequency and urgency every 30 min and urge incontinence.

CASE 7.15 – 'I have been leaking ever since the operation.'

A 38-year-old woman has been continually wet after a vaginal hysterectomy. She did not have any urinary symptoms before the operation.

OSCE Counselling Case

OSCE COUNSELLING CASE 7.7 – 'I keep going to the toilet every 30 min!'

A 34-year-old solicitor has difficulty coping with work because she has to go to the toilet every 30 min; she has day-time frequency and urgency and no nocturia. She has recurrent episodes of cystitis although the urine tests do not grow any organisms. She takes 10 cups of tea every day and about three to four cans of coke. She has no children. She had a normal bladder examination and biopsy.

Key concepts

- Urinary incontinence: involuntary leakage of urine.
- Stress urinary incontinence: loss of urine after increases in intra-abdominal pressure. This is caused by a failure to maintain the normal retropubic position of the bladder neck and posterior urethra during increases in abdominal pressure and/or impaired internal sphincter mechanism.
- Urge incontinence: incontinence associated with urgency; commonly caused by an overactive bladder.
- Total incontinence: may be a result of complete loss of sphincteric control or a fistula (abnormal communication between the urinary tract and the skin). The most common cause of fistulae is iatrogenic and may be ureterovaginal or vesicovaginal.
- An overactive bladder is a symptom complex that includes urinary urgency with or without urge incontinence, urinary frequency (voiding eight or more times in a 24-h period) and nocturia (awakening two or more times at night to void). It is a syndrome with no precise cause and local causes are excluded. The urodynamic evidence of detrusor overactivity is commonly noted in patients with an overactive bladder.

Patients with symptoms of an overactive bladder with underlying mucosal (carcinoma *in situ*, interstitial cystitis, cystitis, bladder stone) or neurological causes (Parkinson's disease, MS, spinal cord injury, diabetic neuropathy etc.) and extrinsic causes (e.g. bladder outlet obstruction) are excluded from the overactive bladder syndrome. The urodynamic diagnosis is confirmed by detrusor overactivity.

Answers

 CASE 7.13 – 'I have a urinary leak every time I cough or strain.'

 Q1: What is the likely differential diagnosis?

A1

- Stress urinary incontinence
- Urge urinary incontinence (with stress-induced contraction and urinary leak)
- Overflow incontinence resulting from neurological causes or anticholinergic effects of drugs
- UTI
- Atrophic vaginitis
- Acute confusional state
- Increased urine output, e.g. heart failure, diuretics, hyperglycaemia.

 Q2: What issues in the given history support/refute a particular diagnosis?

A2

Postmenopausal, complicated obstetric history with instrumental delivery.

 Q3: What additional features would you seek to support a particular diagnosis?

A3

- Lower urinary tract symptoms in keeping with an overactive bladder such as frequency, urgency, nocturia or suprapubic discomfort.
- Voiding diary to identify the amount and type of fluid intake and the frequency of voiding with urinary leaks. Assessment of the number of pads and pad weight (as a measure of severity of leakage).
- The causes of an abnormal urethral support mechanism include congenital weakness and shortness of the vagina, difficult labour, multiparity and menopause. Iatrogenic causes include radical or simple hysterectomy and other types of extensive pelvic surgery.
- Oestrogen deficiency plays a role in the maintenance of the pliability of the urethral mucosa and submucosa and may also present with dyspareunia.
- Chronic inflammatory tissue from previous surgical procedures and radiotherapy also compromises the urethral closure mechanism.
- The sphincteric weakness resulting from damage to the innervation of the urethral musculature may also lead to stress urinary leak: sensory loss and history of neurological dysfunction.

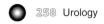

 Q4: What clinical examination would you perform and why?

A4

- A palpable bladder: in overflow incontinence.
- Focused neurological examination: including examination of power and tendon reflexes of the legs and feet, and examination for loss of sensation in legs, feet and perineum. Bulbocavernosus reflex and anal tone.
- Descent of the pelvic floor and anterior vaginal wall is noted with a Valsalva manoeuvre. Loss of urine when the bladder is partially full, and eradication of this leak when the urethra is supported by digital elevation of the urethrovesical junction, suggest that surgical correction would be effective.
- Assessment of the contraction of the pelvic floor muscles, pelvic prolapse and the oestrogen status in the vagina.

 Q5: What investigations would be most helpful and why?

A5

- Urine dipstick and urine culture: rule out urine infection.
- Postvoid residual measurement: helps to identify the treatment procedure and whether further investigations are necessary.
- Urodynamics: rarely necessary and usually performed only before surgical intervention to rule out detrusor overactivity as a cause of incontinence.
- Valsalva leak-point pressure and fluoroscopy may rarely be performed and are useful for identifying the anatomy of the bladder neck and urethra.

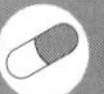 Q6: What treatment options are appropriate?

A6

BEHAVIOUR MODIFICATION

All patients benefit from behavioural modification, weight loss and appropriate fluid management:

- Pelvic floor exercises to strengthen the muscles, called Kegel's exercises
- Voluntary contraction and relaxation of the levator ani musculature, particularly the pubococcygeus muscle
- Use of vaginal cones with weights, vaginal electrical stimulation and biofeedback.

PHARMACOTHERAPY

α-Adrenergic agonists act on the bladder neck and proximal urethra and increase the urethral closure pressure, e.g. ephedrine, phenylpropanolamine.

Newer agents such as duloxetine, which is a dual serotonin (5-HT)/noradrenaline (norepinephrine) re-uptake blocker with antidepressant action, is also useful in stress incontinence.

Tricyclic antidepressants, which inhibit the re-uptake of noradrenaline, and their anticholinergic effects simultaneously inhibit bladder activity and are useful in mixed incontinence.

SURGERY

Stress urinary incontinence caused by urethral hypermobility and descent of the bladder neck may be assessed clinically and correction of the abnormality is sufficient to improve symptoms.

Tension-free vaginal tape placement and colposuspension are useful in correcting urethral hypermobility and have good long-term effects.

CASE 7.14 – 'I have recurrent infections and can't get to the toilet in time.'

Q1: What is the likely differential diagnosis?

A1

- Overactive bladder
- Ingestion of bladder stimulants, e.g. caffeine, alcohol etc.
- Cystitis
- Bladder abnormalities, e.g. bladder stone, interstitial cystitis, bladder cancer
- Obstruction, e.g. in men with prostate enlargement
- Neurological conditions: stroke, MS
- Increased urine output, e.g. diabetes, cardiac failure.

Q2: What issues in the given history support/refute a particular diagnosis?

A2

Frequency, urgency and urge incontinence are symptoms of bladder irritation.

Q3: What additional features would you seek to support a particular diagnosis?

A3

A voiding diary (frequency and volume of voiding including incontinence episodes) and fluid volume chart (record of the amount and type of fluid intake) are crucial to the diagnosis.

An overactive bladder is diagnosed when all the known causes of bladder irritation have been excluded, and when symptoms of frequency and urgency are present. Bladder cancer, urine infection and bladder stones are the common causes of bladder irritation and need to be ruled out by an appropriate history. Neurological conditions are associated with neurological abnormalities.

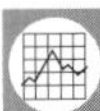 Q4: What clinical examination would you perform and why?

A4

- Examination to rule out a palpable bladder, neurological examination
- Assessment of the contraction of the pelvic floor muscles, pelvic prolapse and the vaginal oestrogen status
- The prostate is assessed in men by DRE.

Q5: What investigations would be most helpful and why?

A5

- Urine dipstick and microscopy: exclude cystitis
- Blood glucose and electrolytes: diabetes and renal impairment
- Urine cytology: useful screen for bladder cancer
- Cystoscopy and/or biopsy: interstitial cystitis and carcinoma *in situ* are identified with a bladder biopsy and appearance on cystoscopy
- Ultrasonography and radiograph: postvoid residual volume, assessment of kidneys and screen for bladder calculi
- Flow rate (in men)
- Urodynamics: diagnose detrusor overactivity.

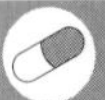 Q6: What treatment options are appropriate?

A6

BEHAVIOURAL MODIFICATION

Appropriate fluid management is commonly sufficient to avoid bladder stimulants, and intake of fluid in the evening should be avoided to prevent nocturia. Pelvic floor exercises are useful as a biofeedback mechanism to treat an overactive bladder.

When urgency is present without significant frequency, timed voiding is useful (a conscious emptying of the bladder on a regular schedule, despite the absence of urgency, every 2–3 h).

Urgency and frequency are treated with 'bladder retraining' by gradually increasing the frequency between voiding.

Biofeedback and electrical stimulation are also useful adjuncts to treatment.

PHARMACOTHERAPY

Anticholinergics acting on the muscarinic receptors are useful to suppress involuntary bladder contractions. The common side effects include dry mouth, constipation and blurred vision, which can be troublesome.

Tricyclic antidepressants also have similar effects on the bladder and often a combination may be required.

SURGERY

- Cystoscopy and biopsy are useful to rule out inflammatory causes of overactive bladder symptoms.
- Hydrodistension of the bladder at a pressure of > 60–100 cmH_2O for 5 min under an anaesthetic may lead to some short-term improvement of symptoms and is more useful in a contracted bladder.
- Augmentation of the bladder using a patch of detubularized bowel or by a detrusor myomectomy.
- Extradural stimulation of S3 nerve root exerts its effect by stimulating the sacral sensory fibres, which have the ability to inhibit the sacral parasympathetic neurons responsible for detrusor contraction.

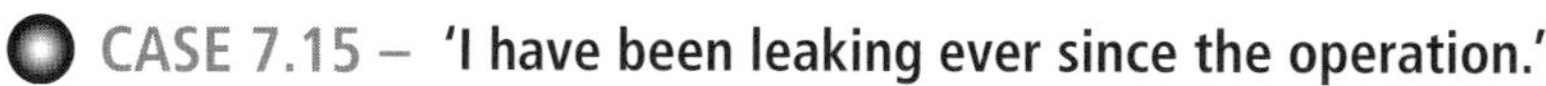

CASE 7.15 – 'I have been leaking ever since the operation.'

Q1: What is the likely differential diagnosis?

A1

- Vesicovaginal fistula/ureterovaginal fistula
- Urethral incontinence.

Q2: What issues in the given history support/refute a particular diagnosis?

A2

- History of operation, no urinary symptoms before surgery.
- Iatrogenic trauma is the most common cause of fistulae in developed countries. Obstructed labour is the most common cause in the developing world.

Q3: What additional features would you seek to support a particular diagnosis?

A3

- The type of operation is important to the aetiology: abdominal hysterectomy, Wertheim's hysterectomy, anterior colporrhaphy or vaginal hysterectomy. The risk of ureteric injury after a standard hysterectomy is 0.5–1.5 per cent and the risk of a fistula is < 1 per cent. The fistula develops soon after the procedure or may be delayed by 2 or more weeks if ischaemic necrosis of the tissues is its cause.

- History of irradiation is an important cause of genitourinary fistulae. They are associated with bladder pain and infection in 40 per cent of cases.
- Direct invasion in late stages of cancer, e.g. cervical cancer.
- Assessment of the severity of urine loss by number of pads and pad weight.

Q4: What clinical examination would you perform and why?

A4

- Examination of the abdomen and genitalia, radiation changes and dermatitis from urinary contact of the skin.
- Three-pad test: performed by inserting three dry cotton-wool swabs into the upper, middle and lower thirds of the vagina. The bladder is adequately distended with methylene blue and any leakage around the catheter is stopped. The swabs in the lower and middle third of the vagina soaking with methylene blue would indicate a vesicovaginal fistula. If the upper third vaginal swab is soaked with clear urine it is likely to be a uretrovaginal fistula (multiple fistulae and vesicouretric reflux may yield false-positive results).
- Direct inspection of the vagina after instillation of dye into the bladder to see the size and site of the fistula.

Q5: What investigations would be most helpful and why?

A5

- Biochemical analysis of the fluid: to confirm urine leak
- IVU: ureteric fistula is associated with ureteric dilatation and/or hydronephrosis and extravasation of contrast
- Cystoscopy and examination under anaesthetic may be helpful to assess the pliability of the tissues and define the fistula.

Q6: What treatment options are appropriate?

A6

Initially insert a catheter and often a small fistula will heal in 3–4 weeks by conservative management.

Surgical repair may become necessary and often the first operation is the best chance to cure the patient, so it must be done by an expert in a specialist centre with appropriate support.

Early repair is in favour because of the improvement in quality of life; if injury to the bladder or ureter is noted intraoperatively, it must be repaired immediately. However, commonly the fistula is not obvious until 2–3 weeks after the procedure. The urine needs to be diverted with either a catheter or a nephrostomy as necessary and the infection treated.

The basic principles of fistula repair are as follows:

- The fistulous tract is excised to healthy, well-vascularized tissue.
- The repair should be tension free and multilayered using absorbable sutures.
- Techniques to improve the viability of the tissue by interposing well-vascularized tissues between the bladder and vagina, e.g. a Martius flap using a flap of labial fibrofatty tissue and the omental flap.

OSCE Counselling Case

OSCE COUNSELLING CASE 7.7 – 'I keep going to the toilet every 30 min!'

Urodynamics: catheterization was painful. It shows a reduced first sensation of filling and a reduced bladder capacity as a result of discomfort. There was no detrusor overactivity or rise in the detrusor pressure during filling.

The patient is worried that she will require major surgery. Counsel her about the various options available.

OVERACTIVE BLADDER SYNDROME WITH FREQUENCY, URGENCY AND NOCTURIA

A voiding diary with a frequency/volume chart is useful to assess severity of symptoms. Day-time frequency not associated with nocturia is typical of a sensory urgency, as opposed to a contracted bladder which produces both nocturia and day-time frequency.

The treatment for a hypersensitive bladder (increased bladder sensation during filling the bladder at urodynamics) is treatment of the cause of the condition, which is often cystitis, urethritis, inflammatory bladder conditions such as interstitial cystitits, post-irradiation cystitis, or chemical or cyclophosphamide cystitis.

When all the causes have been excluded, there is a condition with no evidence of inflammation of the bladder although instrumentation of the urethra is painful. This is referred to as urethral syndrome.

The treatment is to maintain a voiding diary and a fluid volume chart. Reduction in bladder stimulants such as tea and cola would help to improve symptoms. Bladder retraining, use of pelvic floor exercises and biofeedback techniques have a role in management. The involvement of the patient in self-help groups and judicious use of anticholinergics are useful.

Surgery has a minor role.

NEUROPATHIC BLADDER

? Questions for each of the clinical case scenarios given

Q1: What is the likely differential diagnosis?
Q2: What issues in the given history support/refute a particular diagnosis?
Q3: What additional features would you seek to support a particular diagnosis?
Q4: What clinical examination would you perform and why?
Q5: What investigations would be most helpful and why?
Q6: What treatment options are appropriate?

Clinical cases

CASE 7.16 – 'I have leakage and have to go very frequently.'

A 30-year-old T6 paraplegic woman has been performing intermittent self-catheterization (ISC) for 3 years since her accident. She has been on maximum doses of anticholinergics and has been leaking in between her catheterizations. She also notices pain in her loin, recurrent infections and one episode of pyelonephritis. Q1 is not applicable in this case.

CASE 7.17 – 'I am unable to pass urine.'

A 35-year-old woman presented with inability to pass urine, and had loss of power and a tingling sensation in her feet. She also noticed constipation in the last 2 weeks and burning sensation over her genitalia. She had an episode of transient blurring of the vision in her right eye but recovered spontaneously about 2 years ago.

CASE 7.18 – 'I have recurrent infections.'

A 27-year-old who was paraplegic after a road traffic accident has been performing ISC for about 3 years and presents with increasing UTIs. Over the last 6 months he has had over six infections. Q1 only.

Key concepts

- Spinal cord injury
- Sacral/cauda equina lesion
- Detrusor–sphincter dyssynergia (DSD).

Answers

 ## CASE 7.16 – 'I have leakage and have to go very frequently.'

 ### Q2: What issues in the given history support/refute a particular diagnosis?

A2

Urinary leak in between catheterizations would indicate either infrequent catheterizations or improper technique (suggesting that the bladder is not being emptied adequately).

Urine infections are also a common cause of urinary leak.

The history of ascending UTIs is in keeping with incomplete emptying of the bladder with some evidence of reflux.

 ### Q3: What additional features would you seek to support a particular diagnosis?

A3

Spinal cord lesions are commonly associated with DSD: the normal coordinated relaxation of the sphincter to detrusor contraction at the time of voiding is lost. The detrusor contracts against a closed sphincter, thereby generating significant bladder pressures to eventually become transmitted to the kidney. This results in renal damage.

 ### Q4: What clinical examination would you perform and why?

A4

- Examination of the abdomen to rule out a palpable bladder.
- Systemic examination to rule out organomegaly.

 ### Q5: What investigations would be most helpful and why?

A5

- Urine culture and sensitivity
- Urodynamics: detrusor overactivity of neurogenic origin, often associated with DSD
- Ultrasonography of the renal tract: to assess underlying causes of infection, e.g. stone, large residual volume, damage to upper tracts with renal scarring and dilatation
- MAG-3 scan: to assess split function of the renal tract
- Video-urodynamics: would confirm detrusor overactivity, DSD, anatomical abnormalities of the urinary tract and reflux of urine into the upper tracts.

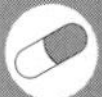 Q6: What treatment options are appropriate?

A6

The urinary symptoms of patients with spinal injuries are commonly managed by intermittent self-catheterization and with anticholinergics. This would ensure that the bladder volumes remain low and reduce the bladder pressure, which is sufficient to retain continence. It also reduces the risk of upper tract damage.

To reduce the bladder pressure it may be necessary to augment the bladder using a patch of detubularized bowel segment onto the bivalved bladder (clam cystoplasty).

If incontinence is still a problem, then improvement in the urethral resistance may be achieved by surgically inserting an artificial sphincter which may be regulated to achieve continence.

A major surgical procedure is to divide the posterior nerve roots (posterior rhizotomy) and insert a surgical implant in the anterior sacral nerve roots (S2–4). This converts the bladder into an areflexic bladder with no sensation. The bladder is drained by stimulating the anterior nerve roots, which may be activated by a subcutaneous transducer.

 CASE 7.17 – 'I am unable to pass urine.'

 Q1: What is the likely differential diagnosis?

A1

- MS
- Spinal cord compression or tumour
- Urethral sphincter overactivity
- Pelvic masses and tumours
- Chronic constipation.

 Q2: What issues in the given history support/refute a particular diagnosis?

A2

Multiple sclerosis is more common in women and the under-40s, and also when there is a previous history of optic neuritis and neurological symptoms.

 Q3: What additional features would you seek to support a particular diagnosis?

A3

- UTIs and constipation
- History of ovarian tumours and pelvic masses.

 Q4: What clinical examination would you perform and why?

A4

- Focused examination of the abdomen and pelvis, and DRE.
- Neurological examination, including assessment of the motor, sensory and tendon reflexes of lower limbs, and perineal sensation, including bulbocavernosus reflex (BCR), to confirm integrity of the sacral reflex arc. A negative BCR would mean that the patient most probably has a spinal cord lesion, whereas a positive BCR does not rule out a cord lesion.

 Q5: What investigations would be most helpful and why?

A5

- Urine dipstick and microscopy
- Ultrasonography of abdomen and pelvis
- MRI of spinal cord and cauda equina.

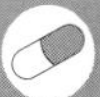 Q6: What treatment options are appropriate?

A6

Referral to a neurologist is appropriate and the immediate treatment consists of relieving the urinary retention.

The long-term outcome depends on progression of the MS.

 CASE 7.18 – 'I have recurrent infections.'

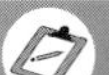 Q1: What is the likely differential diagnosis?

A1

Patients with paraplegia have a tendency to develop urinary tract calculi.

The differential diagnosis is likely to be incomplete emptying of the bladder and re-infection through the use of the wrong technique for ISC.

UPPER TRACT OBSTRUCTION AND RENAL MASS

? Questions for each of the clinical case scenarios given

Q1: What is the likely differential diagnosis?
Q2: What issues in the given history support/refute a particular diagnosis?
Q3: What additional features would you seek to support a particular diagnosis?
Q4: What clinical examination would you perform and why?
Q5: What investigations would be most helpful and why?
Q6: What treatment options are appropriate?

Clinical cases

CASE 7.19 – 'I have pain in my loin when I have a drink.'

A 25-year-old woman presents to her GP with significant pain in her loin and nausea and vomiting after a night out with her friends. She has had a similar episode before and has had an episode of urinary infection in the past.

CASE 7.20 – A 57-year-old man with advanced malignancy has bilateral hydronephrosis.

A 57-year-old man presented with a recurrent colorectal tumour with advanced metastatic disease and a mass in the pelvis. He was unwell with weight loss, loss of appetite and nausea. Ultrasonography revealed bilateral hydronephrosis and a mass in the pelvis.

CASE 7.21 – 'I have lost weight and have a loss of appetite and a lump in my belly.'

A 63-year-old man presents with a rapidly painful swelling of his left testicle, a mass in his abdomen and haematuria. He has had a loss of appetite and lost a stone (about 7 kg) in weight over the last 3 months. He has also been feeling quite tired.

OSCE Counselling Case

OSCE COUNSELLING CASE 7.8 – 'How do I counsel patient for a nephrostomy?'

A 23-year-old woman with fever and confusion and who is systemically unwell undergoes ultrasonography to reveal a right-sided hydronephrosis. There is a stone seen in the renal pelvis. She has previously had significant UTIs. She has been started on antibiotics but she has not improved.

Q1: What would you need to discuss with her before consent for a nephrostomy?

Key concepts

- Upper urinary tract obstruction
- Acute or chronic obstruction.

Hydronephrosis is a descriptive term that is associated with a pathological dilatation of the renal pelvis and calyces. Dilatation may be the result of an obstruction to the urinary tract, which may be unilateral or bilateral, acute or chronic, complete or incomplete.

A PUJ abnormality is caused by a short stenotic segment at the level of the PUJ. In the normal kidney, pacemakers in the minor calyces initiate a contraction wave, which passes down to the lower ureter. The normal spiral muscle of the PUJ and the ureter may be replaced by a localized longitudinal segment which does not allow coordinated proximal contractions to reach the lower ureter. This may also be caused by an abnormal lower-pole vessel crossing the proximal ureter.

Non-obstructive dilatation of the renal pelvis may be vesicoureteric reflux, dysplasia, or problems in the developmental anatomy of the urinary tract.

The most common causes of upper urinary tract obstruction are urinary stone disease, sloughed renal papilla, blood clot, acute retroperitoneal pathology and accidental ligation of the ureter.

Bilateral obstruction of the upper tracts is a result of a lower urinary tract obstruction, with back pressure on to both kidneys, e.g. prostatic obstruction or obstruction to both the ureters caused by a retroperitoneal pathology. Recovery of the obstruction after its relief is initially by the recovery of the tubular function and is followed by a much slower glomerular recovery.

Renal masses

The most common presentation is haematuria and loin pain. An increasing number are being diagnosed incidentally with increasing use of ultrasonography for diagnosis. Thirty per cent note a mass in the abdomen or have symptoms of metastatic disease with weight loss and loss of appetite. The classic triad of 'haematuria, pain and a loin mass' is rare and occurs in about 10 per cent of cases. Involvement of the renal vein and obstruction of the left testicular vein result in presentation with an acute varicocoele.

Renal tumours may mimic a range of conditions as a result of the paraneoplastic syndromes caused by ectopic hormone secretion or mediated by interleukin-6 (common syndromes associated with renal tumours are anaemia, polycythaemia, hypertension, Cushing's syndrome, reversible hepatic dysfunction [Stauffer's syndrome] and pyrexia with night sweats).

Answers

CASE 7.19– 'I have pain in my loin when I have a drink.'

Q1: What is the likely differential diagnosis?

A1

Upper ureteric obstruction may be the result of the following:

- PUJ obstruction.
- Ureteric stone
- Upper ureteric tumour
- Sloughed-off renal papilla
- Ureteric strictures (infective, e.g. tuberculous/iatrogenic/radiation induced)
- Renal pelvis dilatation without obstruction may be the result of reflux of urine into the renal pelvis from the bladder or of a dilated but non-obstructed renal pelvis.

Q2: What issues in the given history support/refute a particular diagnosis?

A2

Commonly associated with increased diuresis, as noted after alcohol intake when an obstruction is precipitated with increased urine output through a fixed obstruction.

Pain in the loin and haematuria are commonly noted.

Q3: What additional features would you seek to support a particular diagnosis?

A3

Sloughed-off renal papilla is associated with diabetics and analgesia abuse.

The upper ureteric tumour was associated with phenacetin-containing analgesic abuse and smoking (phenacetin has consequently been discontinued in the UK). It is more common in males and appears to peak in the seventh decade. These tumours are more common in the distal third of the ureter and are commonly associated with synchronous bladder tumours.

 Q4: What clinical examination would you perform and why?

A4

Loin mass may be palpable.

 Q5: What investigations would be most helpful and why?

A5

- IVU: chronic obstruction is often identified and information about the anatomy is usually obtained. This usually requires a reasonable renal function and glomerular filtration rate (GFR), and is usually not helpful if the creatinine is > 200 mmol/L.
- Ultrasonography: is non-invasive and a useful screening tool; it identifies hydronephrosis and the renal cortical thickness gives a rough assessment of the chronicity of the condition and the possibility of recovery of function.
- Isotope diuresis renography: radioactive tracers are tagged to molecules that are effectively cleared by the first pass through the kidney through a combination of partial filtration and active tubular secretion. Technetium-99m (^{99m}Tc)-labelled mercaptoacetyl triglycine is commonly used intravenously and the renal handling of the radioactive tracer is monitored with gamma scanners over the abdomen and plotted against time. A persistent accumulation of the tracer in the kidney not eliminated by a diuretic is consistent with obstruction. A slow elimination caused by urinary stasis in a dilated renal pelvis responds to an increased urinary flow with a rapid washout of the tracer following the diuretic.

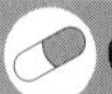 Q6: What treatment options are appropriate?

A6

It is important to note that dilatation does not necessarily mean obstruction.

The following questions are helpful in planning the treatment:

- Is the dilatation the result of an active obstruction or is it a non-obstructive dilatation?
- Is the function of the kidney in obstructed kidneys sufficient to justify correction? A nephrectomy is more appropriate in poorly functioning kidneys.

Defining the anatomical level of the obstruction

It is important to define obstruction before performing an operation for relief of the obstruction. An operation is commonly performed to correct obstruction when there is a deterioration of renal function of the affected renal unit (< 40 per cent of the split function), symptoms of pain, haematuria, and the development of complications from the obstruction.

A PUJ obstruction is a short stenotic segment that may be incised, dilated or excised and re-anastomosed (Anderson–Hynes pyeloplasty).

CASE 7.20 – A 57-year-old man with advanced malignancy has bilateral hydronephrosis.

 Q1: What is the likely differential diagnosis?

A1

- Dehydration: infection may account for deterioration of general health.
- Bilateral hydronephrosis may be the result of an obstruction to the prostate or bladder neck or to both ureters.

 Q2: What issues in the given history support/refute a particular diagnosis?

A2

Advanced malignancy is associated with retroperitoneal pathology and may involve the ureters, causing bilateral hydronephrosis.

 Q3: What additional features would you seek to support a particular diagnosis?

A3

Duration of symptoms may be useful in estimating loss of renal function.

Prognosis from the advanced malignancy and treatment options is available and the patient's choice of treatment needs to be ascertained.

 Q4: What clinical examination would you perform and why?

A4

General assessment to treat dehydration and infection.

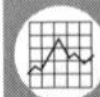 Q5: What investigations would be most helpful and why?

A5

- Renal function
- CT: to assess retroperitoneum and stage disease.

 Q6: What treatment options are appropriate?

A6

Stenting the ureters to remove obstructions is commonly done anterograde after emergency placement of nephrostomies either into both kidneys or into the better-functioning one.

The decision to treat ureters obstructed by malignancy must be discussed openly with the patient because this would prolong life, with the progression of metastatic disease and all the symptoms from that. If a good quality of life can be obtained from treatment of the obstructed kidneys, it may be considered together with the patient, oncologist and palliative consultant.

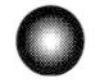 CASE 7.21 – 'I have lost weight and have a loss of appetite and a lump in my belly.'

 Q1: What is the likely differential diagnosis?

A1

Renal masses with weight loss and loss of appetite may be caused by:

- Renal tumour
- Infective granulomatous changes with xanthogranulomatous pyelonephritis
- The paraneoplastic syndromes may mimic a whole range of conditions
- A renal cyst that is infected or haemorrhage in a renal cyst may present with pain and a mass.

 Q2: What issues in the given history support/refute a particular diagnosis?

A2

The renal vein invasion with testicular vein obstruction is associated with a new-onset varicocoele in an adult.

A renal mass with haematuria is commonly associated with an underlying renal tumour.

 Q3: What additional features would you seek to support a particular diagnosis?

A3

History of stone disease with recurrent infections is common with XGPN.

 Q4: What clinical examination would you perform and why?

A4

Examination of the renal mass and test for anaemia.

 Q5: What investigations would be most helpful and why?

A5

- Contrast CT of chest and abdomen: staging of the renal tumour and assessment of the renal vein and inferior vena cava. Distant metastasis and lymph node involvement may also be obtained from this.
- Urine cytology and urine culture: to rule out infection.
- Liver function tests: hepatic dysfunction that is reversible after nephrectomy is described as 'Stauffer's syndrome'
- FBC: polycythaemia or anaemia may occur.

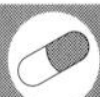 Q6: What treatment options are appropriate?

A6

A radical nephrectomy is the recommended treatment with a curative intent.

Metastatic disease generally has a poor prognosis. The primary tumour should be removed if it is causing symptoms and the patient is fit, and systemic immunotherapy with interleukin-2 or interferon-α may be given; both are associated with severe side effects.

OSCE Counselling Case – Answer

OSCE COUNSELLING CASE 7.8 – **'How do I counsel patient for a nephrostomy?'**

Nephrostomy is associated with 1 per cent mortality and with loss of renal unit as a result of bleeding.

Percutaneous nephrostomy is usually performed by the radiologist using an image intensifier.

The drainage of pus should be sent for culture and sensitivity and appropriate antibiotics started.

Finally, the stone in the renal pelvis would require treatment with either ESWL or ureteroscopy and lithotripsy, or enlarging the nephrostomy port and PCNL.

SCROTAL PAIN, TESTICULAR LUMPS

? Questions for each of the clinical case scenarios given

Q1: What is the likely differential diagnosis?
Q2: What issues in the given history support/refute a particular diagnosis?
Q3: What additional features would you seek to support a particular diagnosis?
Q4: What clinical examination would you perform and why?
Q5: What investigations would be most helpful and why?
Q6: What treatment options are appropriate?

Clinical cases

CASE 7.22 – 'I have noticed a lump in my scrotum. Have I got cancer?'

A 24-year-old man presents with a painless lump in his scrotum that he noticed in the shower. He is fit and well and is a non-smoker.

CASE 7.23 – A 22-year-old man presents with painful swelling of his scrotum.

A 22-year-old man presents with a painful lump in his scrotum. He has mild dysuria and has had treatment for chlamydial urethritis in the past.

CASE 7.24 – 'My son is complaining of a painful scrotum and is not able to walk.'

My son is 9 years old and has woken up with a painful scrotum and is unable to walk; the scrotum is red and tender. He has never had any problems before.

Key concepts

Testicular cancer is common in young men (20–45 years). It is now one of the most curable cancers. Teratomas usually occur at a younger age than seminomas (20–35 versus 35–45 years). It is associated with undescended testis and contralateral testicular tumour. Testicular tumours are associated with HIV infection.

Germ cell tumours are classified as seminomatous or the non-seminomatous (Table 7.2). The latter include teratomas.

Table 7.2 Germ-cell and non-germ-cell tumours

Germ-cell tumours	Non-germ-cell tumours (relatively rare)
Seminoma	Leydig cell tumours
Teratoma	Sertoli cell tumours
Yolk sac tumour	Granulosa cell tumours
Trophoblastic tumour (choriocarcinoma)	Mixed

There are two types of torsion: that inside the tunica vaginalis (intravaginal, most common) and that outside (extravaginal). Testicular torsion is an emergency because irreversible ischaemic damage occurs within 4 h.

In patients who are prone to an intravaginal torsion in the testis, the space between the layers of the tunica vaginalis extends high up into the spermatic cord. This creates an abnormally mobile testis that hangs freely within the space of the tunica (a 'bell-clapper deformity'), allowing the testis to twist in the axis of the cord.

Torsion is recognized by sudden onset of pain and swelling of the testicle. There is often a history of previous severe self-limiting scrotal pain. Dysuria and bladder symptoms are absent. It is worth noting that 90 per cent of adolescents presenting with severe scrotal pain and swelling have a torsion.

Epididymo-orchitis occurs in all age groups and must be differentiated from testicular torsion and testicular tumour. The typical presentation is a gradual onset of testicular pain and swelling associated with scrotal redness and a hydrocoele. In men under 40 years the most common causative organisms are *Chlamydia* spp., gonococci and coliforms. Coliforms and other Gram-negative organisms are more common in those aged over 40 years. The aetiology in children is commonly abacterial (often viral, i.e. mumps).

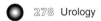

Answers

CASE 7.22 – 'I have noticed a lump in my scrotum. Have I got cancer?'

 Q1: What is the likely differential diagnosis?

A1

Testicular lumps:

- Testicular cancer
- Epididymal cyst
- Hydrocoele
- Hernia
- Varicocoele.

 Q2: What issues in the given history support/refute a particular diagnosis?

A2

Testicular tumours occur in young adults and are often painless.

 Q3: What additional features would you seek to support a particular diagnosis?

A3

- History of an undescended testis is an important risk factor.
- Sperm granulomas with a painful lump in the cord may be present after a vasectomy.
- Hydrocoele is a globular swelling in the scrotum that is not painful.
- A cough impulse is commonly present with a hernia.
- Metastatic disease from testicular cancer may present with shortness of breath, back pain and nipple tenderness.

Q4: What clinical examination would you perform and why?

A4

- Physical examination to reveal supraclavicular lymph nodes, chest signs, hepatomegaly, abdominal mass and lower limb oedema.

- Testicular examination may reveal a hard mass in the testis.
- A hydrocoele is fluctuant and transilluminates.
- The ability to get above the mass at the level of the spermatic cord helps exclude inguinoscrotal hernia.

 Q5: What investigations would be most helpful and why?

A5

- Ultrasonography: distinguishes solid and fluid-filled scrotal lesions
- Testicular tumour markers:
  - β-human chorionic gonadotrophin (β-hCG): 40 per cent of teratomas and 15 per cent of seminomas
  - lactate dehydrogenase (LDH): 10–20 per cent of seminomas
  - α-fetoprotein (AFP): 50–70 per cent of teratomas and yolk sac tumours
- Abdominal and chest contrast CT for staging.

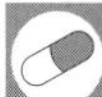 Q6: What treatment options are appropriate?

A6

The primary treatment of all testicular tumours is a radical orchidectomy through a groin incision. Further treatment depends on the staging CT and tumour markers. Systemic disease is commonly treated with combination chemotherapy or radiotherapy.

Residual lymph nodal disease after chemotherapy may be resected by a retroperitoneal lymph node dissection.

CASE 7.23 – A 22-year-old man presents with painful swelling of his scrotum.

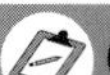 Q1: What is the likely differential diagnosis?

A1

- Epididymo-orchitis
- Testicular torsion
- Testicular tumour with a bleed
- Strangulated hernia.

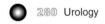

 Q2: What issues in the given history support/refute a particular diagnosis?

A2

A history of previous urethritis may suggest an infective process; an epididymo-orchitis is commonly associated with dysuria and bladder symptoms. The onset of symptoms is more gradual and associated with scrotal redness and may have a moderate hydrocoele.

 Q3: What additional features would you seek to support a particular diagnosis?

A3

- Acute testicular torsion is common in younger patients with sudden onset of symptoms. In addition pain is more prominent than tenderness, whereas in epididymo-orchitis tenderness is the main feature.
- A history of sexual activity and promiscuity. Previous sexually transmitted infections (STIs) and contact tracing are an important aspect of the management.
- A strangulated inguinoscrotal hernia is commonly associated with nausea and vomiting. Patients are often systemically unwell.

Q4: What clinical examination would you perform and why?

A4

Scrotal examination: epididymo-orchitis is associated with a tender swelling of the epididymis. It has a vertical lie and the epididymis is posterior. It may be associated with a small hydrocoele.

Testicular tumour is a hard, non-tender mass involving part or the whole of the testis.

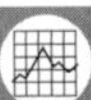 Q5: What investigations would be most helpful and why?

A5

- Urine microscopy and culture: isolate organism
- Urethral swab for *Chlamydia* spp.
- Ultrasonography of scrotum: differentiates solid and cystic masses
- Colour Doppler study: not commonly done but is useful to assess vascularity of the testis.

 Q6: What treatment options are appropriate?

A6

In men aged under 40 years doxycyline or a quinolone for 10 days is appropriate. If gonococci are suspected a single intramuscular dose of ceftriaxone should be added to doxycycline.

In men aged over 40 years a fluoroquinolone for 10 days may be sufficient.

Box 7.3 Key points to note in treatment

- Men rarely develop a UTI and, in the absence of an STI, it is important to investigate the urinary tract to identify other predisposing factors for infection
- Diabetes and factors affecting general immunity
- Factors related to the urinary tract: bladder outlet obstruction, bladder stones, indwelling catheters or urinary stents

CASE 7.24 – 'My son is complaining of a painful scrotum and is not able to walk.'

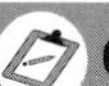 Q1: What is the likely differential diagnosis?

A1

- Testicular torsion
- Torsion of a testicular appendage
- Epididymo-orchitis
- Idiopathic scrotal oedema.

 Q2: What issues in the given history support/refute a particular diagnosis?

A2

Torsion of the testicle on the spermatic cord is common around puberty. The symptoms are sudden in onset with pain and often associated with nausea and vomiting. There may be local redness and the testis may be lying higher in the root of the scrotum.

 Q3: What additional features would you seek to support a particular diagnosis?

A3

A history of sharp intermittent pains that are self-limiting may be present and signify previous intermittent torsions that have resolved.

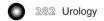

 Q4: What clinical examination would you perform and why?

A4

The testis may be horizontal or retracted up to the root of the scrotum. The testis is usually swollen and exquisitely tender. A cremasteric reflex is often absent and may be a useful indicator.

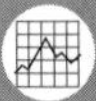 Q5: What investigations would be most helpful and why?

A5

Ultrasound and colour Doppler assessment are operator dependent and may delay prompt surgical intervention; they are considered only if the diagnosis is doubtful.

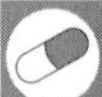 Q6: What treatment options are appropriate?

A6

A manual de-torsion may be attempted but this must not delay an urgent exploration of the testicle. The testis is examined for signs of ischaemia; if normal it is repositioned and fixed to the tunica vaginalis with non-absorbable, non-reactive sutures.

ERECTILE DYSFUNCTION/INFERTILITY

? Questions for each of the clinical case scenarios given

Q1: What is the likely differential diagnosis?
Q2: What issues in the given history support/refute a particular diagnosis?
Q3: What additional features would you seek to support a particular diagnosis?
Q4: What clinical examination would you perform and why?
Q5: What investigations would be most helpful and why?
Q6: What treatment options are appropriate?

Clinical cases

CASE 7.25 – 'I am unable to have erections.'

A 45-year-old man newly diagnosed with diabetes presents with difficulty having erections for the last 6 months. He does not have adequately rigid erections and is unable to maintain them.

CASE 7.26 – 'We have been trying for a child for 3 years.'

A couple have had unprotected intercourse for 3 years and have not conceived. He had repair of an undescended testicle as a child.

CASE 7.27 – 'I have an ulcer on my penis.'

A 78-year-old man has had a foul-smelling discharge from his foreskin for several months and on clinical examination has a fungating mass on the end of his penis.

OSCE Counselling Case

OSCE COUNSELLING CASE 7.8 – Counsel a 35-year-old patient for a vasectomy.

A 35-year-old man has requested a vasectomy; he and his partner have three children, have completed their family and would like a permanent sterilization.

Key concepts

Erectile dysfunction is the inability to obtain a satisfactory erection for sexual intercourse.

The male factors of infertility or subfertility are the following: men with one or both undescended testicles regardless of the age at orchidopexy, mumps or orchitis after puberty, and substance abuse.

Penile carcinoma is uncommon but common in elderly men. The premalignant conditions associated with penile cancers appear as chronic, painless, red or pale patches and include leukoplakia and erythroplasia of Queyrat.

Infections with human papilloma virus (HPV)-16, -18 and -21 are important and associated with cervical cancer in the partner. Circumcision as a neonate may confer some protection against penile cancer, and this may be related to the chronic irritation from the smegma and balanitis in men with poor hygiene.

The most common cancer is a squamous carcinoma which may be preceded by carcinoma *in situ* of the glans or the foreskin. Metastasis is to the inguinal lymph nodes and then to the pelvic lymph nodes. Blood-borne metastasis to the lungs and liver is rare.

The common presentation is a hard painless lump or a malignant ulcer on the penis.

Vasectomy is a permanent form of sterilization. There are several techniques that are used. The principle involves isolating the vas deferens, delivering it through a small skin incision and dividing a portion of it.

Answers

CASE 7.25 – 'I am unable to have erections.'

Q1: What is the likely differential diagnosis?

A1

Psychogenic erectile dysfunction is the most common cause and is associated with stress, performance anxiety and previous sexual relationship problems.

Organic erectile dysfunction may also occur as a result of disruption of nerve conduction caused by neurological processes such as Parkinson's disease, stroke, head trauma and nerve disruption, as in a radical prostatectomy.

Arterial occlusive disease of the pudendal cavernous helicine arteries can reduce arterial inflow to the sinusoids. Common risk factors include hypertension, hyperlipidaemia, cigarette smoking and diabetes.

Drug-induced causes and hypogonadism (pituitary or gonadal).

Q2: What issues in the given history support/refute a particular diagnosis?

A2

Diabetes is a common cause of erectile dysfunction.

Q3: What additional features would you seek to support a particular diagnosis?

A3

Erectile dysfunction that is gradual and insidious in onset is more likely to be organic. It is often associated with loss of spontaneous or early morning erections.

On the contrary, erectile dysfunction related to periods of stress, e.g. marital, financial and psychological stress, is commonly sudden in onset and spontaneous erections are often preserved.

Drug-induced erectile dysfunction is common with centrally acting anti-hypertensives, anti-psychotics and antidepressants.

Chronic alcoholism and smoking are known to affect erection adversely.

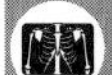

Q4: What clinical examination would you perform and why?

A4

- Examination of the breasts, hair distribution, testes and thyroid to detect an endocrine abnormality.
- Femoral and foot pulses for vascular insufficiency.

- Genital and perineal sensation for neurological deficit and penile abnormalities.

Clinical syndromes such Klinefelter's syndrome are associated with a typical appearance.

 Q5: What investigations would be most helpful and why?

A5

- Hormonal evaluation: serum prolactin, luteinizing hormone (LH), follicle-stimulating hormone (FSH) and testosterone (if evidence of low testosterone on clinical examination), thyroid hormones, liver and renal function tests
- Serum glucose: diabetes.

Tests that are rarely performed:

- Duplex ultrasonography: measures penile blood flow velocity
- Cavernosography: identifies a venous leak, but is fraught with false positives and is rarely performed
- Nocturnal tumescence testing: to access sleep-related erection; useful in differentiating psychogenic erectile dysfunction (where nocturnal erections are preserved) from the organic erectile dysfunction (nocturnal erections are lost). It is performed using a Rigiscan device.

 Q6: What treatment options are appropriate?

A6

- General principles include: stop smoking, reduce alcohol intake, healthy diet and exercise. Remove precipitating factors such as drugs, long-distance cycling.
- If a psychological component is present, refer to a psychosexual counsellor.
- Treatment depends on patient suitability and preference.
- Oral medications: phospodiesterase inhibitors (sildenafil, vardenafil, tadalafil).
- Major side effects are headaches, flushing and dyspepsia, caution with cardiac patients on nitrates (associated with fatal hypotension and arrhythmia).
- Sublingual apomorphine acts on the central dopaminergic receptors and induces erections. The side effects include nausea and vomiting.
- Vacuum device is placed over the penis and a pump produces a vacuum; a constricting ring is placed on the base of the penis to maintain the rigidity after the penis is engorged by the negative pressure. A hinged erection caused by a softer proximal end of the penis, and retained ejaculate and numbness of the penis are some of the side effects.
- Intracavernosal injections: papaverine and alprostadil are used and this is one of the most effective and reliable second-line therapies for erectile dysfunction. There is a risk of persistent erection lasting > 4 h (priapism) that requires urgent decompression.
- Penile prosthesis is implanted into the corpora and replaces the normal erectile tissue; the prosthesis may be solid (rigid or semirigid) and is malleable. The most common prosthesis is the inflatable device with a reservoir and pump, and inflatable rods that are implanted into the corpora.

CASE 7.26 – 'We have been trying for a child for 3 years.'

Q1: What is the likely differential diagnosis?

A1

MALE CAUSES OF PRIMARY INFERTILITY

- Hypothalamic causes: hypogonadotrophic hypogonadism: Kallmann's syndrome
- Pituitary causes: surgery, irradiation, infarction, tumours, infections
- Hormonal excess: anabolic steroids, congenital adrenal hyperplasia, excess oestrogens and prolactinomas
- Chromosomal: Klinefelter's syndrome (XXY)
- Systemic diseases: uraemia, liver failure
- Testicular causes: orchitis (postpubertal), undescended testes, trauma, infections, varicocoele
- Cystic fibrosis: associated with bilateral vasal agenesis.

Q2: What issues in the given history support/refute a particular diagnosis?

A2

History of an undescended testis as a child.

Q3: What additional features would you seek to support a particular diagnosis?

A3

- Duration of infertility and prior pregnancies; details of sexual history and potency and use of lubricants are important.
- History of previous surgery to the vas or pelvis, infections, e.g. mumps, trauma to testis.
- History of diabetes and drug history and family history of cystic fibrosis.

Q4: What clinical examination would you perform and why?

A4

- General examination: body hair distribution, gynaecomastia
- Examination of genitalia, size of the testis, thickening of epididymis
- Penile abnormalities, e.g. hypospadias
- The presence of a vas deferens
- Examine for a varicocoele.

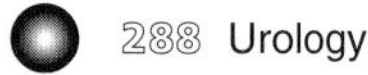

Q5: What investigations would be most helpful and why?

A5

- Urine: microscopy to rule out infection and to assess for sperm (retrograde ejaculation)
- Semen analysis: oligospermia/azoospermia sperm counts
- Asthenospermia
- Hormonal evaluation: LH, FSH, testosterone and prolactin
- Testicular biopsy: in azoospermia to differentiate between obstructive and non-obstructive forms; it is reported as a Johnsen's score 0–10 and a score > 8 would suggest that the sperm is useful for intracytoplasmic sperm injection (ICSI)/in vitro fertilization (IVF)
- In cases of obstructive azoospermia: transrectal ultrasonography to assess the fullness of the seminal vesicles and vasography to identify the level of the block
- Rare tests: postcoital tests/anti-sperm antibodies (in serum, seminal plasma), karyotyping and cystic fibrosis mutation testing.

Q6: What treatment options are appropriate?

A6

A combined cause is noted in 30 per cent of cases and a purely male factor for infertility is noted in 20 per cent of cases.

- For post-testicular causes: after vasectomy or focal obstruction: the block is identified using a vasography. A vasovasostomy or vasoepididymostomy is performed.
- Testicular causes: varicocoele is a common cause for infertility and this is repaired either by an open technique (ligation of spermatic veins) or by a laparoscopic technique.
- Correction of the hormone abnormalities.
- Investigation for a prolactinoma and appropriate management.

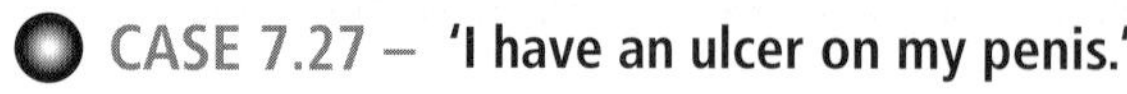

CASE 7.27 – 'I have an ulcer on my penis.'

Q1: What is the likely differential diagnosis?

A1

- Carcinoma of the penis
- Balanitis xerotica obliterans: white patch involving prepuce and glans and also the meatus
- Leukoplakia: rare condition, common in those with diabetes, white plaque involves meatus
- Condyloma acuminata: viral origin – HPV.

 Q2: What issues in the given history support/refute a particular diagnosis?

A2

Carcinoma of the penis is more common in older patients. It may develop as an ulcer (typical shallow erosion/excavated ulcer with rolled-out edges) or an exophytic lesion. It eventually develops into a fungating mass and has a purulent smell.

Circumcision in the neonate is protective and is believed that the presence of smegma and poor hygiene are contributory.

 Q3: What additional features would you seek to support a particular diagnosis?

A3

- The aetiology is linked to HPV-16 and occurs in partners with carcinoma of the cervix (thought to be linked to HPV).
- Smoking is a known risk factor for carcinoma of the penis.
- The metastatic spread of penile carcinoma is to the lymph nodes and then to the distant organs (lungs/liver/bone).
- Carcinoma *in situ* (Bowen's disease, when it appears in the shaft of the penis, and erythroplasia of Queyrat, when it appears as a red velvety lesion with ulceration on the glans penis) is a precursor for squamous carcinoma of the penis.

Q4: What clinical examination would you perform and why?

A4

General examination is needed to assess the nutritional status, hygiene and general well-being of the patient.

The diagnosis is made by clinical examination and in some circumstances a biopsy may be necessary. Assess the ulcer (size, shape, base, edge, site and involvement of the shaft of the penis and bodies of the corpora). Inguinal lymph nodes may be palpable and in 50 per cent of the cases they are enlarged as a result of infection of the ulcer and not as a result of metastatic spread of the cancer.

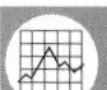 Q5: What investigations would be most helpful and why?

A5

- Culture swab
- Biopsy of the lesion may be necessary in suspicious circumstances
- Primary tumour (corporal involvement): MRI
- Lymph node involvement: CT of groin, pelvis, abdomen and chest
- Bone scan: distant metastases.

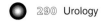

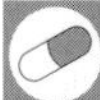 Q6: What treatment options are appropriate?

A6

Prognosis depends on:

- Histological classification (Broder's grade 1–3 with 5-year survival rate of 80 per cent in grade 1 and of 30 per cent in grade 3)
- Depth of invasion
- Pattern of growth (superficial spreading, vertical growing, verrucous and multicentric)
- Vascular invasion.

Carcinoma *in situ* may be treated with penis-conserving treatment: topical chemotherapy, e.g. 5-fluorouracil, or glansectomy with resurfacing.

The primary lesion of carcinoma of the penis is treated by excision. Penis-conserving surgery may be performed for lesions involving only the glans. A tumour that involves the corpus spongiosus or cavernosus (T2), or the urethra and prostate (T3), is treated by excision of the lesion with a margin (partial or total penectomy).

A 4-week course of antibiotics often allows differentiation of the lymph nodes with cancer from the ones that are enlarged as a result of infection.

If no palpable nodes are present a prophylactic lymph node dissection of superficial inguinal lymph nodes, and if the frozen section is positive an ipsilateral deep inguinal and pelvic node dissection, is performed in high-grade G3 tumour and high-stage T2–4 disease.

In low-grade G1–2 tumour and T1 disease with no lymph nodes a protocol for surveillance is acceptable, but with a 2-monthly follow-up.

The presence of nodes after the antibiotic course would require a full dissection of ipsilateral lymph nodes (superficial/deep inguinal/pelvic) and contralateral superficial lymph nodes.

A positive pelvic lymph node is associated with a very poor prognosis: 5-year survival rate of 10 per cent. Chemotherapy is considered for large lymph nodal metastasis and pelvic nodal metastasis.

OSCE Counselling Case – Answer

OSCE COUNSELLING CASE 7.8 – Counsel a 35-year-old patient for a vasectomy.

Vasectomy is a permanent form of sterilization and a decision needs to be made by both partners.

The contraindications for vasectomy are mainly relative: clotting abnormalities, local infections and skin abnormalities. Appropriate counselling of couples with a pregnant partner who request a vasectomy is necessary to take into account the risk of stillbirth or perinatal mortality.

A reversal of vasectomy is not as successful (success depends on time between vasectomy and reversal). Microsurgical techniques have a success rate of 60–80 per cent, with much lower paternity rates.

Vasectomy is not foolproof. Success is confirmed by negative semen analysis in the third and fourth months after vasectomy. Late recanalization after a negative semen analysis may occur up to 15 years after the procedure in 1:2000.

Persistence of semen in the tract will account for positive semen analysis; a guarded clearance may be given for patients with non-motile sperm of < 10 000/mL at least 7 months after the vasectomy.

Technique may be by an open vasectomy or a 'no-scalpel technique' using fine sharp instruments to puncture the skin and deliver the vas for ligature – excising a segment of vas and repositioning the ends of the vas either with or without ligation (open-ended vasectomy).

Complications include the sperm granuloma with a painful nodule on the vas. There is post-vasectomy testicular pain/discomfort in up to 18 per cent of patients (caused by epididymal congestion, often treated by non-steroidal anti-inflammatory drugs and rarely requiring reversal of vasectomy). Local complications of haematoma and wound infection are < 5 per cent.

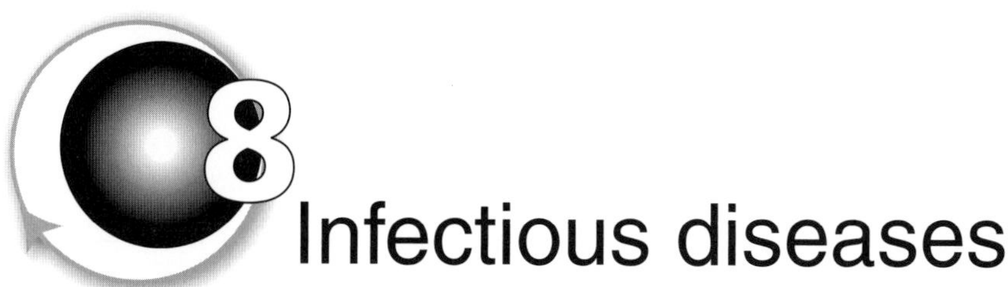

8 Infectious diseases

Chris Ellis

? Questions for each of the clinical case scenarios given

Q1: What is the likely diagnosis or differential diagnosis?
Q2: What investigations should be performed?
Q3: What would be the initial management?
Q4: What is the prognosis?

Clinical cases

CASE 8.1 – A 26-year-old man with fever, headache and confusion.

A 26-year-old executive presents with a 1-week history of headache and 2 days of confusion. He has a temperature of 39°C. He returned 3 weeks previously from a 2-week safari in Kenya. Full blood count (FBC) and biochemical profile are normal; computed tomography (CT) shows no abnormality.

CASE 8.2 – A 30-year-old woman with prolonged fever of unknown origin.

A 30-year-old woman is referred to you with a 6-month history of fever in the evenings, often accompanied by a faint erythematous rash with aches and pain, some of which clearly arise from joints. She has not lost weight. She has already been extensively investigated with a normal chest radiograph and abdominal CT. Rheumatoid antibodies and antinuclear antibodies (ANAs) are both negative. On examination you find a faint macular rash, a temperature of 39°C, a 3-cm smooth liver enlargement and 1-cm glands in both axillae. Cardiovascular examination was unremarkable. Blood cultures yielded no growth.

CASE 8.3 – A woman of 30 who has fainted and who has fever and a rash.

A 30-year-old woman was well until 48 h before presentation. Her illness began with nausea and vomiting and later she felt feverish. On the morning of admission she had got up, then felt faint and briefly lost consciousness. On admission her temperature is 39°C, pulse 110/min, blood pressure 100/60 mmHg supine. There is a diffuse erythematous rash on her face and trunk which blanches on pressure. She is menstruating.

CASE 8.4 – A 30-year-old man with productive cough, feverishness and weight loss.

A 30-year-old Somali man who has lived in the UK for 2 years presents with 1 month of productive cough, feverishness and weight loss. On examination he is thin but otherwise no abnormality is detected. A chest radiograph shows patchy consolidation of the right upper zone. There is no significant past medical history.

CASE 8.5 – A 36-year-old woman with fever, headache and a rash.

A 36-year-old female university lecturer presents with 3 days of fever, headache and a rash that she describes as 'a return of her suntan'. Four weeks earlier she returned from a 2-week holiday in Kenya. She is on no medication. She has several 1-cm diameter glands in her neck, pharyngitis and a maculopapular rash on her trunk. The temperature is 38°C.

CASE 8.6 – A 22-year-old man with persistent diarrhoea and weight loss.

A 22-year-old male medical student presents 6 weeks after returning from his elective period in Nepal. While there he had two episodes of watery diarrhoea and took a single dose of ciprofloxacin on each occasion; his symptoms settled within 48 h. He was well on return but developed watery diarrhoea 1 week later, which has persisted, and he now reports five or six motions a day with some abdominal distension and excessive flatus. He has lost 6 kg in the last 2 weeks.

OSCE Counselling Cases

OSCE COUNSELLING CASE 8.1 – 'I am a 26-year-old builder. Last year I fell off a ladder and had to have my spleen removed. Someone in the pub told me I can die of septicaemia. Was he right and what can I do about it?'

OSCE COUNSELLING CASE 8.2 – 'I am a gay man who has one regular partner but occasionally I have sex with new male acquaintances and, although I try to remember to "play safe", I don't think I have always succeeded. I am fully fit and, as far as I know, none of my partners is HIV positive. Would you advise me to be tested?'

OSCE COUNSELLING CASE 8.3 – 'I am a 24-year-old mother of a 6-month-old baby girl. My widowed mother was recently in hospital for a hip replacement and her wound was infected with MRSA. I love my mother but don't want her in my home as she could infect my baby. In any case, shouldn't she have been kept in hospital?'

Key concepts

The following are definitions of sepsis (often referred to in the literature as SIRS, or systemic inflammatory response syndrome):

- Sepsis: two or more of:
  - temperature > 38°C or < 36°C
  - pulse > 90/min
  - respiratory rate (RR) > 20/min
  - white blood cell count (WBC) > 12 000 or < 4000

- Severe sepsis: sepsis with one or more of:
  - hypotension
  - confusion
  - oliguria
  - hypoxia
  - acidosis
  - disseminated intravascular coagulation (DIC)
- Septic shock: severe sepsis with hypotension despite fluid resuscitation.

Answers

CASE 8.1 – A 26-year-old man with fever, headache and confusion.

Q1: What is the likely diagnosis or differential diagnosis?

A1

Headache, fever and confusion suggest encephalitis but this man is at risk of falciparum malaria, which can produce a picture identical to encephalitis (so-called cerebral malaria). The differential diagnosis therefore includes two conditions for which early treatment can be literally vital – herpes simplex encephalitis and falciparum malaria.

Q2: What investigations should be performed?

A2

A haematological sample should be sent immediately to look for malarial parasites, which will usually be seen as rings within erythrocytes. It is crucial that the request be made specifically because automated cell counters do not detect malarial parasites. The normal CT excludes cerebral swelling so it is safe to perform a lumbar puncture and the cerebrospinal fluid (CSF) may contain lymphocytes and erythrocytes in keeping with a primary encephalitis.

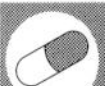

Q3: What would be the initial management?

A3

It would be prudent to cover both the treatable, life-threatening possible diagnoses unless the blood film conclusively confirms falciparum malaria. Malaria should be covered by intravenous quinine (consult the current *British National Formulary* for details and confer with your regional infectious diseases department) whereas intravenous aciclovir will cover herpes encephalitis.

Q4: What is the prognosis?

A4

The prognosis of severe malaria is good, provided that the patient survives the first few days, but during that period the full sepsis syndrome may be encountered with acute renal failure, DIC and adult respiratory distress syndrome (ARDS).

About one-third of patients with herpes encephalitis die; a third survive with varying degrees of permanent brain damage and a third eventually make a virtually complete recovery. Early treatment is crucial to a good outcome but even patients who are treated very promptly may suffer permanent brain damage.

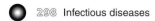

CASE 8.2 – A 30-year-old woman with prolonged fever of unknown origin.

 Q1: What is the likely diagnosis or differential diagnosis?

A1

This is adult systemic Still's disease.

Patients who have been pyrexial for several weeks usually turn out to have:

- occult infection
- occult neoplasm (lymphoma or non-obstructing cancers, e.g. renal)
- a 'connective-tissue' disorder.

This story is typical of systemic Still's disease in young adults.

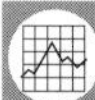 Q2: What investigations should be performed?

A2

First-line investigations for pyrexia of unknown origin (PUO) are: FBC and biochemical profile; blood culture; midstream urine (MSU); and chest radiograph (with malarial parasites [MPs] requested specifically and urgently if the patient has been in a malarial area in the preceding 3 months). If these are unhelpful proceed to anti-nuclear antibody (ANA) and imaging of the abdomen (ultrasonography usually available first but CT necessary if ultrasonography inconclusive and no other diagnosis has emerged).

Adult Still's disease is under-recognized partly because there is no specific test for it. It has definite features, however:

- daily fever (typically early evening)
- arthralgia/arthritis
- negative rheumatoid factor and negative ANA
- plus two out of: leukocytosis; rash-transient erythema, often with fever; serositis (e.g. pleural effusion); hepatomegaly; splenomegaly; generalized lymphadenopathy.

 Q3: What would be the initial management?

A3

A trial of corticosteroids. Clinicians are often reluctant to give steroids to patients for fear of 'lighting up occult infection'. In practice this is almost never a problem. Prolonged steroid therapy can, indeed, lead to activity of dormant tuberculosis but makes little difference to most bacterial infections. Furthermore the response in conditions such as Still's disease is usually rapid and decisive so that, if the patient is not apyrexial and dramatically improved within 3 days, the therapy should be reconsidered.

 Q4: What is the prognosis?

A4

The prognosis is usually good. It may take several months before the patient can be weaned off steroids entirely and relapses are common for about 5 years after the first episode, after which they usually cease. A minority of patients develop an established connective tissue disorder such as a rheumatoid disorder.

 CASE 8.3 – A woman of 30 who has fainted and who has fever and a rash.

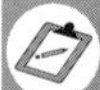 Q1: What is the likely diagnosis or differential diagnosis?

A1

There is enough evidence to justify treating this woman for presumed septic shock. A possible focus of infection could be the genital tract and a tampon should be sought and, if present, removed. Toxic shock syndrome (TSS) is a specific form of septic shock caused by toxins liberated by staphylococci, which may colonize the vagina and multiply on tampons or cause soft tissue infection such as cellulitis.

 Q2: What investigations should be performed?

A2

Any patient with sepsis should be examined carefully for a focus, including careful inspection for evidence of skin or soft-tissue infection, as well as evidence of focal infection in the thorax, abdomen and pelvis. Blood cultures must be taken; a chest radiograph is mandatory because pneumonia may not be apparent clinically and, when appropriate, the vagina should be examined and a tampon or intrauterine contraceptive device (IUCD) removed and cultured.

Sepsis is a clinical diagnosis based on a constellation of abnormalities (see Key concepts). A positive blood culture (bacteraemia) supports it and in this case isolation of a toxin-producing *Staphylococcus aureus* from a tampon would confirm TSS. The critical practical point is, however, that immediate management will not be affected by what the laboratory may report later.

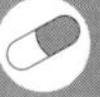 Q3: What would be the initial management?

A3

This is intravenous fluids, which should be given as rapidly as possible, and high-dose, intravenous broad-spectrum antibiotics to ensure specific cover for any likely focus. In this case, standard broad-spectrum cover should be augmented by a potent anti-staphylococcal agent such as flucloxacillin. When pneumonia is suggested clinically or radiologically, augment with cover for atypical pathogens (e.g. a macrolide such as clarithromycin or a quinolone). When appropriate remove a focus of infection (tampon, IUCD, aspirate or drain fluctuant areas in soft-tissue infection).

Q4: What is the prognosis?

A4

The prognosis depends very much on the promptness and thoroughness of immediate intervention. Complete recovery is the aim but, the more the initial intervention is delayed, the more likely is progression to a full sepsis syndrome with circulatory collapse, acute renal failure, ARDS and DIC.

CASE 8.4 – A 30-year-old man with productive cough, feverishness and weight loss.

Q1: What is the likely diagnosis or differential diagnosis?

A1

Pulmonary tuberculosis (TB) is overwhelmingly the most likely diagnosis. Acute bacterial pneumonias typically progress more rapidly. The absence of a previous history makes bronchiectasis unlikely.

Q2: What investigations should be performed?

A2

Sputum should be sent for TB microscopy and culture. If TB is confirmed he should be tested for HIV after appropriate counselling.

Q3: What would be the initial management?

A3

It is common practice for patients with this presentation to receive an antibacterial appropriate for community-acquired pneumonia (e.g. amoxicillin plus a quinolone and/or a macrolide such as clarithromycin), pending confirmation of the diagnosis of TB. There is an argument for avoiding quinolones in this context because they have anti-tuberculous activity and we must avoid promoting resistance to agents that we may wish to use in the future to treat TB. Once confirmed the patient should be treated with a combination of rifampicin, isoniazid, pyrazinamide and ethambutol for 2 months, reducing to rifampicin and isoniazid for a further 4 months. He will need careful supervision to ensure both compliance and recovery. If smear positive (acid-fast bacilli or AFBs seen on Ziehl–Neelsen staining), he will be highly infectious and will remain so until 2 weeks after the start of treatment. Consider isolating him in hospital for this period.

The patient should be officially notified to the consultant in communicable disease control, who will arrange for screening of household contacts and, if appropriate, of acquaintances and colleagues.

 Q4: What is the prognosis?

A4

The prognosis is good. Over 95 per cent of compliant patients with the drug-sensitive strain are cured at the end of the conventional 6-month course of treatment, with a relapse rate of no more than 2 per cent. Most relapses occur within 1 year of stopping treatment. If HIV positive, treatment should still cease at 6 months but the relapse rate will be higher.

 CASE 8.5 – A 36-year-old woman with fever, headache and a rash.

 Q1: What is the likely diagnosis or differential diagnosis?

A1

Falciparum malaria must be considered in any patient with a fever within 3 months of return from an endemic area. It would not cause lymphadenopathy or a rash. This could be a non-specific viral infection, glandular fever (primary Epstein–Barr virus infection) or a primary HIV illness.

 Q2: What investigations should be performed?

A2

These are a blood sample asking for MPs and a glandular fever screen. After discussion the patient agreed to testing for HIV infection, having admitted to unprotected sex during her holiday. Her HIV test was positive. (Modern HIV serology tests for both antigen and antibody, but if the diagnosis is likely a negative test should still be repeated 1 week later.)

Primary HIV infection presents as a glandular fever-like illness, often with a rash, and is one of the HIV presentations most likely to present to accident and emergency departments (A&E) in patients in whom the underlying diagnosis is not yet established. Other 'front-door' presentations include *Pneumocystis carinii* pneumonia (typically 3 or 4 weeks of dry cough with more recent shortness of breath on effort or fever), oral candidiasis and generalized lymphadenopathy.

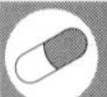 Q3: What would be the initial management?

A3

The patient should be referred for specialist HIV care and would be started on antiretroviral treatment when the CD4 lymphocyte count had fallen to about 250.

 Q4: What is the prognosis?

A4

Provided that the patient is established on antiretroviral therapy at an appropriate stage, the prognosis appears good, with most patients who started modern treatment when it was introduced in 1996 enjoying a good quality of disease-free life 9 years later.

 CASE 8.6 – A 22-year-old man with persistent diarrhoea and weight loss.

 Q1: What is the likely diagnosis or differential diagnosis?

A1

Giardiasis (infection with the protozoon *Giardia lamblia*) is the most likely cause of these symptoms. The most common cause of transient travellers' diarrhoea is probably enterotoxigenic strains of *Escherichia coli* (ETEC), which cause hypersecretions from the small intestine. They have a short incubation period of 1 or 2 days and rarely cause diarrhoea lasting longer than 1 week.

Giardia lamblia multiplies more slowly than bacteria and symptoms commonly start a few days after the traveller has returned from wherever he or she acquired it. Watery diarrhoea is usual for the first 2 or 3 weeks but malabsorption may then develop, with more bulky stools and flatulence from the fermentation of undigested sugars.

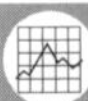 Q2: What investigations should be performed?

A2

Stool should be sent for culture and microscopy, but a negative result does not exclude giardiasis and a therapeutic trial of an anti-giardial agent such as tinidazole is good practice.

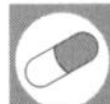 Q3: What would be the initial management?

A3

This is tinidazole as a single dose, repeated after 1 week.

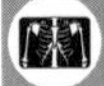 Q4: What is the prognosis?

A4

The prognosis is excellent. Symptoms of giardiasis improve decisively within a few days of starting appropriate treatment. If there is no improvement, small bowel endoscopy should be performed and a biopsy taken. This may reveal less common parasites such as cyclospora or the flat mucosa indicative of coeliac disease.

OSCE Counselling Cases – Answers

OSCE COUNSELLING CASE 8.1 – 'I am a 26-year-old builder. Last year I fell off a ladder and had to have my spleen removed. Someone in the pub told me I can die of septicaemia. Was he right and what can I do about it?'

The spleen protects very specifically against capsulated bacteria. Pneumococci are by far the biggest threat, with fulminating pneumococcal septicaemia about 1000 times more frequent in splenectomized patients than in the intact population. The risk appears to be less in individuals splenectomized after traumatic rupture than in those whose spleen was removed electively, but consensus advice is to offer pneumococcal vaccine and life-long prophylactic penicillin to splenectomized patients.

OSCE COUNSELLING CASE 8.2 – 'I am a gay man who has one regular partner but occasionally I have sex with new male acquaintances and, although I try to remember to "play safe", I don't think I have always succeeded. I am fully fit and, as far as I know, none of my partners is HIV positive. Would you advise me to be tested?'

Yes, the advantages of people at high risk of HIV knowing their status clearly outweighs any disadvantages. For the individual, the main advantage is that, if he tests positive, he can then have his virus load and CD4 lymphocyte count monitored so that antiretroviral therapy can be started as soon as it is clear that his infection has entered a stage when AIDS is inevitable, but before significant attrition of the CD4 lymphocytes. The aim is for the CD4 population to be stabilized at a level above that likely to be associated with life-threatening opportunistic infections such as *Pneumocystis carinii* pneumonia. He should be offered same-day testing to minimize anxious waiting and be seen with the result, not informed of it over the phone. The importance of safe sex must be reinforced, whatever the result of the test.

OSCE COUNSELLING CASE 8.3 – 'I am a 24-year-old mother of a 6-month-old baby girl. My widowed mother was recently in hospital for a hip replacement and her wound was infected with MRSA. I love my mother but don't want her in my home as she could infect my baby. In any case, shouldn't she have been kept in hospital?'

Methicillin-resistant *Staphylococcus aureus* (MRSA) rarely causes clinically significant infection in healthy individuals, including healthy babies. Significant infection in hospital is largely confined to elderly or debilitated people. There is no reason why colonized patients should not go home, if they are fit enough to manage, whereas, if they are admitted to hospital, they may have the depressing experience of being nursed in a side room because there is some evidence that this reduces the likelihood of transmission to others. Common sites for colonization are the nostrils and wounds. If there is no evidence of an inflammatory response, there is no imperative to treat the patient but, if wounds are inflamed, the choice of antibiotic should be guided by sensitivity testing although there may be no alternative to intravenous agents such as vancomycin. Colonization can be treated with topical antiseptics in an attempt to eliminate MRSA if readmission to hospital is likely to be necessary within 1 year.

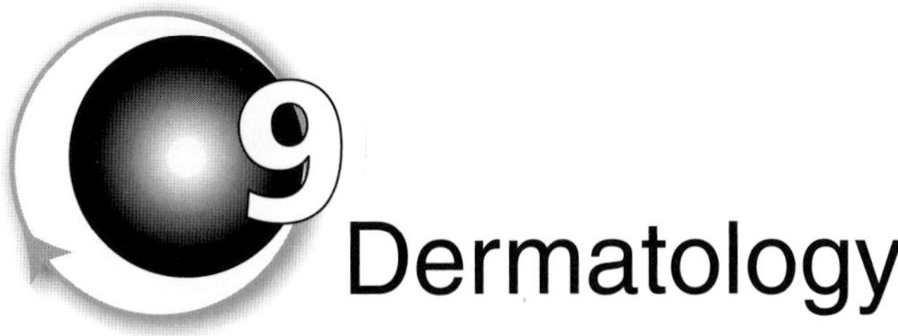

9 Dermatology

Nevianna Tomson

MALIGNANT MELANOMA

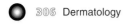

? Questions for each of the clinical case scenarios given

Q1: What is the likely differential diagnosis?
Q2: What issues in the given history support the diagnosis?
Q3: What additional features in the history would you seek to support a particular diagnosis?
Q4: What clinical examination would you perform and why?
Q5: What investigations would be most helpful and why?
Q6: What treatment options are appropriate?

Clinical cases

CASE 9.1 – 'I've developed a brown mark on my leg.'

A 40-year-old woman presented with a 3-month history of a gradually enlarging brown mark over her left shin. It had bled spontaneously on two occasions and appears to have become darker over the last few weeks.

CASE 9.2 – 'The age spot on my forehead is more noticeable.'

An 80-year-old woman attends the accident and emergency department (A&E) after a fall at home. The attending casualty officer incidentally notices a dark brown and black-coloured mark over her forehead. It is entirely asymptomatic and has been present for many years. The patient comments that it has become more noticeable over the last few months.

CASE 9.3 – 'I have developed a brown mark under my thumbnail.'

A 62-year-old African–Caribbean man presents to his GP having developed a dark-brown longitudinal streak under his right thumbnail. It has appeared in the last 2 months and is asymptomatic.

OSCE Counselling Cases

OSCE COUNSELLING CASE 9.1 – 'My mother died of melanoma. Is there anything I should do?'

A 20-year-old woman has come to see you concerned about her risk of developing malignant melanoma. She tells you that her mother died aged 35 from metastatic malignant melanoma and her maternal aunt has recently been diagnosed at the age of 50 with melanoma.

Q1: Does she have an increased risk of developing melanoma?

Q2: What can she do to minimize her risk of melanoma in the future?

OSCE COUNSELLING CASE 9.2 – 'What happens now that I have been diagnosed with malignant melanoma?'

A 49-year-old man has recently had a suspicious mole excised from his back. The histology has confirmed this to be a malignant melanoma. He attends the dermatology clinic today and is told the diagnosis.

Q1: What is the next step in his management?

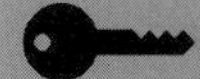

Key concepts

What is malignant melanoma?

Malignant melanoma is an invasive malignant tumour of melanocytes that usually develops anew in skin that was previously normal, but may arise in a pre-existing mole.

Where do they occur?

The leg is the most common site in women and the back in men, although malignant melanoma can affect any site of the body. Acral lentiginous melanoma is the most common melanoma in Oriental and black patients but is rare in white patients. It occurs on palmar and plantar skin and under the nails. Mucosal melanoma may occur in the oral cavity, around the anus or on the genitalia but is rare.

What are the distinguishing features between a benign and a malignant pigmented lesion?

The main diagnostic feature of malignant melanoma is the history of change in a pigmented lesion. The Glasgow Seven Point Check List and the American ABCDE System have been devised to help with diagnosing malignant melanoma. The Glasgow system lists three major features – change in size, irregularity in colour and irregularity of outline – and four minor features – diameter > 6 mm, inflammation, bleeding, itch or change in sensation.

Excision biopsy of the mole is suggested in the presence of one major feature. The presence of minor features adds to the suspicion of melanoma. In the UK, the American ABCDE system is mainly used:

A: **a**symmetry of the shape of the lesion.

B: irregularity of the **b**order

C: variation in **c**olour.

D: **d**iameter of the lesion (most melanomas are > 6 mm in diameter)

E: **e**levation and **e**xamination of other lesions.

A malignant melanoma usually looks different from the patient's other moles.

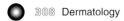

Answers

CASE 9.1 – 'I've developed a brown mark on my leg.'

Q1: What is the likely differential diagnosis?

A1

- Malignant melanoma
- Benign mole
- Seborrhoeic wart
- Dermatofibroma
- Freckle
- Solar lentigo
- Pigmented basal cell carcinoma (BCC).

Q2: What issues in the given history support the diagnosis?

A2

The patient gives a clear history of a pigmented lesion that is changing in size and colour. Both of these features suggest malignant melanoma. Melanomas may appear black or have irregular pigmentation with shades of white, red, blue, brown or black. Associated symptoms such as itching or bleeding can also signify that a melanoma is developing but are less important than change in size, shape and colour.

Q3: What additional features in the history would you seek to support a particular diagnosis?

A3

Establish how the lesion began. Was there a pre-existing mole there and when did it start to change? Determine how the lesion has changed. Is it simply a change in diameter or has its outline become more irregular? Benign moles usually have a symmetrical, even outline, whereas malignant melanomas tend to have an irregular edge with one area advancing more than the rest of the lesion. Finally, determine if there is any family history of skin cancer, in particular malignant melanoma.

Q4: What clinical examination would you perform and why?

A4

Examine the lesion in detail. Remember ABCDE! If a malignant melanoma is suspected, a general examination to look for secondary metastases is mandatory, paying particular attention to any cervical, axillary or inguinal lymphadenopathy.

 Q5: What investigations would be most helpful and why?

A5

A screen for metastatic disease is necessary once the diagnosis of malignant melanoma has been confirmed. This may include a full blood count (FBC), renal and liver function tests, and a chest radiograph. Abdominal ultrasonography or computed tomography (CT) are also occasionally requested. If a lymph node is clinically involved, it should be removed.

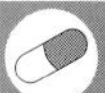 Q6: What treatment options are appropriate?

A6

Surgical excision is the only definitive treatment for malignant melanoma and is performed according to the depth of invasion. A 2-cm excision margin is generally accepted. Chemotherapy is used to treat metastatic disease.

 CASE 9.2 – 'The age spot on my forehead is more noticeable.'

 Q1: What is the likely differential diagnosis?

A1

- Lentigo maligna
- Lentigo maligna melanoma
- Solar lentigo
- Simple or senile lentigo
- Malignant melanoma
- Seborrhoeic keratosis
- Café-au-lait spot.

 Q2: What issues in the given history support the diagnosis?

A2

Lentigo maligna is an *in situ* malignant melanoma. It can closely resemble other pigmented lesions, such as simple or solar lentigos and flat seborrhoeic keratosis. It appears as a flat, pigmented lesion with colours that may vary from light tan to dark brown or black. It gradually enlarges but is otherwise asymptomatic. Its margin is usually irregular. It becomes thickened and nodular as it invades through the basement membrane and is then known as lentigo maligna melanoma.

 Q3: What additional features in the history would you seek to support a particular diagnosis?

A3

Lentigo maligna typically occurs over sun-exposed areas and most patients give a history of significant sunlight exposure throughout their lives. Ask the patient whether the lesion is more noticeable because it has enlarged or developed an irregular border or colour.

 Q4: What clinical examination would you perform and why?

A4

Examine the lesion in detail for irregularity in border and colour, and measure its size. In particular, note any nodularity that may suggest progression to lentigo maligna melanoma. Examine for lymphadenopathy.

 Q5: What investigations would be most helpful and why?

A5

Magnification of the lesion by dermatoscopy can be useful in trying to distinguish lentigo maligna from simple lentigo and early seborrhoeic keratosis. However, biopsy of the lesion is necessary to confirm the diagnosis of lentigo maligna and distinguish it from lentigo maligna melanoma.

Q6: What treatment options are appropriate?

A6

Ideally, lentigo maligna should be excised surgically. However, it usually occurs in elderly people and is often quite sizeable at presentation. Dermatologists sometimes prefer to observe these lesions and monitor with serial photographs. Excision is then undertaken only if the lesion becomes thickened and confirmed on biopsy to have developed into lentigo maligna melanoma. Early lentigo maligna can also be treated with radiotherapy or cryotherapy.

 CASE 9.3 – 'I have developed a brown mark under my thumbnail.'

 Q1: What is the likely differential diagnosis?

A1

- Subungual melanoma
- Trauma

- Linear melanonychia (straight, longitudinal, brown/black, evenly pigmented line – common in the nails of black patients and very rarely in white people)
- Fungal nail infection.

 Q2: What issues in the given history support the diagnosis?

A2

In the absence of a history of trauma, a subungual melanoma must be considered as the most likely diagnosis.

 Q3: What additional features in the history would you seek to support a particular diagnosis?

A3

Ask if the patient recalls any trauma to the nail. Are any of the other nails affected in a similar way?

 Q4: What clinical examination would you perform and why?

A4

Examine the nail carefully. In subungual melanoma the pigment under the nail is deep and often irregular. Deep red/purple colours or pinpoint russet areas suggest haemorrhage from trauma. Look out for Hutchinson's sign: a flat, pigmented and irregular patch of skin over the nail fold, highly diagnostic of subungual melanoma. The nail may also have become deformed and may split as the melanoma underneath thickens. The patient must also be examined for metastatic spread.

 Q5: What investigations would be most helpful and why?

A5

A nail biopsy is the only way to confirm or refute the diagnosis.

 Q6: What treatment options are appropriate?

A6

The melanoma is surgically excised, which frequently necessitates amputation of the digit.

OSCE Counselling Cases – Answers

OSCE COUNSELLING CASE 9.1 – 'My mother died of melanoma. Is there anything I should do?'

The incidence of melanoma is rapidly increasing. In the UK, the incidence is approximately 5 cases per 100 000 population. This is much higher in other countries such as Australia where there are 50 new cases per 100 000. Ultraviolet (UV) light is considered to be the most important factor. Intense and infrequent exposure once or twice a year appears to carry a greater risk than chronic continuous sunlight exposure. Fair-skinned individuals, those with red hair, blue eyes and poor tanning capacity, who burn frequently when exposed to sunlight, have the greatest risk of developing melanoma.

Most malignant melanomas occur sporadically. However, 2–10 per cent of patients diagnosed with malignant melanoma give a positive family history of melanoma in one or more first-degree relatives. This may be a result of inheritance of specific melanoma susceptibility genes or grouping of other known risk factors, e.g. similar skin type, sun exposure and number of pigmented naevi in family members.

Prevention of melanoma is extremely important. Patients must be educated on the dangers of UV radiation and sunburn, and the importance of using photoprotection, including clothing, to cover sun-exposed areas and high-factor sunscreens. Patients should also be educated on the features of malignancy to look out for, in order to help with early detection and treatment of malignant melanoma in the future.

OSCE COUNSELLING CASE 9.2 – 'What happens now that I have been diagnosed with malignant melanoma?'

The patient will need to have the following:

- A full clinical examination to look for metastases.
- Investigations to look for metastatic spread of the melanoma: FBC, renal and liver function tests and a chest radiograph. Abdominal ultrasonography or CT are sometimes requested. If a lymph node is clinically involved it should be removed for histological analysis.
- Further excision of the scar with a 2-cm margin to minimize the risk of local recurrence in the future.
- Follow-up for a minimum of 5 years to exclude recurrence or metastasis. At each visit the patient should have the scar examined and a general examination. He or she should also be taught self-examination of the scar and how to look for lymphadenopathy.

NON-MELANOMA SKIN CANCER

? Questions for each of the clinical case scenarios given

Q1: What is the likely differential diagnosis?
Q2: What issues in the given history support the diagnosis?
Q3: What additional features in the history would you seek to support a particular diagnosis?
Q4: What clinical examination would you perform and why?
Q5: What investigations would be most helpful and why?
Q6: What treatment options are appropriate?

Clinical cases

CASE 9.4 – 'I have a small ulcer on my scalp.'

A 70-year-old man presents with an ulcer over the vertex of his scalp. He has been losing his hair since the age of 30 and noticed the sore appear 6 months ago. It has increased in size and bleeds on minimal trauma.

CASE 9.5 – 'The lump over my cheek is getting bigger.'

A 48-year-old man who works as a landscape gardener presents to his GP, having noticed a small lump appear over his right cheek about 1 year ago. It has been slowly increasing in size but is otherwise asymptomatic

CASE 9.6 – 'Two red patches have appeared on my shin.'

An 82-year-old woman has come to see you with two red, scaly patches over her right shin. She is not sure how long they have been present because they are not giving her any symptoms. Two years ago she had some solar keratosis over her forehead that were treated with cryotherapy.

OSCE Counselling Case

OSCE COUNSELLING CASE 9.3 – 'What can I do to reduce my risk of more skin cancers in the future?'

A 42-year-old woman has recently had two nodular BCCs excised from her face. She attends for a routine follow-up visit.

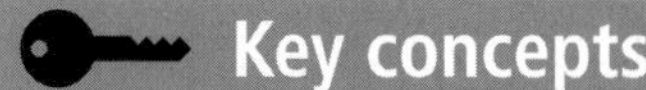

Key concepts

What is an actinic keratosis (solar keratosis)?

These are areas of chronic sun-induced skin damage occurring on exposed sites (face, balding scalp, ears, dorsum of hands); they are also known as solar keratoses. They are usually multiple and appear as clearly demarcated, rough, red, scaly lesions. Small lesions are more easily felt than visualized. They are considered premalignant and have the potential to progress to squamous cell carcinoma. A variety of treatments are available, the most commonly used being cryotherapy, 5-fluorouracil (5FU) cream or curettage.

What is Bowen's disease?

Bowen's disease is another name for intraepidermal squamous cell carcinoma (SCC). It occurs predominantly in elderly people over sun-exposed sites (usually over the lower legs but also the face and neck). Lesions present as a red patch with a variable amount of scale, and enlarge slowly over time. They are typically asymptomatic but may itch, ulcerate or bleed. Often they are misdiagnosed as eczema or psoriasis. In a fifth of patients, multiple lesions occur. Progression to invasive SCC has been reported in about 5 per cent. Treatment of Bowen's disease is with cryotherapy, 5FU cream, photodynamic therapy or surgical excision/curettage.

What is a basal cell carcinoma?

Basal cell carcinoma (BCC) is the most common skin cancer and is also known as a rodent ulcer. It originates from basal cells of the lower epidermis and is locally destructive but rarely metastasizes. It is common on the head and neck and over the back and chest. It presents as an asymptomatic nodule that slowly enlarges and may occasionally bleed. It is often diagnosed incidentally. It may be surgically removed by excision or curettage, or treated by radiotherapy or cryotherapy .

What is a squamous cell carcinoma (SCC)?

This is a malignant tumour that arises from keratinocytes and has the potential to metastasize. It presents on sun-exposed sites (face, ears, balding scalp, dorsum of hands, forearms, lower legs) as a sore or ulcer that enlarges quite rapidly and fails to heal. Surgical excision is the treatment of choice but radiotherapy may also be used.

Answers

CASE 9.4 – 'I have a small ulcer on my scalp.'

Q1: What is the likely differential diagnosis?

A1

- SCC
- Solar keratosis
- Bowen's disease
- Ulcerated BCC
- Keratoacanthoma
- Viral wart.

Q2: What issues in the given history support the diagnosis?

A2

A non-healing ulcer over a sun-exposed area raises the possibility of an SCC. Patients may report that the lesion crusts over, or bleeds when traumatized (e.g. on combing hair) or spontaneously.

Q3: What additional features in the history would you seek to support a particular diagnosis?

A3

Ultraviolet irradiation is the most common cause so ask about previous sun exposure. Has the patient worked outdoors or lived abroad? Has he received PUVA (psoralen and UVA) or used sunbeds in the past? Ask about X-ray irradiation, used in the past to treat tinea capitis, eczema, psoriasis etc., which may have been a predisposing factor. Squamous cell carcinomas are also well known to arise in scars, such as those from previous burns. Immunosuppressants also predispose to non-melanoma skin cancers and SCCs are common in organ transplant recipients. Also, enquire about any family history of skin cancer.

Q4: What clinical examination would you perform and why?

A4

Examine the ulcer and measure its size. The rest of the skin must also be examined for other sun-induced cutaneous premalignant and malignant conditions, such as solar keratosis, Bowen's disease and BCCs. Look also for any clinical signs of metastasis, paying particular attention to the regional lymph nodes.

Q5: What investigations would be most helpful and why?

A5

The lesion must be biopsied to confirm the diagnosis histologically.

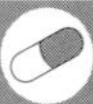

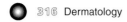

Q6: What treatment options are appropriate?

A6

The treatment of choice is surgical excision with a minimum of 4 mm margin of normal skin excised with the tumour. Radiotherapy is also very effective and typically used for patients who refuse surgery, non-resectable tumours, and where tumour margins are ill defined. Small, well-defined, low-risk tumours are occasionally treated with curettage or cryotherapy. Patients are followed up to look for clinical signs of recurrence.

CASE 9.5 – 'The lump over my cheek is getting bigger.'

Q1: What is the likely differential diagnosis?

A1

- BCC
- Epidermoid cyst
- Sebaceous hyperplasia
- Intradermal naevus
- Seborrhoeic keratosis
- Viral wart
- SCC
- Keratoacanthoma.

Q2: What issues in the given history support the diagnosis?

A2

A BCC must be considered when there is a history of a slowly enlarging lump over a sun-exposed site. It generally starts as an asymptomatic papule that becomes nodular and ulcerates centrally.

Q3: What additional features in the history would you seek to support a particular diagnosis?

A3

Ask about exposure to UV light, X-ray irradiation and use of immunosuppressant medication as you would when an SCC is suspected.

 Q4: What clinical examination would you perform and why?

A4

Examine the lesion and measure its diameter. The lesion classically appears as a pearly papule or nodule with telangiectasia and a raised 'rolled' edge. Basal cell carcinomas are usually subdivided into types:

- Superficial BCCs: flat, red patches usually over the trunk. A rolled, pearly, telangiectatic border may be visible.
- Nodular/cystic BCCs: as described above.
- Multifocal BCCs: these start as nodules that expand with areas of apparent regression between them. However, there are fine strands of tumour connecting the nodules.
- Morphoeic BCC: elevated, smooth, firm plaque that is often misdiagnosed as a scar. It may appear pearly with telangiectasia.
- Pigmented BCCs: as for nodular BCCs but with pigmented margins. A pigmented BCC may be mistaken for malignant melanoma.

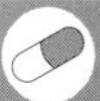 Q5: What investigations would be most helpful and why?

A5

A diagnostic biopsy is performed for histological confirmation of the type of BCC.

Q6: What treatment options are appropriate?

A6

Surgical treatment can be by excision with a 4 mm margin or curettage and cautery for small, multiple and superficial lesions. Cryotherapy is sometimes used for superficial or multiple lesions. Radiotherapy is often more appropriate than surgery in elderly people, and may produce better cosmetic results. Patients need to be followed up to exclude recurrence and look for further premalignant and malignant lesions.

 CASE 9.6 – 'Two red patches have appeared on my shin.'

 Q1: What is the likely differential diagnosis?

A1

- Bowen's disease
- Actinic keratosis
- SCC
- BCC

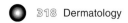

- Eczema
- Psoriasis
- Seborrhoeic keratosis.

 Q2: What issues in the given history support the diagnosis?

A2

A red, scaly patch on the lower leg of an elderly woman is typical of Bowen's disease. Most lesions are asymptomatic and go unnoticed by the patient.

 Q3: What additional features in the history would you seek to support a particular diagnosis?

A3

Lesions of Bowen's disease show gradual radial growth. Ask about symptoms such as bleeding or ulceration, which may occur as the lesion enlarges. Most lesions are caused by chronic UV light irradiation so ask about sun exposure.

 Q4: What clinical examination would you perform and why?

A4

Examine the lesions and record the diameter of each. Look for induration, erosion or ulceration of the plaques which may suggest malignant transformation into SCC. Examine the rest of the skin for other premalignant or malignant lesions.

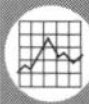 Q5: What investigations would be most helpful and why?

A5

The diagnosis is usually made on clinical examination and can be confirmed by biopsy of the lesion.

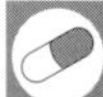 Q6: What treatment options are appropriate?

A6

Cryotherapy with liquid nitrogen or topical 5FU cream is usually used and is very effective, although it may lead to ulceration particularly when treating lesions on the lower limbs of elderly patients. Curettage and cautery or occasionally excision can also be used. Photodynamic therapy is usually reserved for large or multiple lesions.

OSCE Counselling Case – Answer

OSCE COUNSELLING CASE 9.3 – 'What can I do to reduce my risk of more skin cancers in the future?'

Prevention of skin cancer involves education of patients about the disease in order to change their behaviour and lifestyle. Advise the patient to limit her exposure to UV light by wearing suitable clothing to cover her trunk and limbs, and a wide-brimmed hat to protect her scalp, face and ears. She should avoid going outdoors during the middle of the day when the sun is at its strongest. A sunscreen of sun protection factor 25 or above should be applied to any sun-exposed site. She should also be educated to examine her skin regularly for any new lesions so that any skin cancers can be detected early and treated.

ECZEMA

Questions for each of the clinical case scenarios given

Q1: What is the likely differential diagnosis?
Q2: What issues in the given history support the diagnosis?
Q3: What additional features in the history would you seek to support a particular diagnosis?
Q4: What clinical examination would you perform and why?
Q5: What investigations would be most helpful and why?
Q6: What treatment options are appropriate?

Clinical cases

CASE 9.7 – 'I have painful weeping lesions over my face.'

An 18-year-old girl attends A&E complaining of painful weeping lesions over her face. These started 2 days ago over her chin and have now spread to involve her entire face. She has had eczema since she was a baby but it has not been active for the last 2 years. Last week she had a cold sore over her upper lip.

CASE 9.8 – 'My hands have become red and sore.'

A 24-year-old hairdresser has developed painful, red, scaly lesions over the palmar aspect of both hands. She has noticed small blisters and weeping areas when it is very severe. While she was on maternity leave last year her hands improved, but since she has returned to work the condition has flared up again.

OSCE Counselling Case

OSCE COUNSELLING CASE 9.4 – 'Which creams do I use for my baby's eczema?'

A mother comes to see you with her 6-month-old baby. He developed eczema soon after birth, with red dry areas over his cheeks, limb flexures and abdomen, and dry scale (cradle cap) over his scalp. She has been prescribed lots of different creams by different GPs each time she takes him to the surgery and is not sure where to use each cream.

Q1: Explain to her what general measures she can take to help improve the child's eczema.

Q2: Explain to her where and how to use emollients and topical steroids.

OSCE COUNSELLING CASE 9.5 – 'I have been referred for patch testing. What does this involve?'

A 42-year-old man has been referred to the contact dermatitis clinic for patch testing. He is a keen gardener and suspects the eczema over his hands results from contact with plants in the summer months.

Q1: Explain to him what patch testing involves.

Key concepts

What are the different types of eczema?

- Atopic eczema: chronic, pruritic inflammatory disorder, mainly affecting children but may persist into adulthood. Characterized by relapses and remissions. Frequently associated with other atopic disorders such as asthma and hayfever.
- Seborrhoeic eczema: chronic eczematous disorder with erythema and scaling distributed over the face (glabella, alae of the nose, eyebrows, sideburns, ears), scalp, flexures and upper trunk. Typically non-pruritic and associated with overgrowth of the yeast *Pityrosporum ovale*.
- Discoid eczema: coin-shaped raised erythematous lesions occurring over the trunk and limbs. Usually occurs in older individuals but can also present in young adults. Secondary infection with staphylococci is common.
- Pompholyx eczema: pruritic vesicular eruption over the palms, soles and sides of the digits. Usually occurs in young individuals and is associated with excessive sweating and warm weather.
- Varicose eczema: pruritic, red eczematous patches over the shins commonly occur secondary to venous hypertension. Varicose veins are often visible. Other changes may include oedema of the lower limbs, induration, and hyperpigmentation caused by haemosiderin deposition in the skin. Ulceration may be precipitated by minor injury or infection.
- Contact dermatitis: an irritant or allergic eczematous reaction caused by an external substance coming into contact with the skin. Irritant contact dermatitis can affect anyone as long as they are exposed to a sufficient concentration of the irritant agent and for enough time. Allergic contact dermatitis is a delayed-type hypersensitivity allergic reaction that occurs only in predisposed individuals on every encounter with the allergen.

Answers

 CASE 9.7 – 'I have painful weeping lesions over my face.'

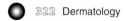

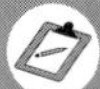 Q1: What is the likely differential diagnosis?

A1

This is eczema herpeticum.

Impetigo caused by staphylococci or streptococci (or combination of these) is also a possibility, although it is more common in childhood.

 Q2: What issues in the given history support the diagnosis?

A2

Eczema herpeticum is the most likely diagnosis in the light of the recent cold sore. Contrary to popular belief this does not occur only when the eczema is in an active phase.

 Q3: What additional features in the history would you seek to support a particular diagnosis?

A3

Start by finding out when, where and how the lesions began, and whether any treatment was given by the GP or if the patient used any over-the-counter medication, and whether there was any improvement or deterioration from this. Are any other members of the family or friends affected in a similar way? Painful and weeping lesions indicate infection, so establish whether the patient has been feeling unwell in any way, e.g. fever, rigors. Finally, find out more about the past medical history and how her eczema was managed in the past.

 Q4: What clinical examination would you perform and why?

A4

Examine the skin and document the extent and morphology of the lesions. Vesicles, yellow crusts or a combination of these is usually present. Look for associated lymphadenopathy. Examine the eyes for any conjunctival involvement.

 Q5: What investigations would be most helpful and why?

A5

Bacterial and viral swabs of the vesicle fluid or crusts will confirm the organism responsible. If the patient is pyrexial, blood cultures must be taken. An FBC may show raised white cell count (WCC) and the C-reactive protein (CRP) will also be elevated in infection.

 Q6: What treatment options are appropriate?

A6

Oral aciclovir 200 mg five times a day for 5 days is the treatment of choice for eczema herpeticum. If the infection is severe, intravenous aciclovir may be used. If the diagnosis is in doubt or secondary bacterial infection is also suspected, it is best to add in flucloxacillin and penicillin. Topical emollients will provide symptomatic relief and, once the infection has been treated, topical corticosteroids are usually necessary to treat the eczema. If there is eye involvement, an urgent assessment by an ophthalmologist is needed to exclude corneal ulceration which may lead to blindness if left untreated.

Patients should be nursed in a side room and warned to avoid close physical contact with friends and family, because the herpes virus is contagious. Once the infection has been treated, it is important to educate the patient on management of her eczema with daily use of emollients and topical corticosteroids over areas of active eczema. Bath oils and soap substitute emollients are useful to prevent dryness of the skin. Antihistamines can also be used to control pruritus.

 CASE 9.8 – 'My hands have become red and sore.'

 Q1: What is the likely differential diagnosis?

A1

- Allergic contact dermatitis
- Irritant contact dermatitis
- Pompholyx eczema
- Tinea
- Psoriasis.

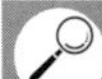 Q2: What issues in the given history support the diagnosis?

A2

Allergic contact dermatitis is a delayed hypersensitivity reaction. Once an individual has been sensitized to a given allergen, dermatitis recurs on every subsequent exposure. Frequently the allergen responsible is encountered in the workplace and the dermatitis remits at weekends or holidays. Lesions are often pruritic or sore and blisters are common with severe reactions. The distribution reflects the areas of contact with the allergen. Industrial dermatitis is commonly seen over the palms of the hands; the dorsum of the hands and wrists are typically affected with allergy to rubber gloves, and the earlobes and navel are affected with allergy to nickel in earrings and metal jeans studs etc.

Q3: What additional features in the history would you seek to support a particular diagnosis?

A3

The history is very important when allergic contact dermatitis is suspected. The distribution of dermatitis may give a clue to the responsible allergen, as indicated above. Common allergens responsible for contact dermatitis include metal (nickel and cobalt in costume jewellery), rubber, perfumes, nail varnish, plants, dyes, cosmetics, and colophony in adhesive dressings such as plasters. Ask about any hobbies that the patient may have where she may come into contact with potential allergens. Find out if she has tried any topical preparations and whether they have improved or exacerbated the problem. Topical anaesthetics, antihistamines and rarely corticosteroids may occasionally be the culprit allergen.

Q4: What clinical examination would you perform and why?

A4

Determine if the dermatitis is confined to the palms of the hands or if other areas are also involved. In palmoplantar psoriasis, the soles of the feet may be similarly involved. There may also be other clues for psoriasis such as scaly plaques over the extensor surfaces of the limbs, scaling of the scalp or pitting and onycholysis of the nails. On the other hand, tinea is almost always unilateral and there may be a history or clinical evidence of athlete's foot as the source of infection.

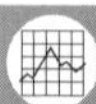

Q5: What investigations would be most helpful and why?

A5

The diagnosis of allergic contact dermatitis can be confirmed by patch testing (see OSCE Counselling Case 9.5 for details about how it is performed). If tinea is suspected, skin scrapings from the lesion can be taken and sent for mycology to look for the presence of fungus. In weeping lesions superimposed infection can be identified by sending skin swabs for microbiology.

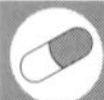

Q6: What treatment options are appropriate?

A6

If possible, the antigen should be completely removed from the patient's environment. This usually leads to complete recovery. However, this is not always possible and patients should be advised to avoid contact with the allergen as much as they possibly can, e.g. by wearing rubber gloves when handling it. Topical corticosteroids will provide symptomatic relief but the dermatitis will recur on exposure to the allergen. In very severe cases, a short course of systemic steroids may be used.

OSCE Counselling Cases – Answers

OSCE COUNSELLING CASE 9.4 – 'Which creams do I use for my baby's eczema?'

A1

Simple measures can help with the management of eczema. Skin contact with irritants such as woollen clothing (the clothing layer next to the skin should always be 100 per cent cotton), fragranced soaps and bubble baths should be avoided. Preventing the child from overheating will help reduce pruritus. This includes ensuring that bath water is not too warm and that the room temperature is controlled.

A2

The daily use of emollients to prevent dryness of the skin is vital. These should be used at least first thing in the morning and after a bath at night, and more frequently in the winter months and if the skin is still dry. A soap substitute such as emulsifying ointment is good to help with skin hydration, and a bath oil can also be added to the bath water. Some emollients, soap substitutes and bath oils also contain an antibacterial agent that is useful in treating and preventing infection, especially in children who often scratch at their eczema. The child should have a bath each night and then have an emollient applied. Olive oil is an effective emollient for the scalp in babies with cradle cap. A topical corticosteroid should be applied to areas of active eczema. Ointment preparations are generally better than creams at hydration, but creams are used in preference over weeping areas, where ointments tend to slide off. A 20-min gap between emollient and steroid application will prevent dilution of the steroid. Topical steroids should not be used over areas of infected eczema. Occasionally a topical antibiotic and corticosteroid combination is prescribed for areas of mildly infected eczema.

OSCE COUNSELLING CASE 9.5 – 'I have been referred for patch testing. What does this involve?'

When allergic contact dermatitis is suspected, patch testing is performed whereby the suspected allergen is placed in direct contact with the skin. About 30 commonly encountered allergens are used in a 'standard battery' to which other potential allergens are added, e.g. a range of plants in suspected plant-induced contact dermatitis, the patient's own cosmetics in facial dermatitis. The allergens are placed in individual aluminium wells and applied to the patient's back with adhesive tape. They are left in place for 48 h and then removed. The skin is inspected at 96 h for areas of dermatitis corresponding to the application site of each allergen. Positive readings are interpreted with the clinical context in mind because they may not be relevant to the patient's symptoms.

PSORIASIS

? Questions for each of the clinical case scenarios given

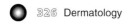

Q1: What is the likely differential diagnosis?
Q2: What issues in the given history support the diagnosis?
Q3: What additional features in the history would you seek to support a particular diagnosis?
Q4: What clinical examination would you perform and why?
Q5: What investigations would be most helpful and why?
Q6: What treatment options are appropriate?

Clinical cases

CASE 9.9 – 'I have dry red patches over my elbows and knees.'

A 33-year-old woman presents with dry, red, scaly patches of skin over the elbows and knees. These have come on gradually over the years and are asymptomatic. She also has dandruff. This has recently become much worse and is causing her great embarrassment.

CASE 9.10 – 'My skin has turned red.'

A 54-year-old man has developed redness and discomfort of the skin over his trunk and limbs. He was diagnosed with chronic plaque psoriasis in his 20s. On examination, he is pyrexial and has confluent erythema over his chest, back, abdomen, arms and legs.

OSCE Counselling Cases

OSCE COUNSELLING CASE 9.6 – 'Can I have some tablets instead of creams for my psoriasis?'

A 40-year-old woman has had chronic plaque psoriasis affecting her trunk, limbs and scalp for 20 years. This has been reasonably well controlled with topical preparations. She has recently read an article in a magazine which described a 'miracle tablet that cures psoriasis'. She tells you that she is fed up with her messy creams and wants to have this tablet.

Q1: What systemic therapies are commonly used to treat psoriasis? When are they used and what does a specialist need to take into consideration when initiating treatment?

Q2: What monitoring is required?

OSCE COUNSELLING CASE 9.7 – 'Can I use a sunbed to treat my psoriasis?'

A 22-year-old woman has recently been diagnosed with psoriasis. She tells you that her aunt also has the condition, which has almost completely cleared with UV treatment given by her specialist. She wants to know if buying a sunbed to use at home will help her psoriasis.

Q1: Explain to her why it is not recommended for her to use a sunbed at home.

Q2: What types of UV treatment are available for the treatment of psoriasis?

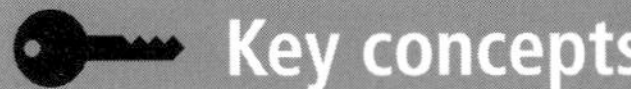

Key concepts

What is psoriasis?

Psoriasis is a common, chronic, hyperproliferative and immunological condition, characterized by well-demarcated, erythematous, silvery scaled plaques, typically in a symmetrical distribution over extensor surfaces and in the scalp.

What are the different types of psoriasis?

- Chronic plaque psoriasis/psoriasis vulgaris: well-defined, usually symmetrical raised red plaques with thick silvery scale, most commonly over the extensor surfaces of the elbows and knees, but may occur at any skin site. The scalp is usually affected and there may be nail involvement.
- Flexural psoriasis: may occur alongside chronic plaque psoriasis. There are well-defined areas of erythema affecting the flexures (groin, perianally, axillae, umbilicus, inframammary folds).
- Guttate psoriasis: usually affects adolescents and young adults, occurring days/few weeks after a severe streptococcal throat infection. However, a history of this is not always obtained. It presents with widespread, drop-like ('guttate'), red papules with silvery scale over the trunk and limbs. It resolves within a few months but may recur in some patients.
- Palmoplantar pustular psoriasis: pustules occur over the palms and soles, on the background of well-defined, red, scaly plaques. It is usually bilateral and there may be psoriasis elsewhere.
- Erythrodermic psoriasis: worsening psoriasis can develop into erythroderma – a term used to describe abnormal reddening of the skin affecting over 90 per cent of the total body surface area. Patients are usually unwell and may be pyrexial. The redness is the result of capillary proliferation. Erythroderma may also be caused by eczema, drugs or cutaneous T-cell lymphoma (also known as mycosis fungoides).
- Generalized pustular psoriasis: an extreme form of psoriasis with extensive, small, sterile pustules and underlying erythema covering the skin. It can be provoked by abrupt cessation of potent steroids or reduction in immunosuppressive treatment for psoriasis, or possibly as a result of concurrent infection, pregnancy or alcohol excess. There is a significant associated mortality.
- Psoriasis of the nails: about a third of patients with psoriasis and a quarter of those with psoriatic arthropathy and psoriasis have nail changes. However, they may occur in isolation and include pitting, onycholysis and subungual hyperkeratosis.
- Psoriatic arthropathy: arthropathy occurs in 8–10 per cent of patients with psoriasis but may occur in the absence of skin changes. It may present in different forms, most commonly asymmetrical arthritis, symmetrical polyarthritis, ankylosing spondylitis and arthritis mutilans.

Answers

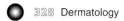

 CASE 9.9 – 'I have dry red patches over my elbows and knees.'

 Q1: What is the likely differential diagnosis?

A1

- Psoriasis
- Eczema
- Tinea.

 Q2: What issues in the given history support the diagnosis?

A2

The distribution of the lesions is characteristic of psoriasis. Apart from its cosmetic appearance, which causes significant distress to some patients, the condition is asymptomatic. Both eczema and tinea are typically pruritic.

 Q3: What additional features in the history would you seek to support a particular diagnosis?

A3

Find out how the condition has progressed until now. Has it gradually got worse over the years or does it come and go? Is it worse at any particular time of year? Most patients find that their psoriasis is worse in the winter and improves with sun exposure in the summer months. Find out if there are any other exacerbating or relieving factors. Alcohol, nicotine, β blockers, lithium and anti-malarial tablets can all make psoriasis worse. Ask about family history because one-third of patients with psoriasis recall a family member with the condition.

 Q4: What clinical examination would you perform and why?

A4

Examine the skin, scalp and nails for changes consistent with psoriasis. Plaques vary in size and shape and may coalesce into large areas. The central area of the plaque clears first on healing, which leaves ring-shaped configurations. The Auspitz sign may be elicited by scraping away the surface of a scaly plaque to reveal tiny bleeding points from the dilated superficial capillaries.

 Q5: What investigations would be most helpful and why?

A5

Psoriasis is a diagnosis made clinically and usually no investigations are necessary. If tinea is suspected, skin scrapings sent for mycology may differentiate between the diagnoses.

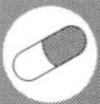 Q6: What treatment options are appropriate?

A6

There are many treatments for psoriasis. Daily emollients are used alongside other topical preparations such as coal tar, dithranol, corticosteroids and vitamin D analogues, some being available in combined preparations. For scalp psoriasis, tar shampoos and topical corticosteroid scalp applications usually achieve good results. Long-wave UV (UVA) radiation exposure after ingestion of psoralen (PUVA) or short-wave UV (UVB) radiation without psoralen can be used for widespread psoriasis. The number of treatments that can be given to a patient during their lifetime is limited because UV radiation increases the risk of skin malignancies. Cytotoxic drugs such as methotrexate, ciclosporin and oral retinoids can be very effective for severe psoriasis but require careful monitoring to avoid complications.

 CASE 9.10 – 'My skin has turned red.'

 Q1: What is the likely differential diagnosis?

A1

Causes of erythroderma include:

- Psoriasis
- Eczema
- Drugs
- Cutaneous T-cell lymphoma (also known as mycosis fungoides).

 Q2: What issues in the given history support the diagnosis?

A2

Erythroderma is a term used to describe abnormal reddening of the skin affecting over 90 per cent of the total body surface area. In this case the patient's psoriasis is most probably the cause.

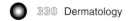

Q3: What additional features in the history would you seek to support a particular diagnosis?

A3

Find out when the symptoms began. Was there a preceding illness (e.g. sore throat) or did he become unwell once the skin erythema developed? What is the extent of his psoriasis normally and how is it managed? Determine if there have been any changes made to his psoriasis treatment recently? Abrupt cessation of topical corticosteroids or oral immunosuppressive medication can precipitate erythroderma. An increase in alcohol consumption can cause an exacerbation of psoriasis.

Q4: What clinical examination would you perform and why?

A4

Erythrodermic psoriasis is deep red in colour. It may also be exfoliative with scaling or peeling of the skin. Thick white/silvery scaly plaques may cover the body or be confined to the extensor surfaces of the elbows and knees. In most psoriatic patients there is also scalp involvement, which may vary from fine flakes to thick scaly plaques. The nails may also be affected with pitting, ridging and/or onycholysis.

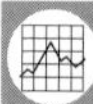

Q5: What investigations would be most helpful and why?

A5

The diagnosis is usually made on history and examination. An FBC may show a leukocytosis, and inflammatory markers such as the CRP or erythrocyte sedimentation rate (ESR) may be raised. An infection screen (blood cultures, chest radiograph etc.) is necessary if there is any history or sign of infection. Monitor renal function because vasodilatation leads to increased percutaneous water loss with consequent decreased urine output, which may lead to renal failure. Liver function must also be measured if the patient admits to excess alcohol consumption.

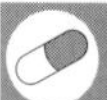

Q6: What treatment options are appropriate?

A6

Correction of hypovolaemia and hypothermia, and treatment of concomitant sepsis, are vital in the early stages of erythroderma. Emollients are applied daily. Systemic therapy (e.g. retinoids, methotrexate) is usually needed to control the underlying psoriasis. Corticosteroids and UV light therapy (narrowband UVB or psoralen and UVA) are usually avoided.

OSCE Counselling Cases – Answers

OSCE COUNSELLING CASE 9.6 – 'Can I have some tablets instead of creams for my psoriasis?'

A1

The decision to start systemic therapy can be difficult and is made by a specialist. It is generally a long-term commitment, using drugs with potential side effects, which require careful monitoring. Patients must be told that it is not a cure for psoriasis and that on cessation of treatment the disease usually returns to its previous state. Drug interactions may occur so a drug history is important before initiating treatment. Systemic therapies are used to treat:

- erythrodermic psoriasis
- generalized pustular psoriasis
- extensive psoriasis (where other therapy has failed/multiple admissions to hospital have been necessary/disease interferes with function or restricts quality of life etc.).

The most commonly used systemic therapies are:

- Methotrexate
- Ciclosporin
- Oral retinoids.

A2

METHOTREXATE

- Given as a once-weekly dose of 0.2–0.4 mg/kg. A test dose of 2.5–5 mg is given before starting therapy to detect idiosyncratic myelosuppression, which may occur within 7–10 days (an FBC is necessary).
- Bone marrow toxicity may occur so the FBC must be monitored.
- Liver function tests are needed regularly because hepatotoxicity may occur. Occasionally a liver biopsy is necessary if hepatic fibrosis is suspected.
- The drug is excreted by the kidneys so renal function is also monitored.
- The drug is teratogenic in early pregnancy and therefore all women need adequate contraception and are told to avoid pregnancy for at least 3 months after cessation of treatment.

CICLOSPORIN

- Low-dose (2.5 mg/kg per day and increased slowly) or high-dose (5 mg/kg per day) regimens are used and are usually well tolerated.
- Risk of nephrotoxicity means that careful monitoring of renal function is vital.
- There is also a risk of hypertension and blood pressure checks are mandatory.

ORAL RETINOIDS – ACITRETIN

- Taken as tablets: 1 mg/kg daily.
- Hyperlipidaemia and hepatotoxicity may occur so monitoring of cholesterol, triglycerides and liver function is necessary.
- It is highly teratogenic and should be avoided in women of childbearing age.

OSCE COUNSELLING CASE 9.7 – 'Can I use a sunbed to treat my psoriasis?'

A1

Ultraviolet treatment can be very beneficial for the treatment of psoriasis. However, it must be initiated by a specialist and given in a controlled manner. The dose given (in joules per square centimetre or J/cm^2) depends on the patient's skin type. There is a risk of cutaneous malignancy, which is cumulative and becomes highly significant after a total dose of 1200 J/cm^2. Psoriasis patients often require repeated courses of UV treatment to keep the disease under control. A record is kept of how much cumulative exposure has been given to each patient and this is kept to a minimum where possible. It is not recommended that patients use sunbeds because there is no monitoring of the dose given.

A2

Long-wave UV (UVA) radiation exposure after ingestion of psoralen (PUVA) or short-wave UV (UVB) radiation without psoralen can be used in the treatment of psoriasis. Psoralens may also be applied topically or added to the bath before UVA exposure (bath PUVA). Treatment is usually given two to three times a week for about 20 treatments to obtain clearance of the disease. Multiple courses of treatment are usually necessary in a patient's lifetime. Patients must be warned of the risks of developing cutaneous malignancies.

PRURITUS

? Questions for each of the clinical case scenarios given

Q1: What is the likely differential diagnosis?
Q2: What issues in the given history support the diagnosis?
Q3: What additional features in the history would you seek to support a particular diagnosis?
Q4: What clinical examination would you perform and why?
Q5: What investigations would be most helpful and why?
Q6: What treatment options are appropriate?

Clinical cases

CASE 9.11 – 'I feel itchy all over.'

A 36-year-old Asian woman presents with 2-month history of generalized pruritus. There is no associated rash. She has been feeling tired for a few months now but has no other symptoms. On examination, she has pale conjunctivae.

CASE 9.12 – 'I have a very itchy rash.'

An 88-year-old man who lives in a residential home has developed a generalized itchy rash. It is particularly bad over his hands, arms, groin and thighs. The itching is worse at night and prevents him from sleeping. Some of the other residents at the home have developed a similar itchy rash.

OSCE Counselling Case

OSCE COUNSELLING CASE 9.8 – 'I have been told I have urticaria. What is this?'

A 33-year-old man has suffered with intermittent episodes of a 'nettle-like' rash over his body for the last 6 months. Each episode lasts for a few hours. He has not identified any triggers but has noticed that the rash becomes less itchy and slowly fades after taking antihistamine tablets. He has been told the diagnosis is urticaria.

Q1: Explain to him what this diagnosis means.

Q2: Are there any investigations he can have to determine the cause?

Key concepts

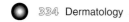

What are the common causes of generalized pruritus?

- **Haematological**
  - iron deficiency anaemia
  - polycythaemia rubra vera
  - paraproteinaemia
- **Hepatic disease**
  - extrahepatic obstructive jaundice
  - primary biliary cirrhosis
  - cholestasis of pregnancy
- **Renal disease**
  - chronic renal failure
- **Endocrine disease**
  - hyper- or hypothyroidism
  - diabetes mellitus
- **Internal malignancy**
  - lymphoma
  - leukaemia
  - abdominal cancer
  - bronchial carcinoma
- **Drugs**
  - oral contraceptive pill (causes cholestasis)
  - opiates (cause histamine release)
  - alcohol and drug withdrawal
- **Psychological.**

What are the common pruritic skin disorders?

- Eczema
- Scabies
- Urticaria
- Insect bites

- Lichen planus
- Drug eruptions
- Bullous pemphigoid
- Dermatitis herpetiformis
- Polymorphic light eruptions.

Answers

CASE 9.11 – 'I feel itchy all over.'

Q1: What is the likely differential diagnosis?

A1

Causes of generalized pruritus must be considered (see Key concepts).

Q2: What issues in the given history support the diagnosis?

A2

The most likely diagnosis is pruritus secondary to iron deficiency anaemia. Patients with anaemia often have non-specific symptoms and complain of lethargy. The pale conjunctivae also suggest anaemia.

Q3: What additional features in the history would you seek to support a particular diagnosis?

A3

Find out if there are any other associated symptoms. The tiredness and pale conjunctivae suggest anaemia, although iron deficiency in the absence of anaemia can also cause pruritus. Is there anything in the history to suggest iron deficiency? Is she a vegetarian or a vegan, and does she eat a balanced diet? Enquire about any history of blood loss (bleeding per rectum, heavy menstrual blood loss etc.). Does the pruritus occur at any specific time? For example, pruritus after a hot bath is classically associated with polycythaemia. Are there symptoms suggesting internal malignancy such as weight loss, haemoptysis, chronic cough, fevers, night sweats etc. Drugs such as opiates and their derivatives may also cause pruritus so ask about medication.

Q4: What clinical examination would you perform and why?

A4

A full general examination is necessary to look for coexisting skin disease or a cause for the pruritus. Often, the only positive findings are the excoriations caused by the patient scratching! Look for scabies burrows in the finger webs or pruritic papules over the genitals. Examine for evidence of chronic liver disease, hypo- or hyperthyroidism, renal failure or malignancy, all of which may present with pruritus.

 Q5: What investigations would be most helpful and why?

A5

An FBC to look for anaemia or polycythaemia rubra vera is necessary. Iron studies (ferritin, total iron-binding capacity) can determine whether iron deficiency is present, and it may be necessary to investigate further for a cause with faecal occult blood, by sigmoidoscopy etc. Liver function tests may indicate cholestasis, renal function tests may reveal uraemia secondary to chronic renal failure as the cause of pruritus, and thyroid function tests may show thyrotoxicosis or hypothyroidism. Diabetes can also cause generalized pruritus so check the fasting glucose.

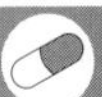 Q6: What treatment options are appropriate?

A6

Treatment is that of the underlying cause. Prevent dryness of the skin that can cause or exacerbate pruritus. Menthol in aqueous cream can be very soothing. Bath oils and emollients used as soap substitutes can also provide symptomatic relief. Antihistamines may provide symptomatic relief. A sedating antihistamine may help the patient sleep at night but a non-sedating one is better for daytime use so as not to interfere with driving and work.

 CASE 9.12 – 'I have a very itchy rash.'

 Q1: What is the likely differential diagnosis?

A1

- Scabies
- Eczema
- Tinea corporis and tinea cruris
- Drug eruption.

 Q2: What issues in the given history support the diagnosis?

A2

Itching that is particularly bad over the hands and groin area and is worse at night suggests a diagnosis of scabies, especially if other members of the family/residential home are also complaining of pruritus. The itch intensifies with time and, apart from sparing the face, affects the whole body.

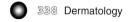

 Q3: What additional features in the history would you seek to support a particular diagnosis?

A3

A very observant patient may have noticed the scabies burrows and describe them as very pruritic. However, usually they go unnoticed. Ask if the patient has any small itchy lumps between the fingers, around the nipples, or on the buttocks and genitalia. Pruritic papules on the penis or scrotum are characteristic of scabies. Find out whether the patient has tried any treatments because topical corticosteroids are often wrongly prescribed if the rash is mistaken for eczema, and they often provide temporary symptomatic relief from itching but make the condition worse.

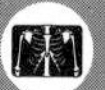 Q4: What clinical examination would you perform and why?

A4

Finding a scabies burrow is diagnostic. Look carefully over the webs of the fingers, dorsum of the hands, around the wrists and on the palms. Multiple, serpiginous, slightly raised, linear tracks of a few millimetres in length are characteristic. The *Sarcoptes scabiei* mite may be just visible as a black dot at one end of the burrow. The pruritus and rash associated with scabies are a result of an allergic reaction to the mite's faeces and present as an extremely itchy erythematous papular eruption. Multiple excoriations are often present and bruising from vigorous scratching may occur.

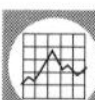 Q5: What investigations would be most helpful and why?

A5

The diagnosis is made on history and examination, although occasionally a mite can be carefully extracted from a burrow using a fine needle and visualized under the microscope.

 Q6: What treatment options are appropriate?

A6

Scabies is easily treatable but the patient must apply the treatment correctly and be warned that the itching (which is caused by the allergic reaction) typically persists for a few weeks after the mite has been eradicated. The treatment should be applied to all the skin areas except the face. Most lotions for scabies need to be applied and left on for 12–24 h before being washed off, and usually two applications are recommended. Permethrin 5 per cent cream or malathion 0.5 per cent lotion are usually used. Close contacts (family members, carers etc.) may also need treatment. Other measures include washing the patient's bedding, towels and undergarments at a high temperature. As the itch and eczema persist for weeks, application of crotamiton (Eurax cream), with or without a topical corticosteroid, and a sedating antihistamine tablet can provide symptomatic relief.

OSCE Counselling Case – Answers

OSCE COUNSELLING CASE 9.8 – 'I have been told I have urticaria. What is this?'

A1

Urticaria is a term used to describe intermittent, transient, itchy, red swellings of the skin that occur secondary to histamine and other vasoactive substances being released from granules within mast cells in blood vessels. Angio-oedema occurs if the mucous membranes are also involved, with swelling around the eyes and of the lips, tongue and larynx. This may be life threatening because of the possibility of asphyxia. Patients often describe the rash as itchy weals and blisters or as 'nettle rash' or 'hives'. They typically appear as raised annular areas with a red periphery and central pallor. It lasts for several hours and the skin appears completely normal afterwards. In most patients a cause is never identified. However, the following are some common causes of urticaria:

- Drugs: aspirin and other non-steroidal anti-inflammatory drugs, antibiotics (especially penicillin and cephalosporins)
- Foods: nuts, dairy products, shellfish, dyes, additives, etc.
- Infection: focal sepsis
- Physical: cold, heat, UV light, pressure
- Blood transfusion reactions.

Treatment involves avoiding any precipitating cause identified, and controlling the symptoms with antihistamines. If there is a history of angio-oedema leading to anaphylaxis, the patient must be provided with an adrenaline autoinjector (EpiPen).

A2

The diagnosis is usually made on the history alone. Investigations are rarely helpful. Blood tests are usually normal and therefore not indicated. It can be helpful to ask the patient to make a list of things ingested in the 24 h before each attack in order to try to identify the trigger. An elimination diet may be worth trying. Skin-prick and radioallergosorbent (RAST) tests are often positive in a non-specific way but the results must be interpreted in the clinical context.

ACNE

? Questions for the clinical case scenario given

Q1: What is the likely differential diagnosis?
Q2: What issues in the given history support the diagnosis?
Q3: What additional features in the history would you seek to support a particular diagnosis?
Q4: What clinical examination would you perform and why?
Q5: What investigations would be most helpful and why?
Q6: What treatment options are appropriate?

Clinical case

CASE 9.13 – 'My spots won't go away!'

A 17-year-old girl presented to her GP complaining of spots over her face for the past 4 years. She has tried multiple over-the-counter acne preparations with no improvement and is very concerned about the scarring left behind.

OSCE Counselling Case

OSCE COUNSELLING CASE 9.9 – 'Can I have Roaccutane for my acne?'

A 23-year-old girl has been treated for acne with various topical preparations and different courses of antibiotics for the past 2 years with little success. Her friend was recently given Roaccutane tablets which have cured her acne. She wishes to have the same treatment.

Q1: What are the indications for prescribing Roaccutane?

Q2: What are the side effects that she needs to know about before starting treatment?

Key concepts

Why does acne occur?

Acne is a chronic disorder of the pilosebaceous apparatus of the skin. It results from overactivity of the sebaceous glands and blockage of its ducts, leading to the formation of open (blackheads) and closed (whiteheads) comedones. The sebaceous glands are under the control of androgens and produce sebum that may be converted into comedogenic and irritant free fatty acids by the anaerobic bacterium *Propionibacterium acnes* within the pilosebaceous duct.

How is it treated?

There are various treatments available for acne and the choice of treatment depends on the disease severity and the individual patient:

- Topical therapy: used for mild acne and as an adjunct to other acne treatments. Includes benzoyl peroxide, retinoic acid, antibiotics and salicylic acid.
- Systemic antibiotics: tetracyclines and erythromycin are the most commonly used antibiotics for acne not responding to topical treatment alone.
- Hormone therapy: a combined preparation of cyproterone acetate and ethinylestradiol (co-cyprindiol or Dianette) reduces sebum production and is helpful in some patients.
- Systemic retinoid therapy: 13-*cis*-retinoic acid (isotretinoin/Roaccutane) is a synthetic derivative of vitamin A. It acts by reducing sebum secretion by 90 per cent, micro-organisms (especially *P. acnes*), plugging of the pilosebaceous duct and inflammation. It also influences epithelial proliferation and differentiation so that the sebaceous glands return to their prepubertal state.

Answers

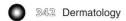

CASE 9.13 – 'My spots won't go away!'

Q1: What is the likely differential diagnosis?

A1

- Acne vulgaris
- Acne rosacea (usually occurs from the fourth decade onwards)
- Perioral/periorbital dermatitis (secondary to misuse of topical corticosteroids).

Q2: What issues in the given history support the diagnosis?

A2

Acne is a very common problem in adolescents. The characteristic lesions and their distribution give the diagnosis away!

Q3: What additional features in the history would you seek to support a particular diagnosis?

A3

Find out when the lesions started and their distribution. Do they affect just the face or are the back, chest or upper arms also involved? Ask the patient to describe the lesions – are they small papules or large cysts? What type of scars do they leave when they resolve? Post-inflammatory hyperpigmentation is common and appears as a brown mark when the lesion resolves. It is not a permanent scar but can take many months to fade away. The colour tends to be more intense in patients with darker skin. Pitted scars (also known as ice-pick scars) may occur after severe nodulocystic acne and are permanent.

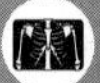

Q4: What clinical examination would you perform and why?

A4

The skin may appear greasy with red papules, pustules, comedones, and sometimes nodules, cysts, post-inflammatory hyperpigmentation and pitted scars. Determine the distribution of the acne.

 Q5: What investigations would be most helpful and why?

A5

The diagnosis is made on history and clinical examination. If the lesions look infected, a swab may be sent for microbiology. Bear in mind that pustules are typically sterile.

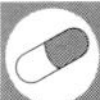 Q6: What treatment options are appropriate?

A6

Topical benzoyl peroxide is antibacterial and comedolytic. Combined preparations with an antibiotic are also available. It can be very drying and cause irritation so the treatment is started at the weakest concentration. Topical antibiotics alone are also used. Topical retinoic acid is a keratolytic agent and useful for comedonal acne and post-inflammatory hyperpigmentation. Salicylic acid can also be used as a keratolytic agent. Systemic antibiotics are the mainstay of acne treatment. Tetracyclines or erythromycin are most effective but need to be prescribed for at least 6 months before a benefit is seen. As a rule, acne over the trunk responds slower than facial acne, and antibiotics may need to be continued for longer. For antibiotic-resistant acne or severe acne leading to scarring, systemic retinoid therapy is the treatment of choice.

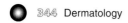

OSCE Counselling Cases – Answers

OSCE COUNSELLING CASE 9.9 – 'Can I have Roaccutane for my acne?'

A1

Isotretinoin (Roaccutane) is used to treat:

- nodulocystic acne: severe, chronic acne that is usually resistant to standard therapy; it is most frequent in males and presents with deep, painful papules and nodules that lead to scars, occasionally with keloid formation
- acne leading to scarring
- antibiotic-resistant acne
- acne causing significant psychological distress to the patient.

A2

Isotretinoin is given as 1 mg/kg per day tablets for 16 weeks. The effect is usually evident within 6 weeks. One course is usually sufficient to clear most patients' acne.

The main side effect noticed by the patient is dryness of the skin and mucous membranes. They must be advised to use an emollient and lip balm to alleviate this. Patients who wear contact lenses are advised to wear spectacles instead during the treatment period. Nosebleeds may also occur in those patients with a predisposition. Isotretinoin is metabolized through the liver and may cause hyperlipidaemia. Liver function tests, cholesterol and triglyceride levels are taken before starting and during treatment. Patients are also warned of the risk of depression. There have been cases of suicide reported in patients receiving treatment and therefore depression is a relative contraindication to starting treatment.

It is vital that patients are informed that the drug is highly teratogenic, especially as most female patients on treatment are of child-bearing age. A pregnancy test is mandatory before starting therapy and adequate contraception should be used during and for at least 3 months after cessation of treatment.

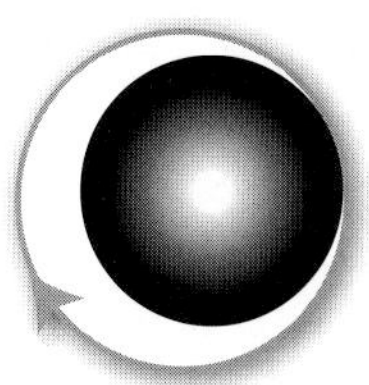

Index

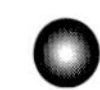